Evidence Report/Technology Assessment

Number 216

Antidepressant Treatment of Depression During Pregnancy and the Postpartum Period

Prepared for:
Agency for Healthcare Research and Quality
U.S. Department of Health and Human Services
540 Gaither Road
Rockville, MD 20850
www.ahrq.gov

Contract No. 290-2007-10057-I

Prepared by:
Pacific Northwest Evidence-based Practice Center
Portland, OR

Investigators:
Marian McDonagh, Pharm.D.
Annette Matthews, M.D., M.C.R.
Carrie Phillipi, M.D., Ph.D.
Jillian Romm, R.N., L.C.S.W.
Kim Peterson, M.S.
Sujata Thakurta, M.P.A.:H.A.
Jeanne-Marie Guise, M.D., M.P.H.

AHRQ Publication No. 14-E003-EF
July 2014

This report is based on research conducted by the Pacific Northwest Evidence-based Practice Center (EPC) under contract to the Agency for Healthcare Research and Quality (AHRQ), Rockville, MD (Contract No. 290-2007-10057-I). The findings and conclusions in this document are those of the authors, who are responsible for its contents; the findings and conclusions do not necessarily represent the views of AHRQ. Therefore, no statement in this report should be construed as an official position of AHRQ or of the U.S. Department of Health and Human Services.

The information in this report is intended to help health care decisionmakers—patients and clinicians, health system leaders, and policymakers, among others—make well informed decisions and thereby improve the quality of health care services. This report is not intended to be a substitute for the application of clinical judgment. Anyone who makes decisions concerning the provision of clinical care should consider this report in the same way as any medical reference and in conjunction with all other pertinent information, i.e., in the context of available resources and circumstances presented by individual patients.

This report may be used, in whole or in part, as the basis for development of clinical practice guidelines and other quality enhancement tools, or as a basis for reimbursement and coverage policies. AHRQ or U.S. Department of Health and Human Services endorsement of such derivative products may not be stated or implied.

This report may periodically be assessed for the urgency to update. If an assessment is done, the resulting surveillance report describing the methodology and findings will be found on the Effective Health Care Program Web site at www.effectivehealthcare.ahrq.gov. Search on the title of the report.

This document is in the public domain and may be used and reprinted without special permission. Citation of the source is appreciated.

Persons using assistive technology may not be able to fully access information in this report. For assistance contact EffectiveHealthCare@ahrq.hhs.gov.

> None of the investigators have any affiliations or financial involvement that conflicts with the material presented in this report.

Suggested citation: McDonagh M, Matthews A, Phillipi C, Romm J, Peterson K, Thakurta S, Guise J-M. Antidepressant Treatment of Depression During Pregnancy and the Postpartum Period. Evidence Report/Technology Assessment No. 216. (Prepared by the Pacific Northwest Evidence-based Practice Center under Contract No. 290-2007-10057-I.) AHRQ Publication No. 14-E003-EF. Rockville, MD: Agency for Healthcare Research and Quality; July 2014. www.effectivehealthcare.ahrq.gov/reports/final.cfm.

Preface

The Agency for Healthcare Research and Quality (AHRQ), through its Evidence-based Practice Centers (EPCs), sponsors the development of systematic reviews to assist public- and private-sector organizations in their efforts to improve the quality of health care in the United States. These reviews provide comprehensive, science-based information on common, costly medical conditions, and new health care technologies and strategies.

Systematic reviews are the building blocks underlying evidence-based practice; they focus attention on the strength and limits of evidence from research studies about the effectiveness and safety of a clinical intervention. In the context of developing recommendations for practice, systematic reviews can help clarify whether assertions about the value of the intervention are based on strong evidence from clinical studies. For more information about AHRQ EPC systematic reviews, see www.effectivehealthcare.ahrq.gov/reference/purpose.cfm.

AHRQ expects that these systematic reviews will be helpful to health plans, providers, purchasers, government programs, and the health care system as a whole. Transparency and stakeholder input are essential to the Effective Health Care Program. Please visit the Web site (www.effectivehealthcare.ahrq.gov) to see draft research questions and reports or to join an email list to learn about new program products and opportunities for input.

We welcome comments on this systematic review. They may be sent by mail to the Task Order Officer named below at: Agency for Healthcare Research and Quality, 540 Gaither Road, Rockville, MD 20850, or by email to epc@ahrq.hhs.gov.

Richard G. Kronick, Ph.D.
Director
Agency for Healthcare Research and Quality

Stephanie Chang, M.D., M.P.H.
Director, EPC Program
Center for Outcomes and Evidence
Agency for Healthcare Research and Quality

Yen-pin Chiang, Ph.D.
Acting Director, Center for Outcomes and Evidence
Agency for Healthcare Research and Quality

Suchitra Iyer, Ph.D.
Task Order Officer
Center for Outcomes and Evidence
Agency for Healthcare Research and Quality

Acknowledgments

The authors gratefully acknowledge the following individuals for their contributions to this project: Tracy Dana, M.L.S., for assistance with literature search strategy development; Leah Williams, B.S., for editorial support; Elaine Graham, M.L.S., for assistance with project management; and Gabriel Valles for article retrieval. We would also like to thank our AHRQ Task Order Officer, Suchitra Iyer, Ph.D., and Denise Dougherty, Ph.D., Children's Health Point of Contact at AHRQ, for their support and guidance in developing this report, and our Associate Editor, Kathleen Lohr, Ph.D., for her review of the report and meaningful comments.

Technical Expert Panel

In designing the review questions and methodology at the outset of this report, the EPC consulted several technical and content experts, reflecting a variety of viewpoints relevant to this topic. Technical experts consulted are expected to have divergent and possibly conflicting opinions. This diversity is helpful in achieving a well-rounded report. The study questions, design, methodological approaches, and/or conclusions do not necessarily represent the views of individual technical and content experts.

Technical Experts must disclose any financial conflicts of interest greater than $10,000 and any other relevant business or professional conflicts of interest. Because of their unique clinical or content expertise, individuals with potential conflicts may be retained. The TOO and the EPC work to balance, manage, or mitigate any potential conflicts of interest identified.

The list of Technical Experts who participated in developing this report follows:

Wendy Davis, Ph.D.
Executive Director
Postpartum Support International
Portland, OR

Adrienne Einarson, R.N.
Assistant Director of Clinical Services
Motherisk
Toronto, Canada

Cathy Emeis, Ph.D., C.N.M.
Assistant Professor & Assistant Program Director for Nurse Midwifery
Oregon Health & Science University
School of Nursing
Portland, OR

RJ Gillespie, M.D., M.H.P.E.
Medical Director, Oregon Pediatric Improvement Partnership
Portland, OR

Kimberly D. Gregory, M.D., M.P.H.
Vice Chair, Women's Healthcare Quality and Performance Improvement, Department of Obstetrics and Gynecology
Cedars Sinai Medical Center
Los Angeles, CA

Susan G. Kornstein, M.D.
Professor of Psychiatry and Obstetrics/Gynecology
Executive Director, Institute for Women's Health
Director of Clinical Research, Department of Psychiatry
Virginia Commonwealth University
Editor-in-Chief, Journal of Women's Health
Richmond, VA

Evan Myers, M.D., M.P.H.
Division of Clinical and Epidemiological Research, Department of Obstetrics and Gynecology
Duke Evidence Synthesis Group, Duke Clinical Research Institute
Duke University School of Medicine
Walter L. Thomas Professor
Duke University Medical Center
Durham, NC

Gail Erlick Robinson, M.D., D.Psych., FRCPC, O.Ont.
Director, Women's Mental Health Program
University Health Network
Professor of Psychiatry and Obstetrics-Gynecology, University of Toronto
Toronto, Canada

Barbara Yawn, M.D., M.Sc., FAAFP
Director of Research, Olmsted Medical Center
Adjunct Professor, Department of Family and Community Health, University of Minnesota
Rochester, MN

Peer Reviewers

Prior to publication of the final evidence report, EPCs sought input from independent Peer Reviewers without financial conflicts of interest. However, the conclusions and synthesis of the scientific literature presented in this report do not necessarily represent the views of individual reviewers.

Peer Reviewers must disclose any financial conflicts of interest greater than $10,000 and any other relevant business or professional conflicts of interest. Because of their unique clinical or content expertise, individuals with potential nonfinancial conflicts may be retained. The TOO and the EPC work to balance, manage, or mitigate any potential nonfinancial conflicts of interest identified.

The list of Peer Reviewers follows:

Matthew A. Broom, M.D., FAAP
Assistant Professor of Pediatrics
Department of Pediatrics
Saint Louis University School of Medicine
Saint Louis, MO

Jocelyn Huang Schiller, M.D.
Associate Professor, Pediatrics
C.S. Mott Children's Hospital
University of Michigan
Ann Arbor, MI

Kimberly A. Yonkers, M.D.
Professor of Psychiatry and of Obstetrics,
Gynecology, and Reproductive Sciences
Director, PMS and Perinatal Psychiatric
Research Program
New Haven, CT

Antidepressant Treatment of Depression During Pregnancy and the Postpartum Period

Structured Abstract

Objectives. To evaluate the benefits and harms of pharmacological therapy for depression in women during pregnancy or the postpartum period.

Data sources. Cochrane Database of Systematic Reviews, the Cochrane Central Register of Controlled Trials, the Cumulative Index to Nursing and Allied Health Literature (CINAHL®), MEDLINE®, Scopus®, ClinicalTrials.gov, and Scientific Information Packets from pharmaceutical manufacturers. Databases were searched from their inception to July 2013.

Review methods. We included studies comparing pharmacological treatments for depression during or after pregnancy with each other, with nonpharmacological treatments, or with usual care or no treatment. Outcomes included both maternal and infant or child benefits and harms. Dual review was used for study inclusion, data abstraction, and quality assessment. We assessed study quality using methods of the Drug Effectiveness Review Project. We graded the strength of the body of evidence according to the methods of the Effective Health Care Program. Direct evidence comprised studies that compared interventions of interest in the population of interest (i.e., depressed women) and measured the outcomes of interest. Studies comparing groups of depressed women with control groups with no evidence of depression were considered indirect.

Results. We included 15 observational studies that provided direct evidence on benefits and harms of antidepressants for depression during pregnancy. We included six randomized controlled trials and two observational studies of antidepressant treatment for depression in postpartum women. Studies of depressed pregnant women primarily compared antidepressant treatment with no treatment, and studies of postpartum women also compared antidepressants alone with combination antidepressant-nonpharmacological treatments. This evidence was insufficient to draw conclusions on the comparative benefits or harms of antidepressants for the outcomes of maternal depression symptoms, functional capacity, breastfeeding, mother-infant dyad interactions, and infant and child development for either pregnant or postpartum women with depression. Low-strength evidence suggests that neonates of women with depression taking selective serotonin reuptake inhibitors (SSRIs) during pregnancy had higher risk of respiratory distress than neonates of untreated women but that risk of preterm birth or neonatal convulsions does not differ between these groups. Direct evidence on the risk of major malformations and neonatal development with exposure to antidepressants in utero was insufficient to draw conclusions. For postpartum women with depression, evidence was insufficient to evaluate the full range of benefits and harms of treatment. Low-strength evidence was unable to show a benefit of adding brief psychotherapy or cognitive behavioral therapy to SSRIs.

To address gaps in the direct evidence, we included an additional 109 observational studies of pregnant women receiving antidepressants for mixed or unreported reasons compared with pregnant women not taking antidepressants whose depression status was unknown. Signals from this indirect evidence suggest that future research should focus on the comparative risk of congenital anomalies and neonatal motor developmental delays. Although the absolute increased risk of autism spectrum disorder or attention-deficit hyperactivity disorder in the child associated with antidepressant use for depression in pregnancy may be very small, this issue also merits attention in future research. Future research should compare available treatments in groups of women with depression and have adequate sample sizes. Investigations should also take into account potential confounding, including age, race, parity, other exposures (e.g., alcohol, smoking, and other potential teratogens), and the impact of dose, severity of depression, timing of diagnosis, or prior depressive episodes.

Conclusions. Evidence about the comparative benefits and harms of pharmacological treatment of depression in pregnant and postpartum women was largely inadequate to allow well-informed decisions about treatment. For pregnant women, this was mainly because comparison groups were not exclusively depressed women. For postpartum women, the lack of evidence arose chiefly from a scarcity of studies. These are major limitations, as depression is known to be associated with serious adverse outcomes. Given the prevalence of depression and its impact on the lives of pregnant women, new mothers, and children, new research to fill this informational gap is essential.

Contents

Executive Summary ES-1
Introduction 1
   Background 1
      Condition 1
      Treatment Strategies 1
   Scope and Key Questions 3
      Key Questions 4
      Analytic Frameworks 5
   Organization of This Report 8
Methods 9
   Search Strategy 9
   Inclusion and Exclusion Criteria 9
      Populations 9
      Interventions 10
      Comparators 10
      Outcomes 10
      Timing 11
      Setting 12
      Study Designs 12
   Study Selection 12
   Data Extraction 13
   Risk of Bias Assessment of Individual Studies 13
   Data Synthesis 14
   Strength of the Body of Evidence 15
   Applicability 15
   Peer Review and Public Commentary 16
Results 17
   Introduction 17
   Results of Literature Searches 17
   Description of Included Studies 19
   Key Question 1. What are the comparative benefits of pharmacological and
   nonpharmacological treatments for women with depression during pregnancy and in the
   postpartum period? 19
      Summary 19
      Detailed Assessment of the Evidence 21
   Key Question 2. What are the comparative harms of pharmacological and nonpharmacological
   treatments for women with depression during pregnancy and in the postpartum period? 37
      Summary 37
      Detailed Assessment of the Evidence 38
   Key Question 3. Is there evidence that the comparative effectiveness of pharmacological and
   nonpharmacological treatments for women with depression during pregnancy and in the
   postpartum period varies based on characteristics such as interventions, populations, and
   providers? 57

    Summary 57
    Detailed Assessment of the Evidence 58
Discussion 60
    Key Findings and Strength of Evidence 60
    Findings in Relationship to What Is Already Known 64
    Applicability 64
    Implications for Clinical and Policy Decisionmaking 65
    Limitations of the Review Process 67
    Gaps in the Research 67
    Conclusion 68
References 69
Abbreviations and Acronyms 81

Tables
Table A. Pharmacological interventions: antidepressant agents ES-7
Table B. Maternal and child benefits and harms outcomes included in the review ES-8
Table C. Key findings of direct-comparison evidence for depression during pregnancy ES-16
Table 1. Pharmacologic interventions: Antidepressant agents 3
Table 2. Maternal and child benefits and harms outcomes included in the review 11
Table 3. Association between antidepressant use during pregnancy and general practitioner visits and hospital admissions; unadjusted relative risk (95% confidence interval) 30
Table 4. Risk of neonatal/postneonatal death for maternal use of a selective serotonin reuptake inhibitor in pregnancy 40
Table 5. Best evidence estimates of risk for major malformations with use of selective serotonin reuptake inhibitors during pregnancy 42
Table 6. Best evidence on risk of cardiac malformations with selective serotonin reuptake inhibitors compared with nonexposure 44
Table 7. Risk of neonatal withdrawal/abstinence syndrome for maternal use of a selective serotonin reuptake inhibitor in pregnancy 46
Table 8. Class compared with class: Risk of congenital malformations 51
Table 9. Risk of persistent pulmonary hypertension with individual selective serotonin reuptake inhibitors 53
Table 10. Key findings and strength of evidence of directly comparative evidence for depression during pregnancy 63

Figures
Figure A. Analytic frameworks for treatment of depression in pregnant and postpartum women
.... ES-4
Figure 1. Analytic frameworks for treatment of depression in pregnant and postpartum women . 7
Figure 2. Literature flow diagram 18
Figure 3. Risk of preterm birth (< 37 weeks gestation) with selective serotonin reuptake inhibitors compared with nonexposure 24
Figure 4. Risk of major malformations with selective serotonin reuptake inhibitors compared with nonexposure 57

Appendixes
Appendix A. Search Strategies
Appendix B. Included Studies
Appendix C. Excluded Studies
Appendix D. Strength of Evidence
Appendix E. Evidence Tables

Executive Summary

Background

Depression is a potentially life-threatening condition. The incidence of depression during pregnancy and the postpartum period is estimated to be anywhere from 5.5 to 33.1 percent, and the American Academy of Pediatrics estimates that more than 400,000 infants are born each year to mothers who are depressed.[1-3]

Depression during pregnancy is known to be associated with harmful prenatal health consequences, such as poor nutrition, poor prenatal medical care, risk of suicide, and harmful health behaviors (e.g., smoking and alcohol or other substance misuse). These circumstances compromise the health of both the woman and her fetus.[4,5] Although causation has not been proven, several obstetric complications have been reported with untreated prenatal depression, including preeclampsia, preterm delivery, low birth weight, miscarriage, small-for-gestational-age babies, low Apgar scores, and neonatal complications. These complications may be more common among women with lower socioeconomic status.[6-8] In addition to being debilitating for the mother, postpartum depression affects maternal-infant interactions and some measures of infant development. In extreme cases, postpartum depression may increase the risk of infant mortality through neglect, abuse, or homicide.[9] It also negatively affects interactions within other members of the family unit and is associated with intimate partner violence.[10]

A 2013 Agency for Healthcare Research and Quality (AHRQ) report found that screening can significantly reduce postpartum depressive symptoms when systems are in place to ensure adequate followup of women with positive results.[11] Management of depression in pregnancy or the postpartum period varies case by case; providers and patients are often concerned about the safety of pharmacological treatment during pregnancy and the postpartum period.[12]

Clinicians can use interventions such as pharmacological treatments, nonpharmacological treatments, and watchful waiting for patients with depression, both during pregnancy and in the postpartum period; they may also elect not to provide any intervention at all. Pharmacological treatments approved by the U.S. Food and Drug Administration (FDA) for treating depression are listed in Table A. Antidepressant medications have been shown to be effective at reducing the symptoms of depression in nonpregnant adults.[13,14] In general, medications that are effective in treating conditions outside of pregnancy are often presumed to remain effective in pregnancy, but the developing fetus and changes in maternal physiology raise questions about safety and dosing of various agents. For safety of the fetus, the FDA Pregnancy Category of antidepressant medications taken during pregnancy is category C ("animal reproduction studies have shown an adverse effect on the fetus and there are no adequate and well-controlled studies in humans, but potential benefits may warrant use of the drug in pregnant women despite potential risks"), with the exception of paroxetine, which is category D ("there is positive evidence of human fetal risk based on adverse reaction data from investigational or marketing experience or studies in humans, but potential benefits may warrant use of the drug in pregnant women despite potential risks"). However, evidence on how the risk of one antidepressant compares with that of another when taken during pregnancy is not well understood. Antidepressant medications are used to treat a variety of other indications, including anxiety disorders such as generalized anxiety disorder, panic attacks, obsessive compulsive disorder, depressed phase of bipolar disorder, and neuropathic pain.

A wide array of nonpharmacological interventions can be used to treat depression, including various psychotherapies, electroconvulsive therapy, repetitive transcranial magnetic stimulation, and acupuncture.[15-19] Some of these may be used during pregnancy, whereas others may be reserved for use in the postpartum period (e.g., electroconvulsive therapy). Decisionmaking surrounding treatment of depression in pregnancy is complex because the harms of treatments must be balanced against the potential harms to mother and fetus of untreated depression.

Objectives

The objective of this systematic review was to evaluate the benefits and harms of various pharmacological treatment options for depression during pregnancy and the postpartum period compared with each other, with nonpharmacological treatments, and with usual care or no treatment.

Key Question 1. What are the comparative benefits of pharmacological and nonpharmacological treatments for women with depression during pregnancy and in the postpartum period?

a. How do pharmacological treatments affect maternal and child[a] outcomes when compared with placebo or no active treatment or usual care?
b. How do pharmacological treatments affect maternal and child outcomes when compared with each other (drug A vs. drug B)?
c. How do pharmacological treatments affect maternal and child outcomes when compared with active nonpharmacological treatments?
d. How does combination therapy affect maternal and child outcomes? The combinations include:
   i. Using a second drug to augment the effects of the primary drug and comparing this treatment with monotherapy with a single drug
   ii. Combining pharmacological treatments with nonpharmacological treatments and comparing them with nonpharmacological treatments alone
   iii. Comparing pharmacological treatments alone with pharmacological treatments used in combination with nonpharmacological treatments

Key Question 2. What are the comparative harms of pharmacological and nonpharmacological treatments for women with depression during pregnancy and in the postpartum period?

a. How do pharmacological treatments affect maternal and child[a] outcomes when compared with placebo or no active treatment or usual care?
b. How do pharmacological treatments affect maternal and child outcomes when compared with each other (drug A vs. drug B)?
c. How do pharmacological treatments affect maternal and child outcomes when compared with active nonpharmacological treatments?
d. How does combination therapy affect maternal and child outcomes? The combinations include:
   i. Using a second drug to augment the effects of the primary drug and comparing

---

[a] A child is defined as a fetus, infant, or child younger than age 18.

    this treatment with monotherapy with pharmacological treatment
  ii. Combining pharmacological treatments with nonpharmacological treatments and comparing them with nonpharmacological treatments alone
  iii. Comparing pharmacological treatments alone with pharmacological treatments used in combination with nonpharmacological treatments
e. In babies born to women who become pregnant while taking medications to treat depression, what is the comparative risk of teratogenicity?

Key Question 3. Is there evidence that the comparative effectiveness (benefits or harms) of pharmacological and nonpharmacological treatments for women with depression during pregnancy and in the postpartum period varies based on characteristics[b] such as:

a. Patient characteristics—race, age, socioeconomic status, family history of depressive or mood disorders, prior use of antidepressive drugs (for treatment or prevention), severity of symptoms, situation at home, unplanned pregnancy, and marital or partner status?
b. Patient comorbidities (e.g., anxiety diagnoses)?
c. Intervention characteristics—dosing regimens and duration of treatments?
d. Coadministration of other psychoactive drugs—specifically, antipsychotics, antianxiety agents (e.g., benzodiazepines), and drugs for insomnia?
e. Medical provider characteristics (primary care physician, obstetrician, pediatrician, psychiatrist, nurse, midwife, or community worker)?
f. Medical care environment (community, private, or public clinic or hospital)?
g. Characteristics of diagnosis—whether depression was detected during screening or not, time of diagnosis, method of diagnosis, and when treatment commenced relative to the onset of symptoms?

Analytic Frameworks

  The analytic frameworks (Figure A) illustrate the population, interventions, outcomes, and adverse effects studied and their relationship to the Key Questions. Framework 1a relates to pregnant women with depression who receive treatment. Treatment leads to health outcomes, shown in the box on the far right of the figure and connected by the overarching line. This evidence is the topic of Key Question 1, as marked on the line. Treatment may lead to intermediate outcomes, such as changes in level of depression symptoms, or adverse events, both noted separately on the diagram. The evidence showing that better intermediate outcomes (e.g., symptoms) improve health outcomes (e.g., reduced risk of suicide) is represented by a dotted line between boxes; we did not review that literature in this report. Framework 1b relates to postpartum women with depression, and again the outcomes that may result from treatment are depicted in relationship to each other, the treatments, and Key Questions. The outcomes considered differed from those considered for pregnant women.

---

[b] Other factors will be considered as they are identified within the comparative studies.

Figure A. Analytic frameworks for treatment of depression in pregnant and postpartum women

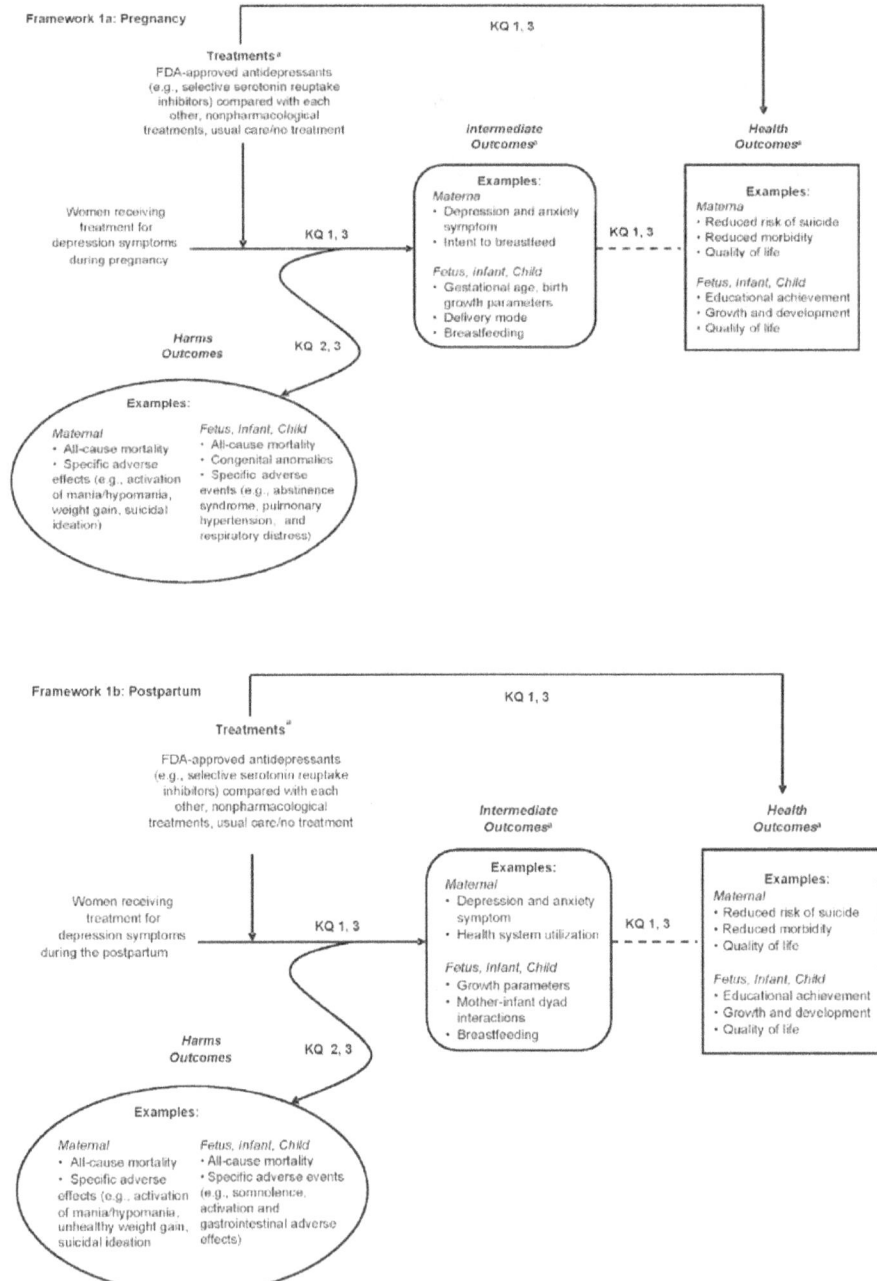

[a] The interventions and outcomes are too numerous to illustrate in their entirety in this diagram. See the Methods section below (Inclusion and Exclusion Criteria), for complete details on interventions and outcomes.
FDA = U.S. Food and Drug Administration; KQ = Key Question.

Methods

The methods for this Comparative Effectiveness Review follow the methods suggested in the AHRQ "Methods Guide for Effectiveness and Comparative Effectiveness Reviews" (available at www.effectivehealthcare.ahrq.gov/methodsguide.cfm).[20] The methods reported here reflect the protocol elements established for Comparative Effectiveness Reviews and methods mapping to the PRISMA (Preferred Reporting Items for Systematic Reviews and Meta-Analyses) checklist.[21] All methods and analyses were determined a priori. The research protocol was posted on the AHRQ Effective Health Care Program Web site (www.effectivehealthcare.ahrq.gov), and we registered the protocol in the systematic review registry, PROSPERO (www.crd.york.ac.uk/NIHR_PROSPERO/; record # CRD42013004493).

Literature Search Strategy

To identify studies relevant to each Key Question, the librarian searched the Cochrane Database of Systematic Reviews (CDSR) from 2005 to July 2013, the Cochrane Central Register of Controlled Trials (CCRCT) from 1980 to July 2013, the Cumulative Index to Nursing and Allied Health Literature (CINAHL®) from 1941 to July 2013, Ovid MEDLINE® and Ovid OLDMEDLINE® (1946 to July 2013), PsycINFO® (1806 to July 2013), and Scopus® (1974 to July 2013). ClinicalTrials.gov was searched for gray literature. The AHRQ Scientific Resource Center solicited Scientific Information Packets from industry stakeholders.

Inclusion and Exclusion Criteria

Populations

We defined the populations of interest as pregnant women and women during the first 12 months after delivery, who received treatment for a depressive episode, including:
- Women with a diagnosis for major depressive disorder according to the 4th edition of the Diagnostic and Statistical Manual of Mental Disorders (DSM-IV)[22]
- Women with subthreshold depressive symptoms

This report focuses chiefly on women diagnosed with depression during pregnancy or the postpartum period, rather than those with a continuing episode. The one exception is for Key Question 2e, regarding teratogenicity of antidepressant drugs taken during the conception period.

Based on input from experts, we also included studies with populations of pregnant women receiving antidepressant drugs for unknown or mixed reasons. We used these studies to provide evidence when no evidence was available on women with known depression or depressive symptoms (gaps in the evidence). To differentiate these populations, in this report we refer to studies of women with known depression as "treated" or "untreated" populations. We refer to studies of women with mixed or unknown diagnoses in terms of "maternal exposure" when receiving antidepressants (at typically unknown doses) and "maternal nonexposure" when not receiving antidepressants.

Interventions

Interventions include commonly used antidepressant drugs listed in Table A. We used the therapeutic classifications used in previous AHRQ comparative effectiveness reviews:[13,14] selective serotonin reuptake inhibitor (SSRI), serotonin norepinephrine reuptake inhibitor

(SNRI), selective serotonin norepinephrine reuptake inhibitor, and tricyclic antidepressant (TCA), except that we classified trazodone and nefazodone as norepinephrine reuptake inhibitors (NRI) for this report.

Table A. Pharmacological interventions: antidepressant agents

Drug Category	Generic Name	Trade Name[a]
Selective serotonin reuptake inhibitor	Citalopram	Celexa®, various generics
	Escitalopram	Lexapro®
	Fluoxetine	Prozac®, various generics Prozac Weekly® Sarafem®
	Fluvoxamine	Luvox®, various generics Luvox CR®
	Sertraline	Zoloft®, various generics
	Paroxetine	Paxil®, various generics Paxil CR®
	Vilazodone	Viibryd®
Serotonin norepinephrine reuptake inhibitor	Desvenlafaxine	Pristiq®
	Venlafaxine	Effexor XR®
	Mirtazapine	Remeron®, various generics Remeron SolTab®
Selective serotonin norepinephrine reuptake inhibitor	Duloxetine	Cymbalta®
Tricyclic antidepressant	Amitriptyline	Various generics
	Desipramine	Norpramin®, various generics
	Imipramine	Tofranil®, various generics
	Nortriptyline	Aventyl hydrochloride® Pamelor™ Various generics
Norepinephrine reuptake inhibitor	Nefazodone	Various generics (previously available as Serzone®)
	Trazodone	Desyrel®, various generics
Other	Bupropion	Wellbutrin® Wellbutrin SR® Wellbutrin XL® Forfivo XL® Aplenzin®

[a] CR, SR, XL, and XR abbreviations all refer to extended-release formulations.

Comparators

The comparators were:
- Placebo or no treatment.
- Usual care.
- The drugs in Table A compared with each other.
- Any nonpharmacological treatment. We recognize the important differences between these treatments and consider them separately when compared with pharmacological treatments, rather than as a group.

Outcomes

Table B presents the included maternal, fetal, infant, and child benefits and harms outcomes.

Table B. Maternal and child benefits and harms outcomes included in the review

Benefit or Harm	Mother	Fetus, Infant, Child
Benefit Outcomes	<ul><li>Danger to self—suicidal and nonsuicidal behaviors</li><li>Danger to infant—infanticidal behavior, abuse, or neglect</li><li>Depression symptomatology as scored using validated scales measuring depression: response, remission, speed and duration of response or remission, relapse, recurrence</li><li>Anxiety symptoms as scored as a subscale item using validated scales measuring depression or validated scales used to measure anxiety symptoms</li><li>Functional capacity<ul><li>Quality of life using validated scales—e.g., Medical Outcomes Survey 36-item Short Form (SF-36)</li><li>Caring for self, infant, and family</li><li>Mother-father dyad interaction success, including reduced violence among intimate partners</li><li>Work productivity</li></ul></li><li>Delivery and postpartum parameters<ul><li>Breastfeeding</li><li>Shared decisionmaking around delivery choices (e.g., cesarean) and delivery mode</li><li>Mother-infant dyad interaction patterns</li><li>Pregnancy weight gain within or outside of 1990 Institute of Medicine Guidelines</li></ul></li><li>Social services use; prevention of child protective service involvement</li><li>Maternal health system resource use, including emergency department use, hospitalizations, and office visits</li><li>Adherence or persistence with treatment regimen</li></ul>	<ul><li>Parameters at birth and up to 12 months of age: preterm birth (e.g., < 32 weeks, < 37 weeks); appropriate growth (height, weight, and head circumference); gestational age (e.g., small for gestational age with race or ethnicity taken into consideration); birth hospitalization length of stay; infant attachment; developmental screening—Ages and Stages Questionnaire, Denver, Modified Checklist for Autism in Toddlers, Bayley Scales of Infant Development</li><li>Growth and development after 1 year of age<ul><li>Developmental screening and diagnoses; growth parameters, such as height, weight, and body mass index percentile according to sex and age</li><li>Learning (e.g., linguistic, cognitive, and social-emotional skills) and educational achievement; kindergarten readiness; age at kindergarten entry; third grade testing outcomes; other standard testing outcomes (eighth grade, etc.)</li><li>Intelligence tests (any), individualized education plans, use of school services</li><li>School failure or dropout rate, high school graduation rate, missed school days</li></ul></li><li>Stress-related chronic disease; mental and chronic illness</li><li>Infant health system visits (e.g., well-baby visits); health care use, including primary care, emergency department, hospitalization</li><li>Social services use—Women, Infants, and Children Program (WIC), community health nurse, social worker, State Department of Health and Human Services, free or reduced-price lunch, and Food Stamps</li><li>Community resource use</li><li>Social and emotional development; quality of life</li><li>Contact with juvenile justice system</li></ul>

Table B. Maternal and child benefits and harms outcomes included in the review (continued)

Benefit or Harm	Mother	Fetus, Infant, Child
Harm Outcomes	• Death, including suicide, all-cause mortality, and cause-specific death (e.g., cardiac death) • Specific adverse effects or withdrawals due to specific adverse events related to treatment (e.g., hyponatremia, activation of mania or hypomania, seizures, suicidal ideation, hepatotoxicity, weight gain, metabolic syndrome, gastrointestinal symptoms, and loss of libido) • Overall adverse-event reports, adverse events associated with discontinuation of treatment, and serious adverse events • Withdrawals from study and discontinuation of treatment due to adverse events	• All-cause mortality • Congenital anomalies (any) stratified into major and minor with further grouping by organ system or type of anomaly • Other specific adverse events, such as withdrawal symptoms (neonatal abstinence symptoms), pulmonary hypertension, respiratory distress, neonatal convulsions, and heart defects

Study Designs

For effectiveness, we used a "best evidence" approach. Top-tier evidence included randomized controlled trials (RCTs) and systematic reviews comparing pregnant women receiving pharmacological treatments for depression during pregnancy with control groups of pregnant women with depression who were treated with nonpharmacological treatments or untreated. If we found no or only very few RCTs, we included observational study evidence and studies that had control groups of nonexposed pregnant women.

For harms, in addition to RCTs and systematic reviews, we included observational studies comparing women receiving pharmacological treatments for depression during pregnancy with control groups of pregnant women with depression who were treated with nonpharmacological treatments or had no treatment. If insufficient evidence was found, studies that compared with control groups of nonexposed pregnant women were included.

Case reports, case series, and single-group studies were excluded.

Study Selection

Two reviewers independently assessed titles and abstracts of publications identified through literature searches using the criteria described above for inclusion and exclusion of studies. Two reviewers assessed potentially relevant full text. Disagreements were resolved by consensus or a third-party arbitrator.

Data Extraction

Key study characteristics were abstracted from included studies into evidence tables. One reviewer abstracted study data and a second reviewer did random checking. Intention-to-treat results were recorded if available.

Risk-of-Bias Assessment of Individual Studies

We assessed the risk of bias (internal validity) based on predefined criteria established by the Drug Effectiveness Review Project.[23] We rated the internal validity of observational studies based on the adequacy of the patient selection process, whether important differential loss to followup or overall high loss to followup occurred, the adequacy of exposure and event ascertainment, whether acceptable statistical techniques were used to minimize potential confounding factors, and whether the duration of followup was reasonable to capture investigated events.

All assessments resulted in a rating of high, medium, or low risk of bias, primarily at the study level. In some cases, the reviewers determined that validity varied by outcome and rated risk of bias for different outcomes separately. Studies that had serious flaws were rated high risk of bias, studies that met all criteria were low risk of bias, and the remainder were medium risk of bias. All studies were rated by one reviewer and checked by another reviewer. All disagreements were resolved through consensus.

Based on input from experts, we identified as key for all outcomes four potential confounding factors to be adjusted for in analyses of observational studies—age, race, parity, and other exposures (e.g., alcohol, smoking, and other potential teratogens). In some cases, additional confounders were considered based on their particular relevancy to specific outcomes. Low or moderate risk-of-bias studies that adjusted for these confounders were considered the best evidence if no RCTs were available.

Data Synthesis

We preferred direct comparisons over indirect comparisons, so they are the focus of our synthesis. We considered three types of directness: populations, intervention comparisons, and outcomes. Direct evidence consists of studies that (1) included the population of interest—depressed pregnant or postpartum women—in both intervention and control groups; (2) made the comparisons of interest—pharmacological treatments compared with each other, nonpharmacological interventions, or no treatment; and (3) measured outcomes of interest directly and did not use proxy measures (e.g., laboratory values). In this report, direct evidence included studies (trials or observational studies) that compared pregnant or postpartum women with depression who received antidepressant treatment with pregnant or postpartum women with depression who were not treated.

Indirect evidence included studies (trials or observational studies) of pregnant or postpartum women treated with antidepressants without specifying that the women had depression. Similarly, studies that compared pregnant or postpartum women who took an antidepressant drug with pregnant or postpartum women who did not take such medications but also were not known to have a diagnosis of depression (a general population) were considered indirect evidence. Indirect comparisons can be difficult to interpret for several reasons; in the case of comparison with a general population, the issue is primarily heterogeneity of underlying risk of the populations.

The underlying risk of untreated depression during pregnancy or the postpartum period is an important factor in assessing the relative benefits and harms of potential treatments. We used data from indirect comparisons when no other directly applicable evidence existed, but readers should interpret findings with caution because comparisons with a generally healthy population without depression rather than with a depressed population may underestimate the benefits and overestimate the harms of treatment.

We generally did not use data from high risk-of-bias studies in our main analysis, except to undertake sensitivity analyses for meta-analyses or when high risk-of-bias studies constituted the only evidence for an important outcome. To determine the appropriateness of meta-analysis, we considered the risk of bias of the studies and the heterogeneity among studies in design, patient population, interventions, and outcomes. We generally used random-effects models to estimate pooled effects; when only two studies were being pooled, we applied a fixed-effect model.[24,25] We calculated the Q statistic and the I^2 statistic to assess heterogeneity in effects between studies.[26,27] When we found statistical heterogeneity, we explored reasons for this by using subgroup analysis. When we could not perform meta-analysis, we summarized the data qualitatively, grouping studies by similarity of population, intervention characteristics, or both.

Strength of the Body of Evidence

We used the methods outlined in the original Chapter 10 of the AHRQ "Methods Guide for Effectiveness and Comparative Effectiveness Reviews"[20,28] to grade strength of evidence. Domains considered in grading the strength of evidence were risk of bias, consistency, directness, and precision. Based on this assessment, reviewers assigned the body of evidence a strength-of-evidence grade of high, moderate, or low. A rating of *high* means that we have high confidence that the evidence reflects the true effect and that further research is very unlikely to change our confidence in the estimate of effect, while a rating of *low* means that we have low confidence that the evidence reflects the true effect and that further research is likely to change our confidence in the estimate of the effect and to change the estimate.[20,28] In cases in which evidence did not exist, was sparse, or contained irreconcilable inconsistency, we assigned a grade of insufficient evidence. A rating of *insufficient* means that the evidence either is unavailable or does not permit estimation of an effect.

We consulted our technical experts to help us set priorities for the outcomes for grading. Specific outcomes selected for rating included the following for any comparison with at least moderate risk-of-bias evidence. For maternal outcomes, we graded danger to self or infant, depression symptomatology (response and remission), breastfeeding intention and duration, number with adverse events, discontinuation due to adverse events, and weight gain. For infant outcomes, we graded preterm birth, small for gestational age, neonatal mortality, congenital malformations, persistent pulmonary hypertension, infant and child neurodevelopment, intellectual function, educational outcome and school performance, mental health, and health care or social service use.

Applicability

We assessed applicability by examining the characteristics of the enrolled populations compared with those of target populations, characteristics of the interventions, and characteristics of the comparators. Technical experts identified items of particular interest that may affect applicability, which are reflected in the subgroups specified in Key Question 3.

Results

Results of Literature Searches

Based on electronic searches (3,405 citations), manual searches (53 citations), and scientific information packets (Forest Pharmaceuticals, Inc.; Jazz Pharmaceuticals; and Sanofi Aventis, U.S.), we identified a total of 3,458 potentially relevant citations. From these, we included 130 eligible unique studies in this report. The majority of the evidence was from observational studies (124 unique studies); we included only 6 RCTs.

Six RCTs and 15 observational studies provided direct evidence comparing treatments in groups of pregnant or postpartum women with depression. This is the primary evidence for this report. We included indirect evidence from 109 observational studies that included pregnant or postpartum women receiving an antidepressant drug for any reason and making comparisons with women who were not receiving an antidepressant drug during pregnancy or the postpartum period. Studies generally did not note the depression status of women in the intervention or control groups, although a few included depression as a confounder that investigators controlled for in analyses. This evidence is indirect for this report. We reported findings from these studies only for important outcomes for which evidence in pregnant women with depression did not exist or was sparse, particularly for serious harms for which even such indirect evidence may be useful in guiding clinical decisions. No studies compared an antidepressant drug with a nonpharmacological treatment; only a few had an intervention that involved use of a nonpharmacological treatment as an add-on to drug therapy.

Key Question 1

The overarching finding for Key Question 1 was that little evidence exists on the maternal benefits of antidepressant therapy specifically during pregnancy or the postpartum period. Studies were generally not designed to measure benefits (e.g., effect on depressive symptoms) when women were treated during pregnancy, and evidence did not allow comparisons among either the specific classes or individual drugs. Evidence on key outcomes and comparisons is lacking. Similarly, we have no information on the most effective dose of antidepressant drugs in pregnant women based on severity of symptoms or on either pharmacokinetic or pharmacodynamic alterations during pregnancy.

Maternal Benefits

Comparative evidence on depressive symptom response, anxiety, functional capacity, healthy maternal weight gain, and breastfeeding outcomes is insufficient to draw conclusions about the effects of antidepressant drugs in women with depression during pregnancy. Based on direct evidence from two very small observational studies, we found inconsistent results on the benefit of SSRI treatment on depressive symptoms during pregnancy and no evidence for other drug classes. A small observational study reported that depressed women treated with SSRIs continuously during pregnancy had higher scores on the SF-12 Mental Component Scale than did untreated women with depression throughout pregnancy (scores of 45 and 35, respectively, on a scale of 0 to 100), but the timing of measurement was not clear. We found no direct evidence of the effects of antidepressant drugs on other important depression outcomes, such as anxiety symptoms in women with depression during pregnancy. No direct evidence was available regarding pregnancy weight gain, intention to breastfeed, uptake of breastfeeding, or duration of breastfeeding.

Studies of pregnant women with unknown depression status provided indirect evidence on weight gain and breastfeeding outcomes. Such evidence was insufficient to draw conclusions about these outcomes in pregnant women with depression, but it may provide insight into directions for future research. Among pregnant women with unknown depression status, weight gain was slightly above recommended limits for women taking SSRIs but within recommended limits for women who did not receive SSRIs. Indirect evidence also suggested that, in pregnant women with unknown depression status, SSRI treatment during pregnancy was associated with fewer women intending to or initiating breastfeeding than among women not receiving such treatment during pregnancy; this probably reflects concerns or uncertainty about potential harms to the breastfed child. No evidence was available for comparative benefits of other pharmacological treatments in pregnant women with depression.

Evidence on maternal benefits from pharmacological treatments for depression during the postpartum period was insufficient. Direct evidence was limited to one small placebo-controlled trial that we rated as high risk of bias; indirect evidence came from a small observational study in pregnant women with unknown depression status rated medium risk of bias.

Evidence on the combination of antidepressant therapy with nonpharmacological interventions was insufficient to draw conclusions because of inconsistency and imprecision; it generally suffered from lack of adequate sample sizes.

Child Benefits

The potential benefits of treatment of depressed women during pregnancy to their children include parameters at birth (e.g., birth weight), child development, diagnosis of chronic diseases, and health care use. Direct evidence was available only for preterm birth and some developmental outcomes. Low-strength evidence from two small observational studies (N = 266 total) suggested that SSRIs have no statistically significant effect on rates of preterm birth (defined as <37 weeks gestation).[29,30] Pooled-analysis yielded an odds ratio (OR) of 1.87 (95% confidence interval [CI], 0.89 to 3.89). Indirect evidence suggested increased risk of preterm birth for women treated with SSRIs, TCAs, SNRIs, or NRIs during pregnancy compared with the risk for women not treated with antidepressants during pregnancy and with unknown depression status. For SSRIs, this finding was consistent across studies; however, the magnitude of risk associated with specific timing of maternal exposure during pregnancy was unclear. Risk may be higher with citalopram or escitalopram than with fluoxetine, paroxetine, and sertraline; however, direct comparisons of the drugs in women with depression are needed to confirm these findings. Evidence on fetal growth was limited to indirect evidence; we found no apparent increased risk associated with exposure to SSRIs or TCAs.

Direct evidence on infant and child development was limited to two very small studies. This evidence was insufficient to draw conclusions about the risk of delayed development in children of mothers taking SSRIs for depression during pregnancy compared with the risk in children of mothers whose depression was not treated with antidepressants. Indirect evidence did not indicate increased risk of motor, language, or cognitive development that is outside of the normal range for age.

Comparative evidence on the risk of diagnosis of attention-deficit hyperactivity disorder (ADHD) in children of mothers treated for depression during pregnancy was insufficient; we had no direct evidence on this concern. Indirect evidence suggested that, compared with children not exposed during pregnancy, diagnosis by the age of 5 years among exposed children was associated with bupropion use (OR, 3.63; p<0.02), particularly for exposure in the second trimester. In contrast, a diagnosis of ADHD was not associated with use of SSRIs or other antidepressants during pregnancy. Filling a prescription for an SSRI after pregnancy (timing not defined) was statistically significantly associated with increased risk of ADHD diagnosis in the child by age 5 (OR, 2.04; p<0.001). These analyses controlled for parental mental health diagnoses; a diagnosis of depression in the mother during pregnancy was statistically significantly associated with the diagnosis of ADHD in the child (OR, 2.58; p<0.001).

Whether autism spectrum disorder (ASD) in the child is associated with depression during pregnancy, antidepressant treatment, or an interaction of the two was not clear. We found no direct evidence on the risk of different treatments for depression during pregnancy on development of ASD in the child. We found indirect evidence, based on two large population-based case-control studies with low and medium risk of bias, that suggested that maternal use of SSRIs is statistically significantly associated with diagnosis of ASD in the child after controlling for maternal depression diagnosis during pregnancy (pooled OR, 1.82; 95% CI, 1.14 to 2.91).[31,32] Both studies also examined antidepressant drugs other than SSRIs: one found an increased risk with TCAs and the other found no increased risk with TCAs combined with SNRIs or NRIs. Although these results controlled for depression, the comparison groups were children of women who did not receive an antidepressant during pregnancy rather than women with untreated known depression; moreover, neither study reported the proportion of women with a diagnosis of depression for either group.

In one of these studies, results of subgroup analyses suggested that depression itself may contribute to ASD diagnosis. Compared with the risk for ASD in children of pregnant women without depression or antidepressant use, the risk for ASD in the children of pregnant women with depression and antidepressant use was statistically significantly elevated (OR, 3.34; 95% CI, 1.50 to 7.47). In contrast, the risk in pregnant women taking an antidepressant for another indication was lower than the risk in children of pregnant women without depression or antidepressant use and not statistically significant (OR, 1.61; 95% CI, 0.85 to 3.06).

We found no evidence comparing drug therapy with nondrug therapy. Evidence for other outcomes or comparisons for exposure either during pregnancy or in the postpartum period was not found or was insufficient.

Key Question 2

Maternal Harms

We found no direct evidence on maternal harms of pharmacological treatments for depression during pregnancy. The main reasons are that, for this population, we had only observational evidence and the studies did not report harms outcomes of interest for this report, such as rates of specific adverse effects (e.g., suicidal ideation, hepatotoxicity, and loss of libido). The risk of mortality may have been reported sporadically, but most of these retrospective observational studies would have excluded women who died during pregnancy, and the remaining studies did not have explicit methodology to ascertain death and other serious harms.

Child Harms

Evidence on harms to the child of a mother treated for depression during pregnancy was limited by the comparison groups that most studies selected—namely, pregnant women who did not take an antidepressant and with unknown depression status. As with comparative benefits to the child, the direct evidence was very limited and was mostly insufficient for drawing conclusions. Indirect evidence may be valuable for harms such as mortality and congenital anomalies, because signals for increased risk of harm may be used to direct future studies. The findings for maternal treatment with antidepressants during pregnancy reflected evidence of greater risk for some serious infant harms associated primarily with exposure to SSRIs, but the contributory role of depression in these outcomes is mostly unstudied.

We had no direct evidence for the risk of infant mortality with maternal use of antidepressant drugs to treat depression during pregnancy. Indirect evidence, based on large population-based cohort studies, was inconsistent; study findings indicated an increased risk of infant death over the first year of life with exposure to SSRIs (OR, 1.81; 95% CI, 1.26 to 2.60), but not when we evaluated early and late death separately. A single cohort study reported no increased risk of neonatal mortality with SNRI or NRI use during pregnancy.

Direct evidence on the association of major congenital malformations with use of SSRIs for depression during pregnancy was insufficient, based on two small studies (N = 282 total) that reported only one or zero events. No comparative evidence on the risk of cardiac malformations in women treated for depression during pregnancy was found. A substantial amount of indirect evidence about the incidence of major congenital malformations was available from 15 cohort studies; they reported on incidence associated with the use of either any SSRI or specific SSRIs among depressed women during pregnancy compared with no use of SSRIs among women who were not known to be depressed. Although exposure to SSRIs as a group did not result in increased risk of major malformations in infants, evidence indicated small but statistically significant risk with exposure to fluoxetine (OR, 1.14; 95% CI, 1.01 to 1.30) or paroxetine (OR, 1.17; 95% CI, 1.02 to 1.35), but not the other SSRIs individually. Timing of exposure was primarily in the first trimester, although our sensitivity analyses removing studies that may have included exposures at other timepoints did not alter these results. Results were similar for cardiac malformations, except that limiting our analyses to the highest quality studies of fluoxetine yielded a nonsignificant increase in risk. The increased risk with paroxetine was 1.49 (95% CI, 1.20 to 1.85). TCAs were also significantly associated with increased risk for major malformations (OR, 1.31; 95% CI, 1.04 to 1.65) and cardiac malformations (OR, 1.58; 95% CI, 1.10 to 2.29). Evidence for other antidepressants was not available.

We found no direct evidence on the risk of neonatal withdrawal symptoms or pulmonary hypertension with maternal use of antidepressant drugs to treat depression during pregnancy. Indirect evidence suggested greater risk of neonatal withdrawal symptoms with fluoxetine use for any reason (indications not specified or mixed) during the first trimester compared with women who did not use an antidepressant during pregnancy but whose depression status was unknown (relative risk, 8.7; 95% CI, 2.9 to 26.6). Risk was also found to be increased with SSRIs or venlafaxine in late pregnancy, but no difference in risk was found between SSRIs and SNRIs (as a group) in neonatal withdrawal symptoms. Indirect evidence suggested that persistent pulmonary hypertension in the child was statistically significantly associated with maternal SSRI use during late pregnancy (OR, 2.72; 95% CI, 1.63 to 4.54).

Based on three studies, there was low-strength evidence that, compared with untreated maternal depression during pregnancy, SSRI treatment was associated with a statistically significant increase in risk of respiratory distress in infants (pooled unadjusted OR, 1.91; 95% CI, 1.63 to 2.24; $I^2 = 0\%$). Direct evidence was not available to assess the risk with TCAs, SNRIs, or NRIs; however, indirect evidence suggested an increase in risk with TCAs used late in pregnancy (adjusted OR, 2.11; 95% CI, 1.57 to 2.83).

Low-strength direct evidence suggested no statistically significant associations between maternal use of SSRIs during pregnancy and neonatal convulsions compared with infants of untreated depressed pregnant women. Indirect evidence was in conflict with this finding, indicating an increased risk of convulsions for children whose mother used SSRIs for any indication during pregnancy compared with the risk for children of women who did not take an SSRI during pregnancy and were not known to be depressed.

Only a few well-designed studies examined the risk for teratogenicity with exposure to antidepressants specifically during the conception period; the evidence was insufficient.

Numerous other studies examined congenital malformations with exposure in early pregnancy but did not report on exposure during the conception period (i.e., pre-existing treatment). These studies contributed to the evidence on potential harms with treatment during pregnancy.

Key Question 3

In Key Question 3, we attempted to examine a wide range of subgroups defined by patient and intervention characteristics. Given the difficulty we had in identifying evidence for the first two Key Questions with appropriate control and intervention groups, it is not surprising that we found very little direct evidence to address these questions. Based on the direct evidence, with comparisons between treated and untreated pregnant women with depression and data stratified into continuous use and use during only one trimester, the duration of treatment did not appear to influence the risk of preterm birth. We found that, in the postpartum period, multiple sessions of cognitive behavioral therapy were not superior to a single session when both were combined with fluoxetine. Depressive symptom response to dynamic psychotherapy, with or without sertraline, did not vary based on depression severity level. For all other subgroups (including those based on coadministration of other drugs, medical provider characteristics, medical care environments, and characteristics of diagnosis), the evidence was limited. Studies that used a definite diagnosis of depression in all comparison groups and that had medium or low risk of bias provided only insufficient evidence to draw conclusions about variation in treatment effects.

Discussion

Table C highlights the findings based on studies that were designed to compare directly the benefits or the harms of pharmacological treatments for depression in pregnant or postpartum women. As noted, we regarded the results of these investigations as direct evidence. We believe that this is the best evidence for the Key Questions posed for this review.

Table C. Key findings of direct-comparison evidence for antidepressant treatment of depression during pregnancy or postpartum

Time of Treatment, Intervention, and Potential Benefits and Harms	Comparison	Outcome	Strength of Evidence; Conclusions
Pregnancy			
Potential Benefits:			
SSRIs + psychotherapy	Psychotherapy alone	Depressive symptoms	Insufficient; no conclusions drawn
SSRIs: fluoxetine	No treatment	Depressive symptoms	Insufficient; no conclusions drawn
SSRIs	No treatment	Functional capacity	Insufficient; no conclusions drawn
SSRIs + psychotherapy	Psychotherapy alone	Breastfeeding	Insufficient; no conclusions drawn
SSRIs	No treatment	Preterm birth	Low; risk not increased
SSRIs + psychotherapy	Psychotherapy alone	Infant and child development: Bayley Scales	Insufficient; no conclusions drawn
SSRIs	No treatment	Infant and child development: Brazelton Neonatal Behavioral Assessment Scale	Insufficient; no conclusions drawn

Table C. Key findings of direct-comparison evidence for antidepressant treatment of depression during pregnancy or postpartum (continued)

Time of Treatment, Intervention, and Potential Benefits and Harms	Comparison	Outcome	Strength of Evidence; Conclusions
Potential Harms:			
SSRIs	No treatment	Major malformations	Insufficient; no conclusions drawn
SSRIs + psychotherapy	Psychotherapy alone	Major malformations	Insufficient; no conclusions drawn
SSRIs	No treatment	Neonatal convulsions	Low; risk not increased
SSRIs	No treatment	Neonatal respiratory distress	Low; risk higher with SSRIs
SSRIs	TCA: nortriptyline	Neonatal respiratory distress	Insufficient; no conclusions drawn
Postpartum			
Potential Benefits:			
Sertraline + brief dynamic psychotherapy	Brief dynamic psychotherapy	Depressive symptoms	Low; no difference in response or remission
Sertraline	Sertraline + interpersonal psychotherapy	Depressive symptoms	Insufficient; no conclusions drawn
Paroxetine	Paroxetine + cognitive behavioral therapy	Depressive symptoms.	Low; no difference in response or remission
Potential Harms:			
Sertraline + brief dynamic psychotherapy	Brief psychodynamic therapy	Adverse events	Insufficient; no conclusions drawn
Sertraline	Sertraline + interpersonal psychotherapy	Adverse events	Insufficient; no conclusions drawn
Fluoxetine + cognitive behavioral therapy	Cognitive behavioral therapy	Adverse events	Insufficient; no conclusions drawn

SSRI = selective serotonin reuptake inhibitor, TCA – tricyclic antidepressant

While the focus of this report is women with a new episode (not necessarily the first) of depression during pregnancy or postpartum, rather than a continuing episode, most studies simply identified women based on treatment status during pregnancy or postpartum (i.e., treated with antidepressants or not).

As reported in Table C, evidence for virtually all outcomes was insufficient. Only the outcomes of neonatal convulsions and respiratory distress in infants of women who took SSRIs as a class during pregnancy compared with those outcomes in infants of women with depression who did not take an antidepressant had low strength of evidence. The risk of convulsions was not higher with SSRIs; in contrast, the risk of respiratory distress was higher. For women with postpartum depression, only the evidence for depression symptom improvement with the comparison of adding brief dynamic psychotherapy or cognitive behavioral therapy to sertraline and paroxetine, respectively, was low strength, while the evidence for other outcomes was insufficient. Adding these nonpharmacological treatments did not improve the response or remission of depression symptoms. The primary reason for the other direct evidence leading to a strength of evidence grade of insufficient—and thus our inability to draw any meaningful conclusions from this evidence—was that these were small studies. They may not have had adequate statistical power to identify differences when they existed and were not as methodologically strong as is necessary to draw firm conclusions.

Not shown are outcomes for which we had only indirect evidence. These included studies that compared outcomes for women who took an antidepressant during pregnancy for any reason with those for women who did not take an antidepressant during pregnancy; the proportions of women with depression in either group were rarely reported and never analyzed. The applicability of indirect evidence of findings from studies of pregnant women with unknown depression status is unclear.

Findings in Relationship to What Is Already Known

Putting these findings into the context of prior comparative effectiveness evidence reviews was difficult; we did not identify any other studies with as broad a scope as ours or other reviews that applied comparable methodologies. For example, a review by Bromley et al.[33] assessed fetal and child outcomes and SSRIs only, but those authors did not limit their comparison group to women with depression, so our results are quite different from theirs. Additionally, we formally assessed the risk of bias in individual studies and graded the strength of evidence for the body of evidence for each key outcome, which other reviews did not.[33-45]

Applicability

The evidence on the benefits and harms of pharmacological treatment during pregnancy was limited to observational studies that generally met criteria for effectiveness studies.[46] The evidence on benefits and harms of pharmacological treatment for postpartum depression came almost entirely from RCTs that met criteria for efficacy studies. These studies were limited by several factors: exclusion of patients with common comorbidities, such as drug and alcohol misuse or abuse, other Axis I disorders, and suicidal ideation; lack of health outcomes and comprehensive assessment of adverse events; short study durations; and small sample sizes.

Only a small group of studies included pregnant women known to be depressed and compared treated and untreated groups, providing direct evidence. In these studies, however, we did not have further information on the diagnosis timing, prior history, or severity of symptoms. As maternal depression is widely recognized as a risk factor for poorer pregnancy outcomes, the findings from all the studies that do not account for maternal depression likely have very low applicability to our target population of pregnant women with depression.

With respect to other variables, the mean maternal age ranged from 26 years to 34 years. Few studies reported race or socioeconomic status. In the studies that reported race, the populations were predominantly white. When reported, a medium socioeconomic status level was most common. The data sources for these studies typically did not include access to information such as depressive symptom severity, coexisting anxiety diagnoses, and other mental health or medical conditions; family history of depressive or other mood disorders; prior use of antidepressant drugs; situation at home; unplanned pregnancy; and marital or partner status. Therefore, we know very little about these important patient characteristics.

Very little evidence was available to assess the benefits and harms of nonpharmacological treatment modalities, and what we found was limited to treatment during the postpartum period. The clinical relevance of the nonpharmacological treatment modalities was difficult to assess because of a general lack of detail about the characteristics of these interventions. Likewise, the clinical relevance of the pharmacological treatment regimens was difficult to assess because of a general lack of information about dose, duration, and cointerventions.

Only approximately 30 percent of included studies were conducted in the United States. Findings from many of the studies done in the United States and Canada may not be reflective of the general population in North America because of their reliance on highly selected samples who voluntarily called teratogen information services, had specific health plan membership, or attended specific community prenatal clinics.

Overall, the applicability of this evidence to programs such as the Children's Health Insurance Program (CHIP) is somewhat limited because of the issues noted above. The large number of studies conducted in health care settings outside the United States and in samples of women with medium socioeconomic status likely limits how well this evidence applies to children served by the CHIP program.

Implications for Clinical and Policy Decisionmaking

Depression during pregnancy and postpartum can have adverse consequences for both mother and child. Knowing the best course of action when a woman is diagnosed with depression during these times is extremely important. For multiple reasons, the evidence base at present is extremely limited in the specific guidance it can provide.

Our overall findings were based on insufficient or low-strength evidence. This means that future studies are very likely to alter the findings in a meaningful way. The implications for decisionmaking for women with depression during pregnancy are unclear. Without better evidence specific to this population, the balance of benefits and harms is uncertain.

Although we believe that treating depressed women with antidepressants is likely to improve some symptoms based on evidence derived from studies of nonpregnant patients, individual drugs may have varying effects in pregnant women because of differences in pharmacokinetic parameters between these two types of patient populations. Current evidence is insufficient to address comparative efficacy in pregnant women. The evidence on functional outcomes for the mother is also insufficient, although it leans toward better outcomes in women treated with an SSRI than in untreated pregnant women. Evidence for other health outcomes in pregnant women is missing.

Women taking antidepressants during pregnancy or in the postpartum period may be less likely to breastfeed or may breastfeed for shorter durations than women who are not taking an antidepressant. Clinicians know that, for women treated with antidepressants, decisions about breastfeeding can be problematic; thus, early discussion and support for maternal intention to breastfeed is warranted. Women who receive prenatal education and professional encouragement or who report that their health care provider encouraged them to breastfeed are more likely to initiate and sustain breastfeeding.[47-49] Antidepressants are widely used in postpartum women. For most antidepressants, no or only negligible amounts are passed from mother to baby through breast milk (fluoxetine and citalopram may be exceptions, but the amount varies with dose and frequency of dosing); no evidence exists of adverse events in babies.[50-52]

Evidence on the comparative benefits of treating depression during pregnancy (compared with not treating) is expected to include benefits in developmental achievement in the child. Our review indicates that use of SSRIs did not result in differences on most measures. Although the direct evidence did not indicate higher rates of preterm birth with use of SSRIs during pregnancy (unadjusted OR, 1.87; 95% CI, 0.63 to 4.42), it was insufficient to guide clinical decisions.

It has been suggested that numerous potentially serious harms may be associated with use of antidepressants during pregnancy. In the comparison of treated and untreated depressed women, however, we found only the risk for neonatal respiratory distress to be associated with SSRIs (as a drug class). The fact that different conclusions may be drawn for some other outcomes based on a large body of evidence that we consider indirect for our questions highlights the importance of making clinically relevant comparisons.

An example is the risk of ASD in children of women treated for depression during pregnancy. The increasing prevalence of ASD diagnosis, likely in part attributable to increased detection, temporally parallels an increasing tendency to prescribe antidepressants in pregnancy. Based on indirect evidence, whether ASD in the child is associated with maternal depression during pregnancy, treatment with antidepressants, or a combination of the two remains unclear. Although we found that ASD was associated with maternal exposure to antidepressants, particularly SSRIs, compared with maternal nonexposure (depression status unknown), we did not find clear evidence on the risk when untreated depressed women were the comparison group. Any suggestion of increased risk for ASD is very concerning. In studies comparing antidepressant use with maternal nonexposure, although researchers controlled for depression, the relationship between depression, antidepressant use, and risk of ASD remained unclear. The small but statistically significant risk of ASD diagnosis with antidepressant use or depression or both is important to understand better, because treatment could mitigate this risk if severe depression underlies the association with ASD. One study examined the risk of having a diagnosis of ASD in the child, finding statistically significantly increased odds in women who were depressed during pregnancy (with and without known treatment) and a nonsignificant increase in mothers without depression during pregnancy. An interaction between depression and antidepressant treatment is possible, but it has not been fully elucidated. Nevertheless, women should be informed about the risk of ASD in their offspring if antidepressants are found more conclusively to increase this risk. Because the fraction of cases of ASD that could potentially be attributed to antidepressants in these studies is exceedingly small (0.6% to 2.5% of the study populations), prenatal antidepressant use is not a major risk factor for ASD and does not explain the increasing prevalence of autism.

Evidence on the benefits or harms of treatment of depression in the postpartum period is insufficient to draw conclusions. Women and clinicians are currently left with only evidence on nonpregnant populations and evidence on intermediate outcomes (e.g., which drugs are passed into breast milk) to guide treatment choices.

Limitations of the Review Process

Methodological limitations of the review within the defined scope included the exclusion of studies published in languages other than English and lack of a specific search for unpublished studies. The review process and results could have benefited from further refinement of the scope to limit inclusion of studies to pregnant or postpartum women with depression in both the intervention and control groups.

Gaps in the Research

A major caveat to interpreting the findings of the majority of studies of exposure during pregnancy is the role of depression itself. Most of the studies specified that women were taking an antidepressant for any reason; few reported the proportions of women with depression and even fewer used this information in their analyses. Studies of women who were taking an antidepressant during or after pregnancy but were not known to be depressed are problematic; a major drawback is that we do not know the differential baseline risk of various outcomes for the various indications for which antidepressants can be used. We know, however, that some baseline risks are associated with depression during pregnancy; this fact underscores the importance of limiting the treated group to women with depression.[4,5]

Some clinicians or investigators may still hesitate to conduct RCTs in pregnant women.[53] Nevertheless, the assumption that the comparative effectiveness of interventions in nonpregnant populations is directly applicable to pregnant women may not be valid for various reasons (e.g., differences in pharmacokinetics of the drugs); moreover, trials in nonpregnant populations do not measure outcomes specific to pregnant or postpartum women. Various groups advocate for RCTs in pregnant women;[54,55] furthermore, the U.S. Department of Health and Human Services outlines detailed rules on protecting pregnant women research subjects and their fetuses.[56] Because clinicians already prescribe antidepressants on a regular basis to pregnant women, RCTs comparing treatments and adequately measuring appropriate outcomes, with measurement of depression severity at baseline and during followup among such populations, do not necessarily increase risk to either the women or their fetuses. Comparisons of specific treatments in pregnancy are badly needed to better uncover variation in risk across drugs, even within a class. Ascertainment of exposure, including both timing and dose, must be done in a way that ensures accuracy and reliability. Outcomes should be determined by blinded evaluators, which is possible for nearly all outcomes considered here. Randomization would be the best approach to minimize potential confounding, but observational studies could also be done in a way that addresses the gaps in the research. For example, studies could identify women being treated for depression as the study population and make comparisons across treatments (including no treatment). These studies should adjust for important prognostic factors such as pre-existing illness, depression history, depression severity, age, race, parity, socioeconomic status, and other exposures (e.g., alcohol, smoking, and other potential teratogens).

Nonpharmacological treatments are generally thought to have fewer risks than antidepressants. Nonetheless, evidence is almost entirely lacking on this point or on the question of the effectiveness of combinations of drug and nondrug treatments. Newer approaches to nonpharmacological interventions using technology such as Internet-based therapies, Web-camera counseling, and mobile phone applications are emerging. These may offer pregnant and postpartum women alternatives to more established treatments, particularly in lower income or rural populations.[57-59]

Studies of women in the postpartum period are both small and methodologically weak. These limitations leave a large gap in knowledge about treatments for a group of patients in whom RCTs could be undertaken. In addition to comparative efficacy (e.g., effects on symptoms), little is known about the benefits of treatments on important outcomes such as improving the mother-infant dyad, enhancing breastfeeding outcomes, or reducing domestic violence. The need for specifically designed research that addresses these problems is substantial.

The current evidence base is insufficient to inform clinical decisionmaking fully, because it requires knowing both benefits and harms and being able to determine the tradeoffs that individual patients might make. For example, if a medication has a lower adverse event profile but is also less effective for a given condition, prescribing it for a patient who needs therapy for that particular condition just because of a lower adverse event profile is not a reasonable therapeutic strategy. We know that depression during pregnancy and the postpartum period can lead to serious adverse outcomes for both mother and child, such that treatment is important.

Research in this area needs to measure both benefits and harms simultaneously, so that results can better inform the tradeoffs that women and clinicians need to weigh.

References

1. Norwitz ER, Lye SJ. Chapter 5: Biology of parturition. In: Creasy RK, Resnick R, Iams JD, eds. Creasy and Resnik's Maternal-Fetal Medicine: Principles and Practice. 6th ed., Philadelphia: Saunders/Elsevier; 2009:69-86.

2. Dietz PM, Williams SB, Callaghan WM, et al. Clinically identified maternal depression before, during, and after pregnancies ending in live births. Am J Psychiatry. 2007 Oct;164(10):1515-20. PMID: 17898342.

3. Halbreich U, Karkun S. Cross-cultural and social diversity of prevalence of postpartum depression and depressive symptoms. J Affect Disord. 2006 Apr;91(2-3):97-111. PMID: 16466664.

4. Hallberg P, Sjoblom V. The use of selective serotonin reuptake inhibitors during pregnancy and breast-feeding: a review and clinical aspects. J Clin Psychopharmacol. 2005 Feb;25(1):59-73. PMID: 15643101.

5. Nonacs R, Cohen LS. Assessment and treatment of depression during pregnancy: an update. Psychiatr Clin North Am. 2003 Sep;26(3):547-62. PMID: 14563097.

6. Alder J, Fink N, Bitzer J, et al. Depression and anxiety during pregnancy: a risk factor for obstetric, fetal and neonatal outcome? A critical review of the literature. J Matern Fetal Neonatal Med. 2007 Mar;20(3):189-209. PMID: 17437220.

7. Henry AL, Beach AJ, Stowe ZN, et al. The fetus and maternal depression: implications for antenatal treatment guidelines. Clin Obstet Gynecol. 2004 Sep;47(3):535-46. PMID: 15326416.

8. Grote NK, Bridge JA, Gavin AR, et al. A meta-analysis of depression during pregnancy and the risk of preterm birth, low birth weight, and intrauterine growth restriction. Arch Gen Psychiatry. 2010 Oct;67(10):1012-24. PMID: 20921117.

9. Murray L, Cooper PJ. Postpartum depression and child development. Psychol Med. 1997 Mar;27(2):253-60. PMID: 9089818.

10. Ludermir AB, Lewis G, Valongueiro SA, et al. Violence against women by their intimate partner during pregnancy and postnatal depression: a prospective cohort study. Lancet. 2010 Sep 11;376(9744):903-10. PMID: 20822809.

11. Myers E, Aubuchon-Endsley N, Bastian L, et al. Efficacy and Safety of Screening for Postpartum Depression. Comparative Effectiveness Review 106. (Prepared by the Duke Evidence-based Practice Center under Contract No. 290-2007-10066-I.) AHRQ Publication No. 13-EHC064-EF. Rockville, MD: Agency for Healthcare Research and Quality; 2013. www.effectivehealthcare.ahrq.gov/reports/final.cfm.

12. Hayes RM, Wu P, Shelton RC, et al. Maternal antidepressant use and adverse outcomes: a cohort study of 228,876 pregnancies. Am J Obstet Gynecol. 2012 Jul;207(1):49 e1-9. PMID: 22727349.

13. Gartlehner G, Hansen RA, Morgan LC, et al. Comparative benefits and harms of second-generation antidepressants for treating major depressive disorder: an updated meta-analysis. Ann Intern Med. 2011 Dec 6;155(11):772-85. PMID: 22147715.

14. Gartlehner G, Hansen, RA, Morgan, LC, et al. Second-Generation Antidepressants in the Pharmacologic Treatment of Adult Depression: An Update of the 2007 Comparative Effectiveness Review. (Prepared by the RTI International–University of North Carolina Evidence-based Practice Center under Contract No. 290-2007-10056-I.) AHRQ Publication No. 12-EHC012-EF. Rockville, MD: Agency for Healthcare Research and Quality; 2011. www.effectivehealthcare.ahrq.gov/reports/final.cfm.

15. Freeman MP, Fava M, Lake J, et al. Complementary and alternative medicine in major depressive disorder: the American Psychiatric Association Task Force report. J Clin Psychiatry. 2010 Jun;71(6):669-81. PMID: 20573326.

16. Kayser S, Bewernick BH, Grubert C, et al. Antidepressant effects, of magnetic seizure therapy and electroconvulsive therapy, in treatment-resistant depression. J Psychiatr Res. 2011 May;45(5):569-76. PMID: 20951997.

17. Cuijpers P, Geraedts AS, van Oppen P, et al. Interpersonal psychotherapy for depression: a meta-analysis. Am J Psychiatry. 2011 Jun;168(6):581-92. PMID: 21362740.

18. Ishak WW, Ha K, Kapitanski N, et al. The impact of psychotherapy, pharmacotherapy, and their combination on quality of life in depression. Harv Rev Psychiatry. 2011 Dec;19(6):277-89. PMID: 22098324.

19. Nieuwsma JA, Trivedi RB, McDuffie J, et al. Brief psychotherapy for depression: a systematic review and meta-analysis. Int J Psychiatry Med. 2012;43(2):129-51. PMID: 22849036.

20. Methods Guide for Effectiveness and Comparative Effectiveness Reviews. AHRQ Publication No. 10(12)-EHC063-EF. Rockville, MD: Agency for Healthcare Research and Quality; April 2012. Chapters available at: www.effectivehealthcare.ahrq.gov.

21. Moher D, Liberati A, Tetzlaff J, et al. Preferred reporting items for systematic reviews and meta-analyses: the PRISMA statement. PLoS Med. 2009;6(7). PMID: 1000097.

22. Diagnostic and Statistical Manual of Mental Disorders: DSM-IV-TR. 4th ed., text revision ed. Washington: American Psychiatric Association; 2000.

23. McDonagh MS, Jonas DE, Gartlehner G, et al. Methods for the Drug Effectiveness Review Project. BMC Med Res Methodol. 2012;12:140. PMID: 22970848.

24. Guyatt GH, Norris SL, Schulman S, et al. Methodology for the development of antithrombotic therapy and prevention of thrombosis guidelines. Chest. 2012 Feb 1;141(2 Suppl):53S-70S. PMID: 22315256.

25. Sutton AJ, Abrams KR, Jones DR, et al. Methods for Meta-Analysis in Medical Research. Chichester, UK: John Wiley & Sons, Inc.; 2000.

26. Higgins JP, Thompson SG, Deeks JJ, et al. Measuring inconsistency in meta-analyses. BMJ. 2003;327(7414):557-60. PMID: 12958120.

27. Higgins JPT, Thompson SG. Quantifying heterogeneity in a meta-analysis. Stat Med. 2002;21(11):1539-58. PMID: 12111919.

28. Owens DK, Lohr KN, Atkins D, et al. AHRQ series paper 5: Grading the strength of a body of evidence when comparing medical interventions--Agency for Healthcare Research and Quality and the Effective Health Care Program. J Clin Epidemiol. 2010 May;63(5):513-23. PMID: 19595577.

29. Wisner KL, Bogen DL, Sit D, et al. Does fetal exposure to SSRIs or maternal depression impact infant growth? Am J Psychiatry. 2013 May 1;170(5):485-93. PMID: 23511234.

30. Yonkers KA, Norwitz ER, Smith MV, et al. Depression and serotonin reuptake inhibitor treatment as risk factors for preterm birth. Epidemiology. 2012;23(5):677-85. PMID: 22627901.

31. Croen LA, Grether JK, Yoshida CK, et al. Antidepressant use during pregnancy and childhood autism spectrum disorders. Arch Gen Psychiatry. 2011 Nov;68(11):1104-12. PMID: 21727247.

32. Rai D, Lee BK, Dalman C, et al. Parental depression, maternal antidepressant use during pregnancy, and risk of autism spectrum disorders: population based case-control study. BMJ. 2013 Apr 19;346:f2059. PMID: 23604083.

33. Bromley RL, Wieck A, Makarova D, et al. Fetal effects of selective serotonin reuptake inhibitor treatment during pregnancy: immediate and longer term child outcomes. Fetal Matern Med Rev. 2012;23(3-4):230-75.

34. Ross EL, Grigoriadis S, Mamisashvili L. Selected pregnancy and delivery outcomes after exposure to antidepressant medication: a systematic review and meta-analysis. JAMA Psychiatry. 2013:1-8. PMID: 23446732.

35. 't Jong GW, Einarson T, Koren G, et al. Antidepressant use in pregnancy and persistent pulmonary hypertension of the newborn (PPHN): a systematic review. Reprod Toxicol. 2012;34(3):293-7. PMID: 22564982.

36. Sockol LE, Epperson CN, Barber JP. A meta-analysis of treatments for perinatal depression. Clin Psychol Rev. 2011 Jul;31(5):839-49. PMID: 21545782.

37. Gentile S. Neonatal withdrawal reactions following late in utero exposure to antidepressant medications. Curr Womens Health Rev. 2011;7(1):18-27.

38. Wurst KE, Poole C, Ephross SA, et al. First trimester paroxetine use and the prevalence of congenital, specifically cardiac, defects: a meta-analysis of epidemiological studies. Birth Defects Res Part A Clin Mol Teratol. 2010 Mar;88(3):159-70. PMID: 19739149.

39. Ng RC, Hirata CK, Yeung W, et al. Pharmacologic treatment for postpartum depression: a systematic review. Pharmacotherapy. 2010 Sep;30(9):928-41. PMID: 20795848.

40. Kendall-Tackett K, Hale TW. The use of antidepressants in pregnant and breastfeeding women: a review of recent studies. J Hum Lact. 2010 May;26(2):187-95. PMID: 19652194.

41. Santone G, Ricchi G, Rocchetti D, et al. Is the exposure to antidepressant drugs in early pregnancy a risk factor for spontaneous abortion? A review of available evidences. Epidemiol Psichiatr Soc. 2009;18(3):240-7. PMID: 20034202.

42. Myles N, Newall H, Ward H, et al. Systematic meta-analysis of individual selective serotonin reuptake inhibitor medications and congenital malformations. Aust N Z J Psychiatry; 2013 Nov:47(11):1002-12. Epub 2013 Jun 12. PMID 23761574.

43. Grigoriadis S, VonderPorten EH, Mamisashvili L. Antidepressant exposure during pregnancy and congenital malformations: is there an association? A systematic review and meta-analysis of the best evidence. J Clin Psychiatry. 2013 Apr;74(4):e293-e308. PMID: 23656855.

44. Grigoriadis S, VonderPorten EH, Mamisashvili L. The effect of prenatal antidepressant exposure on neonatal adaptation: a systematic review and meta-analysis. J Clin Psychiatry. 2013 Apr;74(4):e309-e20. PMID: 23656856.

45. Painuly N, Heun R, Painuly R, et al. Risk of cardiovascular malformations after exposure to paroxetine in pregnancy: meta-analysis. Psychiatrist. 2013 Jun 1;37(6):198-203.

46. Gartlehner G, Hansen RA, Nissman D, et al. A simple and valid tool distinguished efficacy from effectiveness studies. J Clin Epidemiol. 2006 Oct;59(10):1040-8. PMID: 16980143.

47. Lu M, Lange L, Slusser W, et al. Provider encouragement of breast-feeding: evidence from a national survey. Obstet Gynecol. 2001;97(2):290-5. PMID: 11165597.

48. Philipp BL, Malone KL, Cimo S, et al. Sustained breastfeeding rates at a US baby-friendly hospital. Pediatrics. 2003 Sep;112(3 Pt 1):e234-6. PMID: 12949318.

49. Su LL, Chong YS, Chan YH, et al. Antenatal education and postnatal support strategies for improving rates of exclusive breast feeding: randomised controlled trial. BMJ. 2007 Sep 22;335(7620):596. PMID: 17670909.

50. Hale TW. Medications and Mother's Milk 2012: A Manual of Lactational Pharmacology. 15th ed. Amarillo, TX: Hale Publishing LP; 2012.

51. Lanza di Scalea T, Wisner KL. Antidepressant medication use during breastfeeding. Clin Obstet Gynecol. 2009 Sep;52(3):483-97. PMID: 19661763.

52. Lawrence RA, Lawrence RM. Breastfeeding: A Guide for the Medical Profession. 7th ed. St. Louis, MO: Saunders; 2011.

53. Howland RH. Update on St. John's wort. J Psychosoc Nurs Ment Health Serv. 2010 Nov;48(11):20-4. PMID: 21053786.

54. The Second Wave Initiative. Toward the Responsible Inclusion of Pregnant Women in Research. www.secondwaveinitiative.org/. Accessed February 2, 2014.

55. Moyer M. Why Pregnant Women Deserve Drug Trials. Body Politic [Blog]. January 6, 2011. http://blogs.plos.org/bodypolitic/2011/01/06/why-pregnant-women-deserve-drug-trials/. Accessed February 2, 2014.

56. Research involving pregnant women or fetuses [45 CFR Part 46B Section 204]. In Code of Federal Regulations. Title 45: Public Welfare. Part 46: Protection of Human Subjects. Subpart B: Additional Protections for Pregnant Women, Human Fetuses and Neonates Involved in Research. Washington: U.S. Department of Health & Human Services. Revised January 15, 2009. Effective July 14, 2009. www.hhs.gov/ohrp/humansubjects/guidance/45cfr46.html#46.204. Accessed February 2, 2014.

57. Aguilera A, Munoz RF. Text messaging as an adjunct to CBT in low-income populations: a usability and feasibility pilot study. Profess Psychol Res Pract. 2011;42(6):472-8.

58. Boschen MJ, Casey LM. The use of mobile telephones as adjuncts to cognitive behavioral psychotherapy. Profess Psychol Res Pract. 2008;39(5):546-52.

59. Moritz S, Schilling L, Hauschildt M, et al. A randomized controlled trial of internet-based therapy in depression. Behav Res Ther. 2012;50(7-8):513-21. PMID: 22677231.

Introduction

Background

Condition

Depression is a potentially life-threatening condition. With an incidence during pregnancy and the postpartum period estimated to be anywhere from 5.5 to 33.1 percent, the American Academy of Pediatrics estimates that more than 400,000 infants are born each year to mothers who are depressed.[1-5] During the postpartum period, up to 85 percent of women experience some type of mood disturbance.[3-6]

Depression during pregnancy is known to be associated with harmful prenatal health consequences such as poor nutrition and poor prenatal medical care, risk of suicide, and harmful health behaviors, such as smoking and alcohol or other substance misuse. These circumstances compromise the health of both the woman and her fetus.[7,8] Although causation has not been proven, several adverse obstetric complications have been reported with untreated prenatal depression, including pre-eclampsia, preterm delivery, low birth weight, miscarriage, small-for-gestational-age babies, low Apgar scores, and neonatal complications.[9,10] These complications may be more common among women with lower socioeconomic status.[9-11] In addition to being debilitating for the mother, postpartum depression affects maternal-infant interactions and some measures of infant development. In extreme cases postpartum depression may increase the risk of infant mortality through neglect, abuse, or homicide.[12] It also negatively affects interactions within other members of the family unit and is associated with intimate partner violence.[13]

Depression during pregnancy and the postpartum period has a range of presentations, including continuation or relapse of a pre-existing mood disorder, development of changes in mood during pregnancy and the postpartum period, and postpartum "baby blues." Differentiating the correct diagnosis can be complex. Problems with mood are often accompanied by co-existing anxiety and occasionally by potentially life-threatening psychosis.[14]

General risk factors for depression include female sex, previous depression, family history of depression, poor social support, and substance abuse. Additional factors associated with depression in pregnant women include younger age, being without a partner, traumatic events within the previous 12 months, and pregnancy complications.[2,15] A 2013 Agency for Healthcare Research and Quality (AHRQ) report found that screening can significantly reduce postpartum depressive symptoms when there are systems in place to ensure adequate followup of women with positive results.[16]

Treatment Strategies

Decisionmaking surrounding treatment of depression in pregnancy is complex because the potential harms of treatments must be balanced against the potential harms to mother and fetus of untreated depression. Management of mood disorders in pregnancy or the postpartum period varies case by case. In women with existing depression, the tactic may be to stabilize symptoms before attempting pregnancy. But providers and patients are often concerned about the safety of continued pharmacological treatment to the fetus during pregnancy and the postpartum period, particularly if the prospective mother is considering breastfeeding.[17] This makes information about the comparative effectiveness of nonpharmacological treatments for depression during pregnancy of high interest. Treatment choice, or dosing, may vary by the severity of depression, for example, whether the symptoms meet criteria for a diagnosis of major depressive disorder according to the 4th edition of the Diagnostic and Statistical Manual of Mental Disorders (DSM IV),[18] are subclinical (symptoms are present but not meeting these criteria), or whether there are other co-existing psychiatric symptoms (most typically anxiety). Thus clear and accurate diagnosis, and reporting of diagnosis, is important to understanding the benefits and harms of treatment.

Interventions for depression both during pregnancy and in the postpartum period can include pharmacological treatments, nonpharmacological treatments, and watchful waiting or no intervention. Pharmacological treatments approved by the U.S. Food and Drug Administration (FDA) for treating depression are listed in Table 1. Antidepressant medications are also used to treat a variety of other indications, including anxiety disorders (e.g., generalized anxiety disorder, panic attacks, obsessive compulsive disorder, depressed phase of bipolar disorder, and neuropathic pain).

Antidepressant medications have been shown to be effective at reducing the symptoms of depression in nonpregnant adults.[19,20] In general, medications that are effective in treating conditions outside of pregnancy are often presumed to remain effective in pregnancy, but the developing fetus and changes in maternal physiology raise questions about safety and dosing of various agents. The FDA Pregnancy Category for safety to the fetus of antidepressant medications taken during pregnancy is category C ("animal reproduction studies have shown an adverse effect on the fetus and there are no adequate and well-controlled studies in humans, but potential benefits may warrant use of the drug in pregnant women despite potential risks"), with the exception of paroxetine which is category D ("there is positive evidence of human fetal risk based on adverse reaction data from investigational or marketing experience or studies in humans, but potential benefits may warrant use of the drug in pregnant women despite potential risks"). However, evidence on how the risk of one antidepressant compares to another when taken during pregnancy is not well understood. In the postpartum period, depressed mothers often have concerns regarding the use of antidepressants while breastfeeding. Providers can offer encouragement by educating women as to the well-documented benefits of breastfeeding and guide their choice of an individual antidepressant by considering the degree to which each antidepressant is known to pass into breast milk.[21-23]

There are also a wide array of nonpharmacological interventions that can be used to treat depression, including various psychotherapies, electroconvulsive therapy, transmagnetic stimulation, and acupuncture.[24-28] Some of these may be used during pregnancy, while others may be reserved for use in the postpartum period (e.g., electroconvulsive therapy).

Table 1. Pharmacologic interventions: Antidepressant agents

Drug Category	Generic Name	Trade Name
Selective serotonin reuptake inhibitor (SSRI)	Citalopram	Celexa®, various generics
	Escitalopram	Lexapro®
	Fluoxetine	Prozac®, various generics Prozac Weekly® Sarafem®
	Fluvoxamine	Luvox®, various generics Luvox CR®
	Sertraline	Zoloft®, various generics
	Paroxetine	Paxil®, various generics Paxil CR®
	Vilazodone	Viibryd®
Serotonin norepinephrine reuptake inhibitor (SNRI)	Desvenlafaxine	Pristiq®
	Venlafaxine	Effexor XR®
	Mirtazapine	Remeron®, various generics Remeron Soltab®
Selective serotonin norepinephrine reuptake (SSNRI)	Duloxetine	Cymbalta®
Tricyclic antidepressants (TCAs)	Amitriptyline	Various generics
	Desipramine	Norpramin®, various generics
	Imipramine	Tofranil®, various generics
	Nortriptyline	Aventyl hydrochloride® Pamelor™ Various generics
Norepinephrine reuptake inhibitors (NRIs)	Nefazodone	Various generics (previously available as Serzone®)
	Trazodone	Desyrel®, various generics
Other	Bupropion	Wellbutrin® Wellbutrin SR® Wellbutrin XL® Forfivo XL® Aplenzin®

Scope and Key Questions

Previous reviews broadly evaluated infant and child outcomes following all-purpose maternal use of antidepressants during pregnancy,[29-41] but they did not focus on specific populations of women with depression. The objective of this systematic review was to compare the benefits and harms of various pharmacological treatment options, to each other and to nonpharmacological treatments, for depression during pregnancy or the postpartum period. The focus was on women who develop depression during pregnancy or the postpartum period, rather than those with a continuing episode. We assessed factors that might impact maternal and child outcomes, including patient, provider, or environmental factors and a prior history of depression. Negative effects of untreated disease and exposure to antidepressive drugs were evaluated, highlighting the treatment dilemmas confronting women with depression during pregnancy or the postpartum period. Finally, we identified issues that future studies should address so that women, health care providers, and other stakeholders can make optimally informed decisions based on balancing benefits and harms.

Key Questions

The Agency for Healthcare Research and Quality wrote preliminary Key Questions based on input from the topic nominator. The Pacific Northwest Evidence-based Practice Center (EPC) revised the Key Questions and developed eligibility criteria to identify the populations, interventions, comparators, outcomes, timing, and study designs of interest. The EPC solicited additional input from the Technical Expert Panel (TEP).

Key Question 1. What are the comparative benefits of pharmacological and nonpharmacological treatments for women with depression during pregnancy and in the postpartum period?

a. How do pharmacological treatments affect maternal and child[a] outcomes when compared with placebo or no active treatment or usual care?
b. How do pharmacological treatments affect maternal and child outcomes when compared with each other (drug A vs. drug B)?
c. How do pharmacological treatments affect maternal and child outcomes when compared with active nonpharmacological treatments?
d. How does combination therapy affect maternal and child outcomes? The combinations include:
   i. Using a second drug to augment the effects of the primary drug and comparing this treatment with monotherapy with a single drug
   ii. Combining pharmacological treatments with nonpharmacological treatments and comparing them with nonpharmacological treatments alone
   iii. Comparing pharmacological treatments alone with pharmacological treatments used in combination with nonpharmacological treatments

Key Question 2. What are the comparative harms of pharmacological and nonpharmacological treatments for women with depression during pregnancy and in the postpartum period?

a. How do pharmacological treatments affect maternal and child[a] outcomes when compared with placebo or no active treatment or usual care?
b. How do pharmacological treatments affect maternal and child outcomes when compared with each other (drug A vs. drug B)?
c. How do pharmacological treatments affect maternal and child outcomes when compared with active nonpharmacological treatments?
d. How does combination therapy affect maternal and child outcomes? The combinations include:
   i. Using a second drug to augment the effects of the primary drug and comparing this treatment with monotherapy with a single drug
   ii. Combining pharmacological treatments with nonpharmacological treatments and comparing them with nonpharmacological treatments alone
   iii. Comparing pharmacological treatments alone with pharmacological treatments

---
[a] A child is defined as a fetus, infant, or a child up to age 18.

       used in combination with nonpharmacological treatments
  e. In babies born to women who become pregnant while taking medications to treat depression, what is the comparative risk of teratogenicity?

Key Question 3. Is there evidence that the comparative effectiveness (benefits or harms) of pharmacological and nonpharmacological treatments for women with depression during pregnancy and in the postpartum period varies based on characteristics[b] such as:

a. Patient characteristics—race, age, socioeconomic status, family history of depressive/mood disorders, prior use of antidepressive drugs (for treatment or prevention), severity of symptoms, situation at home, unplanned pregnancy, and marital/partner status?
b. Patient comorbidities (e.g., anxiety diagnoses)?
c. Intervention characteristics—dosing regimens and duration of treatments?
d. Co-administration of other psychoactive drugs, specifically, antipsychotics, anti-anxiety agents (e.g., benzodiazepines), and drugs for insomnia?
e. Medical provider characteristics (primary care physician, obstetrician, pediatrician, psychiatrist, nurse, midwife, or community worker)?
f. Medical care environment (community/private/public clinic or hospital)?
g. Characteristics of diagnosis—whether depression was detected during screening or not, time of diagnosis, method of diagnosis, and when treatment commenced relative to the onset of symptoms?

Analytic Frameworks

The analytic frameworks (Figure 1) illustrate the population, interventions, outcomes, and adverse effects studied and their relationship to the Key Questions. The first framework relates to pregnant women with depression (far left) who receive treatment. This population was intended to be women with an episode of depression beginning during pregnancy, rather than a continuing episode. The exception was Key Question 2e, for which the population was intended to be taking an antidepressant during the time of conception. Treatment leads to health outcomes in the box on the far right of the figure, connected by the overarching line. This evidence is the topic of Key Question 1, as marked on the line. Treatment may lead to intermediate outcomes, such as changes in level of depression symptoms, or adverse events, both noted as separate boxes on the diagram. The evidence showing that better intermediate outcomes (e.g., symptoms) improves health outcomes (e.g., reduced risk of suicide) is represented by a dotted line between boxes; we did not review that literature in this report. The second framework relates to postpartum women with depression (far left), and again the outcomes that may result from treatment are depicted in

---

[b]Other factors will be considered as they are identified within the comparative studies.

relationship to each other, the treatments, and the Key Questions. The outcomes considered for postpartum women with depression differed from those considered for pregnant women.

Figure 1. Analytic frameworks for treatment of depression in pregnant and postpartum women

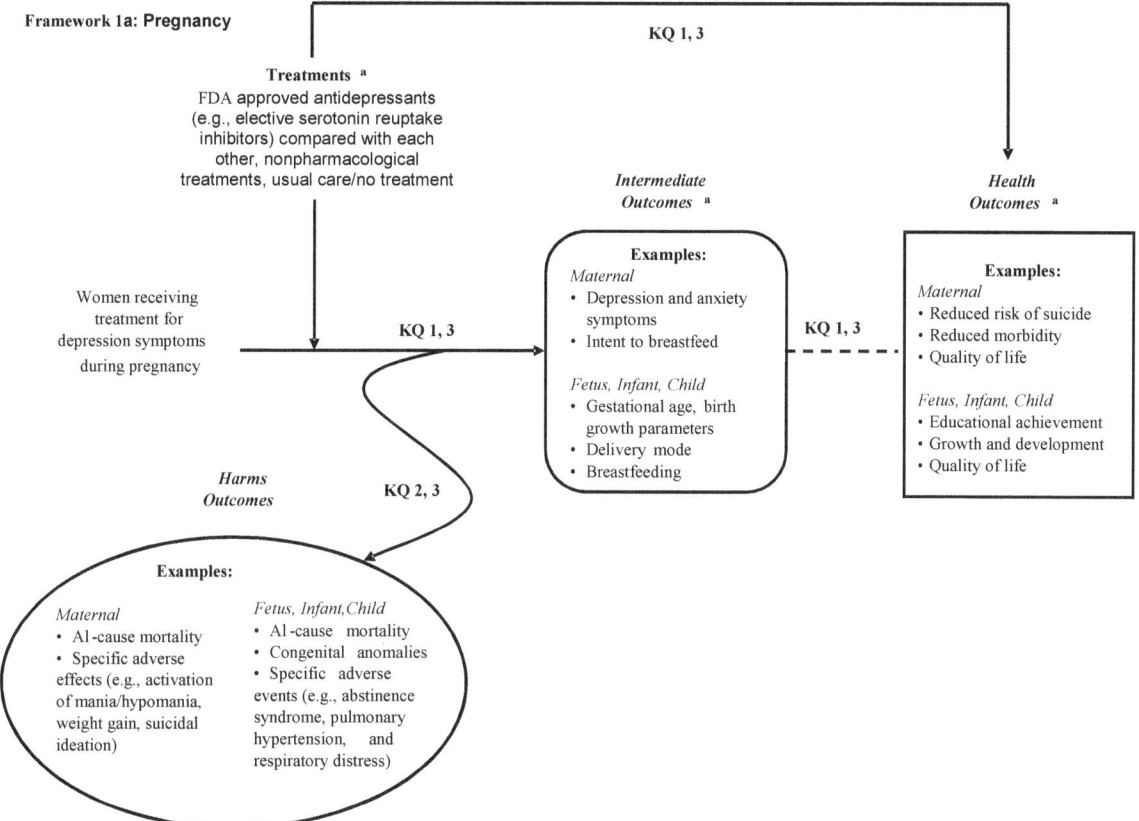

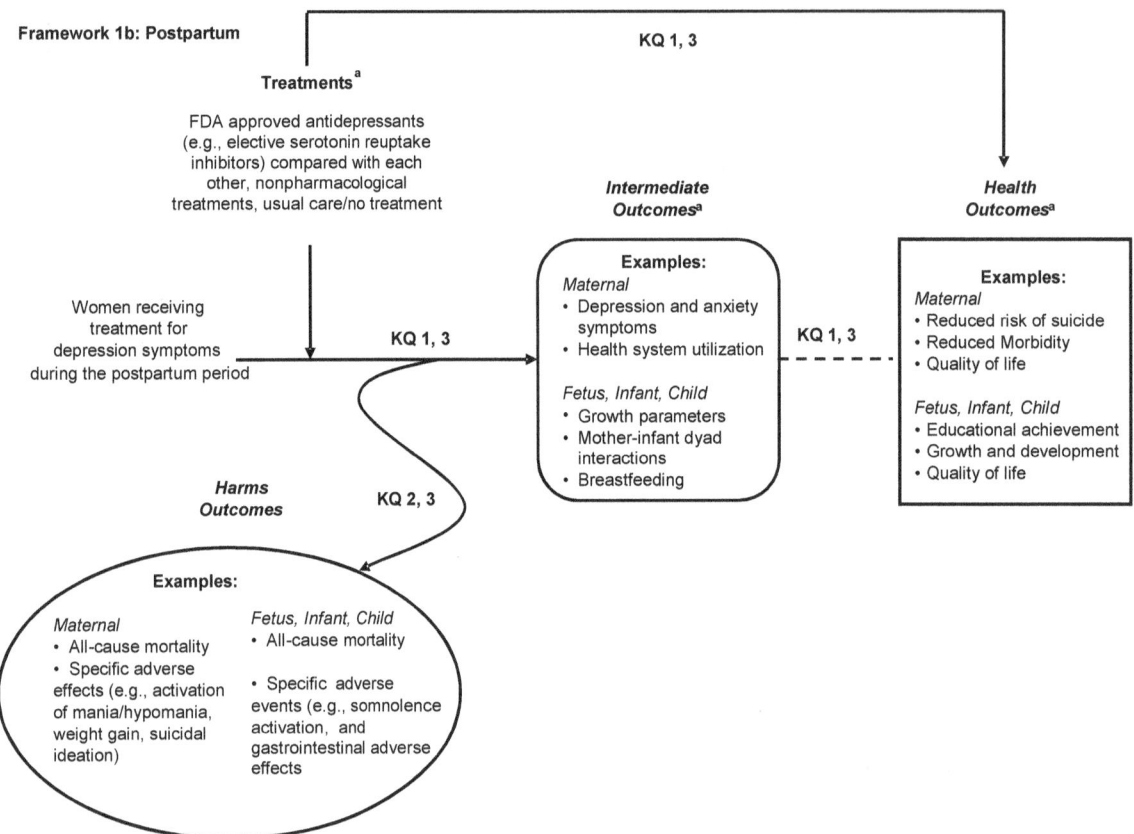

[a] The interventions and outcomes are too numerous to illustrate in their entirety in this diagram. See the Methods section, Inclusion and Exclusion Criteria, for complete details on interventions and outcomes. FDA = U.S. Food and Drug Administration; KQ = Key Question

Organization of This Report

The evidence below is organized first by Key Question, then by the subquestions of the Key Questions, then by pregnancy status at the time of exposure—during pregnancy or postpartum. Within those categories the evidence is presented by pharmacological class with all outcomes for a given class presented together, then by comparisons of pharmacological and nonpharmacological or combination therapy. Under each intervention individual outcomes are assessed; outcomes listed in the inclusions criteria (above) for which *no* evidence was found are not itemized below.

Methods

The methods for this comparative effectiveness review follow the methods suggested in the ARHQ "Methods Guide for Effectiveness and Comparative Effectiveness Reviews."[42] The main sections in this chapter reflect the protocol elements established for the comparative effectiveness review; certain methods map to the PRISMA checklist.[43] All methods and analyses were determined a priori. The research protocol was posted on the AHRQ Effective Health Care program Web site (http://www.effectivehealthcare.ahrq.gov), and we registered the protocol in the systematic review registry, PROSPERO (http://www.crd.york.ac.uk/NIHR_PROSPERO/).

Search Strategy

To identify articles relevant to each Key Question, the librarian searched the Cochrane Database of Systematic Reviews (CDSR) from 2005 to July 2013, the Cochrane Central Register of Controlled Trials (CCRCT) July 2013, the Cumulative Index to Nursing and Allied Health Literature (CINAHL®) from 1941 to July 2013, Ovid MEDLINE® and Ovid OLDMEDLINE® from 1946 to July 2013, PsychINFO® from 1996 to July 2013, and Scopus® from 1974 to July 2013. Search dates and exact search strings are provided in Appendix A. Date restrictions are not placed on database searches. ClinicalTrials.gov was searched for gray literature. Scientific Information Packets were solicited from industry stakeholders through the Scientific Resource Center.

Inclusion and Exclusion Criteria

Populations

We defined the populations of interest as pregnant women and women during the first 12 months after delivery, who received treatment for a depressive episode, including:
- Women who met the diagnostic criteria for a major depressive disorder as described in the 4th edition of the Diagnostic and Statistical Manual of Mental Disorders (DSM-IV)[18]
- Women with subthreshold depressive symptoms that became the subject of clinical attention

We excluded populations of women who met the DSM-IV diagnosis for bipolar depression, psychotic depression, a mood disorder secondary to a general medical condition, or a mood disorder secondary to substance abuse.

This report focuses chiefly on women diagnosed with depression during pregnancy or the postpartum period, rather than on those with a continuing episode. The one exception is for Key Question 2e regarding teratogenicity of antidepressant drugs taken at the time of conception or in early pregnancy. Based on input from experts, we also included studies with populations of pregnant women receiving antidepressant drugs for unknown or mixed reasons. These studies were used to provide evidence when no evidence was available in women with known depression or depressive symptoms (gaps in the evidence). To differentiate these populations, in this report we refer to studies of women with known depression as "treated" or "untreated" populations, and studies of women with mixed or unknown diagnoses as "exposed" populations when receiving antidepressants (typically at unknown doses) or "nonexposed" populations when not receiving antidepressants.

Interventions

Interventions included commonly used antidepressant drugs (see Table 1). Drugs no longer commonly used (e.g., monoamine oxidase inhibitors) were not included. We used the therapeutic classifications used in previous AHRQ Comparative Effectiveness Reviews,[19,20] except that trazodone and nefazodone were classified as norepinephrine reuptake inhibitors for this report.

Comparators

Comparators were:
- The drugs listed in Table 1 when compared with each other
- Placebo or no treatment
- Usual care: We defined usual care as receiving pregnancy and postpartum care similar to those with normal risk pregnancies. When "usual care" was the comparator, two reviewers with experience in delivering postpartum health care (JR and JMG) separately determined if it was "usual," and if they believed it not to be usual, it was included as a separate "greater than usual care" comparator.
- Other active pharmacological treatments used to augment drugs with a U.S. Food and Drug Administration indication for unipolar or bipolar depression
- Any nonpharmacological treatment, including but not limited to over-the-counter treatments, osteopathic or naturopathic treatments, herbal remedies and vitamins, all forms of psychotherapy, case management, electroconvulsive therapy, nonrepetitive and repetitive transcranial magnetic stimulation, vagal nerve stimulation, exercise, meditation, and touch therapies. We recognized the important differences between these treatments and considered them separately when compared with pharmacological treatments, rather than as a group.

Outcomes

Details on the maternal and child benefits and harms outcomes included in the review appear in Table 2.

Table 2. Maternal and child benefits and harms outcomes included in the review

Maternal Benefits	Fetus, Infant, Child Benefits
<ul><li>Danger to self—suicidal and nonsuicidal behaviors</li><li>Danger to infant—infanticidal behavior, abuse, or neglect)</li><li>Depression symptomatology as scored using validated scales measuring depression: response, remission, speed and duration of response or remission, relapse, recurrence</li><li>Anxiety symptoms as scored as a subscale item using validated scales measuring depression, or validated scales used to measure anxiety symptoms</li><li>Functional capacity<ul><li>Quality of life using validated scales, e.g., Medical Outcomes Survey 36-Item Short Form (SF-36)</li><li>Caring for self, infant, and family</li><li>Mother-father dyad interaction success, including reduced violence among intimate partners</li><li>Work productivity</li></ul></li><li>Delivery and postpartum parameters<ul><li>Breastfeeding</li><li>Shared decision making around delivery choices (e.g., cesarean) and delivery mode</li><li>Mother-infant dyad interaction patterns</li><li>Pregnancy weight gain within or outside of 1990 Institute of Medicine Guidelines</li></ul></li><li>Social services utilization; prevention of child protective service involvement</li><li>Maternal health system resource utilization including emergency department use, hospitalizations, and office visits</li><li>Adherence or persistence with treatment regimen</li></ul>	<ul><li>Parameters at birth and up to 12 months of age: preterm birth, e.g., < 32 weeks, < 37 weeks; appropriate growth (height, weight, and head circumference); gestational age, e.g., small for gestational age with race or ethnicity taken into consideration; birth hospitalization length of stay; infant attachment; developmental screening—Ages and Stages Questionnaire, Denver, Modified Checklist for Autism in Toddlers, Bayley Scales of Infant Development</li><li>Growth and development after 1 year of age<ul><li>Developmental screening and diagnoses; growth parameters, such as height, weight, and body mass index percentile according to sex and age</li><li>Learning, e.g., linguistic, cognitive, and social-emotional skills, and educational achievement; kindergarten readiness; age at kindergarten entry; third grade testing outcomes; other standard testing outcomes (eighth grade, etc.)</li><li>Intelligence tests (any), individualized education plans, use of school services</li><li>School failure or dropout rate, high school graduation rate, missed school days</li></ul></li><li>Stress-related chronic disease, mental and Chronic illness</li><li>Infant health system visits, e.g., well baby visits); health care utilization, including primary care, emergency department, hospitalization</li><li>Social services utilization—Women, Infants, and Children Program (WIC), community health nurse, social worker, State Department of Health and Human Services, free or reduced-price lunch, and food stamps</li><li>Community resource utilization</li><li>Social and emotional development, quality of life</li><li>Contact with juvenile justice system</li></ul>
Maternal Harms	**Fetus, Infant, Child Harms**
<ul><li>Death, including suicide, all-cause mortality, and cause-specific death (e.g., cardiac death)</li></ul>	<ul><li>All-cause mortality</li></ul>
<ul><li>Specific adverse effects or withdrawals due to specific adverse events related to treatment, e.g., hyponatremia, activation of mania or hypomania, seizures, suicidal ideation, hepatoxicity, weight gain, metabolic syndrome, gastrointestinal symptoms, and loss of libido</li></ul>	<ul><li>Congenital anomalies (any) Stratified into major and minor with further grouping by organ system or type of anomaly</li></ul>
<ul><li>Overall adverse-event reports, adverse events associated with discontinuation of treatment, and serious adverse events</li><li>Withdrawals from study and discontinuation of treatment due to adverse events</li></ul>	<ul><li>Other specific adverse events, e.g., withdrawal symptoms (neonatal abstinence symptoms), pulmonary hypertension, respiratory distress, neonatal convulsions, and heart defects</li></ul>

Timing

- All followup periods were eligible.

Setting

- Studies conducted in economically advanced countries, as designated by the International Monetary Fund (http://www.imf.org/external), were included: Australia, Austria, Belgium, Canada, Cyprus, the Czech Republic, Denmark, Finland, France, Germany, Greece, Hong Kong, Iceland, Ireland, Israel, Italy, Japan, South Korea, Luxembourg, Malta, The Netherlands, New Zealand, Norway, Portugal, Singapore, the Slovak Republic, Slovenia, Spain, Sweden, Switzerland, Taiwan, the United Kingdom, and the United States.

Study Designs

- For efficacy or effectiveness, a "best evidence" approach was used. Randomized controlled clinical trials and systematic reviews comparing pharmacologic treatments for depression during pregnancy to control groups of pregnant women with depression who were treated with nonpharmacologic or no treatment were included as the top-tier evidence. If insufficient evidence was found with these study designs, we included observational study evidence (defined as cohort studies comparing at least two concurrent treatment groups, case-control studies, and time-series studies) and studies that had control groups of nonexposed pregnant women.
- For harms, in addition to randomized controlled clinical trials (RCTs) and systematic reviews, observational studies (defined as cohort studies comparing at least two concurrent treatment groups, case-control studies, and time-series studies) comparing pharmacologic treatments for depression during pregnancy to control groups of pregnant women with depression who were treated with nonpharmacologic or no treatment were included. If insufficient evidence was found with these designs, studies comparing to control groups of nonexposed pregnant women were included.
- The criteria for systematic reviews required that the review (1) searched at least two databases and (2) discussed methodology of quality assessment and data abstraction. In accordance with established methodologies, any included systematic reviews would be used in place of de novo analysis and synthesis of the included studies whenever possible, depending on the details of how closely the review matched our report scope and how recent the review was.[44,45] We excluded case reports, case series, and single-group studies.

Study Selection

Two reviewers independently assessed titles and abstracts of publications identified through literature searches using the criteria described above for inclusion and exclusion of studies. We retrieved full text articles of potentially relevant citations and two reviewers assessed these for inclusion and exclusion. Disagreements were resolved by consensus or a third-party arbitrator. Results published *only* in abstract form were not included because they do not provide enough information to assess the risk of bias of the study. At the full text level of review, we excluded studies if they met one or more of the following exclusion reasons: published in a language other than English; the intervention, outcome, population, and study design did not meet inclusion criteria; or they were letters, editorials, or nonsystematic reviews. Appendix B lists all studies included at full text review, and Appendix C lists all studies excluded at full text review, along with the exclusion reasons. All citations and screening decisions for each citation were entered in an electronic database (Endnote® X3, Thomson Reuters).

Data Extraction

The following data were abstracted from included studies: design; setting (community, private, or public clinic or hospital); population characteristics (race, age, socioeconomic status, family history of depressive/mood disorders, prior use of antidepressive drugs, severity of symptoms, situation at home, unplanned pregnancy, marital/partner status, comorbidities); study eligibility and exclusion criteria; characteristics of diagnosis (whether depression was detected during screening or not, time of diagnosis, method of diagnosis, and when treatment commenced relative to the onset of symptoms); intervention characteristics (dose, duration, and co-interventions); comparisons; medical provider characteristics (primary care physician, obstetrician, psychiatrist, nurse, midwife, community worker, and pediatrician visits); numbers of patients enrolled; and results for each outcome. One reviewer abstracted study data, and a second reviewer checked a random selection of data abstractions. Intention-to-treat results were recorded if available. Appendix E contains evidence tables for data abstraction of trials and observational studies. Studies that were considered high risk of bias were not abstracted as they were not included in the evidence synthesis.

Risk of Bias Assessment of Individual Studies

We assessed the risk of bias (internal validity) of RCTs and cohort and case control studies based on predefined criteria established by the Drug Effectiveness Review Project.[44] For trials, these criteria were based initially on the criteria used by the U.S. Preventive Services Task Force and the National Health Service Centre for Reviews and Dissemination (United Kingdom).[46,47] In rating the risk of bias of trials, we evaluated methods used for randomization, allocation concealment, and blinding; the similarity of compared groups at baseline; maintenance of comparable groups; adequate reporting of dropouts, attrition, crossover, adherence, and contamination; loss to followup; and the use of intention-to-treat analysis.

We rated the risk of bias of observational studies based on the adequacy of the patient selection process, whether there was important differential loss to followup or overall high loss to followup, the adequacy of exposure and event ascertainment, whether acceptable statistical techniques were used to minimize potential confounding factors, and whether the duration of followup was reasonable to capture investigated events. Based on input from experts, we identified as key for all outcomes four potential confounding factors—age, race, parity, and other exposures (e.g., alcohol, smoking, and other potential teratogens)—factors to be adjusted for in analyses of observational studies. Low or moderate risk of bias studies that adjusted for these factors were considered best evidence if no RCTs were available.

All assessments resulted in a rating of high, medium or low risk of bias, primarily at the study level. In some cases, however, the reviewers determined that internal validity varied by outcome and rated risk of bias for different outcomes separately. Studies that have a fatal flaw were rated high risk of bias; studies that meet all criteria are rated low risk of bias; the remainder are rated medium risk of bias. As the medium risk of bias category is broad, studies with this rating vary in their strengths and weaknesses: The results of some medium risk of bias studies are *likely* to be valid, while others are only *possibly* valid. The results of a high risk of bias study are not valid; the results are at least as likely to reflect flaws in the study design as a true difference between the compared interventions. A fatal flaw is detected by failure of a study to meet combinations of items of the risk of bias checklist.

All studies were first rated by one reviewer and then checked by another reviewer, with disagreements resolved by consensus.

Data Synthesis

Evidence tables were constructed to show the study characteristics, quality ratings, and results for all included studies. A hierarchy-of-evidence approach was used, where the best evidence is the focus of our synthesis for each question, population, intervention, and outcome addressed. Based on input from experts, we stratified our assessment of congenital anomalies into major and cardiovascular categories. Most cardiovascular malformations are considered to be major malformations in congenital anomaly classification systems and were included in our evaluation of major congenital anomalies as a whole. But due to our experts' particular concern for cardiovascular malformations with depression and/or pharmacologic therapy for depression, we also separately evaluated subsets of cardiovascular anomalies as reported in the studies. Data from high risk of bias studies were generally excluded from the synthesis, except to undertake sensitivity analyses or to note where high risk of bias studies constitute the only evidence for an important outcome.

We preferred direct comparisons over indirect comparisons, so they are the focus of our synthesis. We considered three types of directness: populations, intervention comparisons, and outcomes. Direct evidence consists of studies that (1) included the population of interest (depressed pregnant or postpartum women) in both intervention and control groups, (2) made the comparisons of interest (pharmacological treatments compared with each other, nonpharmacological interventions or no treatment), and (3) measured outcomes of interest directly (not using proxy measures, e.g. laboratory values). In this report, direct evidence included studies (trials or observational studies) that compared pregnant or postpartum women with depression who received antidepressant treatment with pregnant or postpartum women with depression who were not treated.

Indirect evidence included trials or observational studies of pregnant or postpartum women treated with antidepressants without specifying that the women had depression. Similarly, studies that compared pregnant or postpartum women who took an antidepressant drug with pregnant or postpartum women who did not take such medications but also were not known to have a diagnosis of depression (a general population) were considered indirect evidence. Indirect comparisons can be difficult to interpret for several reasons; in the latter case the issue is primarily heterogeneity of underlying risk of the populations. The underlying risk of untreated depression during pregnancy or the postpartum period is an important factor in assessing the relative benefits and harms of potential treatments. We used data from indirect comparisons when no other directly applicable evidence exists, but readers should interpret findings with caution because comparisons with a generally healthy population without depression rather than with a depressed population may underestimate the benefits and overestimate the harms of treatment.

We generally did not use data from high risk of bias studies in our main analysis, except to undertake sensitivity analyses for meta-analyses or when high risk of bias studies constituted the only evidence for an important outcome. (High risk of bias studies are not presented in the data evidence tables, but they are included in the risk of bias assessment evidence tables in Appendix E.) To determine the appropriateness of meta-analysis, we considered the internal validity of the studies and the heterogeneity among studies in design, patient population, interventions, and outcomes. Appropriate measures are chosen based on the type of data for meta-analysis, according to the guidance for the EPC program.[48] Random-effects models were used to estimate pooled effects, except when only two studies were being pooled we used a fixed effect model.[49,50] The Q statistic and the I^2 statistic (the proportion of variation in study estimates due to heterogeneity) were calculated to assess heterogeneity in effects between studies.[51,52] When statistical heterogeneity was found, we explored the reasons by using subgroup analysis. For rare events, such as congenital malformations, relative risks would be similar to odds ratios. In meta-analysis, we combined relative risks and odds ratios for such outcomes. Where adjusted summary measures (e.g., odds ratios) were reported by individual studies, we combined summary measures using the 95% confidence intervals to estimate variance.

When meta-analysis could not be performed, the data were summarized qualitatively, grouping studies by similarity of population and/or intervention characteristics.

Strength of the Body of Evidence

We used the methods outlined in the original chapter 10[53] of the AHRQ "Methods Guide for Effectiveness and Comparative Effectiveness Reviews" (an edited version of the chapter has also been published in the Journal of Clinical Epidemiology[54]) to grade strength of evidence. Domains considered in grading the strength of evidence included consistency, directness, precision, and risk of bias. Based on this assessment, the body of evidence was assigned a strength-of-evidence grade of high, moderate, or low.

A rating of *high* means that we have high confidence that the evidence reflects the true effect and that further research is very unlikely to change our confidence in the estimate of effect, while a rating of *low* means that we have low confidence that the evidence reflects the true effect and that further research is likely to change our confidence in the estimate of the effect and to change the estimate. In cases in which evidence did not exist, was sparse, or contained irreconcilable inconsistency, we assigned a grade of insufficient evidence. A rating of *insufficient* means that the evidence either is unavailable or does not permit estimation of an effect.

We consulted our technical experts to help us set priorities for the outcomes for grading. For any comparison with at least moderate risk-of-bias evidence, we selected specific outcomes for rating as follows. For maternal outcomes, we graded danger to self or infant, depression symptomatology (response and remission), breastfeeding intention and duration, number with adverse events, discontinuation due to adverse events, and weight gain. For infant outcomes, we graded preterm birth, small for gestational age, neonatal mortality, congenital malformations, persistent pulmonary hypertension, infant and child neurodevelopment, intellectual function, educational outcome and school performance, mental health, and health care or social service utilization.

Applicability

We assessed applicability by examining study eligibility criteria, characteristics of the enrolled population in comparison to the target population, characteristics of the intervention and comparator used in comparison with care models currently in use, and clinical relevance and timing of the outcome measures. Technical experts identified items of particular interest that contribute to heterogeneity and impact applicability. In general, these included the subgroups specified in Key Question 3: population characteristics—race, age, socioeconomic status, family history of depressive or mood disorders, prior use of antidepressant drugs, severity of symptoms, situation at home, unplanned pregnancy, and marital/partner status; comorbid anxiety diagnoses and other comorbidities; characteristics of diagnosis—whether depression was detected during screening or not, time of diagnosis, method of diagnosis, and when treatment commenced relative to the onset of symptoms; intervention characteristics—dose, duration, and co-interventions; comparisons; and medical provider characteristics—primary care physician, obstetrician, pediatrician, psychiatrist, nurse, midwife, or community worker. We also considered how the evidence may be used by health care funders such as the Federal Children's Health Insurance Program (CHIP) to inform the development of quality measures.

Peer Review and Public Commentary

Experts in treating and studying depression during pregnancy and postpartum, along with individuals representing stakeholder and user communities, provided external peer review of a draft of this comparative effectiveness review; AHRQ and an EPC associate editor also provided comments. The draft report was posted on the AHRQ Web site for 4 weeks to elicit public comments. All comments were reviewed and addressed in a disposition of comments report that will be made available 3 months after the Agency posts the final report of the review on the AHRQ Web site (www.effectivehealthcare.ahrq.gov).

Results

Introduction

We begin by describing the results of our literature searches. We then provide a brief description of the included studies. The remainder of the chapter is organized by Key Question. A list of abbreviations and acronyms is provided at the end of the report.

Results of Literature Searches

Figure 2 depicts the flow of articles through the literature search and screening process.[43] Searches of Ovid MEDLINE®, CDSR®, CCRCT®, CINAHL®, Scopus® and PsycINFO® yielded 3,405 citations. Manual searching and peer review identified 53 additional citations, but searches of ClinicalTrials.gov did not reveal relevant completed or on-going studies. We received scientific information packets from Jazz Pharmaceuticals, Forest Pharmaceuticals, Inc., and Sanofi Aventis, U.S. Based on all these sources, a total of 3,458 abstracts were screened, of which 319 articles were retrieved and assessed for eligibility. Of those, 130 unique studies were included in this report.[55-193] No systematic reviews were found to be eligible for evidence synthesis. The majority of the evidence is from observational studies with 130 articles describing 124 unique studies. Very few trials met inclusion criteria for this report; we included nine articles describing six unique trials. Appendix B provides a listing of all included studies and Appendix C provides a complete list of articles excluded at full text, along with the reasons for exclusion.

Few studies included only pregnant women with depression—most compared pregnant women who received an antidepressant drug for any reason (i.e., maternal exposure) with pregnant women who did not receive an antidepressant drug during pregnancy (i.e., maternal nonexposure). There were no studies comparing an antidepressant drug with a nonpharmacological treatment, and only a few studies in which nonpharmacological treatment was used as an add-on to drug therapy. Using a "best evidence" approach, we focused our findings and conclusions on evidence in pregnant women with depression. We included 6 RCTs and 15 observational studies that focused on women with depression. To address gaps in the direct evidence, we included indirect evidence from an additional 109 observational studies of women receiving antidepressant drugs for mixed or unknown reasons compared with pregnant or postpartum women not taking an antidepressant. Findings from these studies were reported only for important outcomes when there was no better evidence, particularly for serious harms for which even such indirect evidence may be useful in guiding clinical decisions.

Figure 2. Literature flow diagram[a]

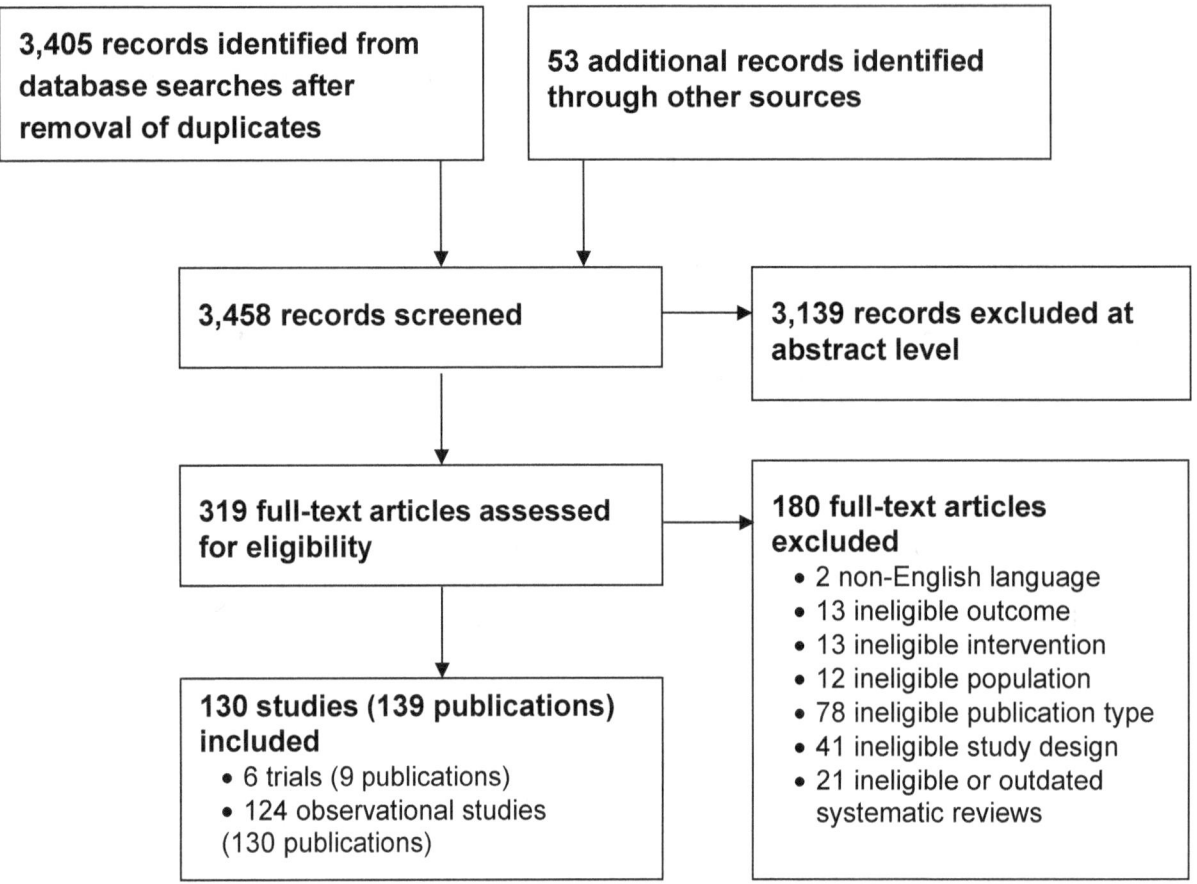

[a] This is a modified PRISMA flow diagram.[43,194]

Description of Included Studies

Of the 130 studies that were included, one-third were conducted in the United States. Four additional studies were conducted in multiple countries, and included sites in the United States and Canada. The remainder were conducted outside the United States.

Of the 124 included observational studies, 39 (30 percent) were rated high risk of bias,[64,68,72,75,78,84,85,88-92,94,98,101,111,112,114,123,126-128,134,137,139,140,144-146,153-155,164,173,174,177,180,185] were rated low risk of bias (9 percent),[74,82,93,104,105,110,125,136,161,169,171,192] and the rest of the observational studies were rated medium risk of bias.[55-57,59-63,66,67,69-71,73,76,77,79-81,83,86,87,95-97,99,100,102,103,106-109,113,115,117-120,122,124,129-131,133,135,138,141-143,147-152,156-160,162,163,165-168,172,175,176,178,179,181,182,184,186,187,189,190,193] For two high risk of bias studies,[98,140] we found secondary publications that we rated medium risk of bias for the specific additional outcomes reported.[120,141] High risk of bias studies suffered from potentially biased selection of patients, lack of assessment of comparability of subjects at baseline, uncertain accuracy of exposure or outcome ascertainment, and lack of appropriate statistical analysis, including controlling for potential confounding. These observational studies largely examined outcomes and associations of exposures during pregnancy, with few evaluating treatment in the postpartum period. The designs of the studies included cohort and case control, with large, linked databases providing data for most of the larger studies, including several population-based cohort studies from Nordic countries. Prospective cohort studies, including data collected by teratology information services around the world, constituted a smaller set of studies with smaller sample sizes. The control groups in most of these observational studies were pregnant women without exposure to an antidepressant drug. The indication for treatment with an antidepressant drug was reported infrequently. In a few studies, depression in either intervention or control groups was controlled for in a way that allowed comparison of treatment groups or examination of the effect on outcomes of treatment. See Appendix E, Evidence Table 2 for individual study risk of bias ratings.

All six of the included RCTs examined women in the postpartum period. Three of these RCTs were rated medium risk of bias,[58,65,132] while three were considered high risk of bias due to problems with uncertain randomization, allocation concealment, or blinding methods combined with lack of an intention-to-treat analysis and/or a high rate of missing data.[170,188,191] None of the trials were rated as having a low risk of bias. Further details on studies are provided below. See Appendix E, Evidence Table 4 for individual study risk of bias ratings.

Key Question 1. What are the comparative benefits of pharmacological and nonpharmacological treatments for women with depression during pregnancy and in the postpartum period?

Summary

We found no clinical trials to provide direct evidence on the comparative benefit or harms of antidepressant drugs used to treat depression in pregnancy. Direct evidence was limited to 16 observational studies of pharmacological treatments given at unknown dosages. Indirect evidence consisted of studies of women taking an antidepressant during pregnancy for any reason compared with women who did not take an antidepressant during pregnancy, with unknown depression status in either group.

- Direct evidence was sparse on the maternal and infant/child benefits associated with pharmacological and nonpharmacological treatment for depression during pregnancy and the postpartum period, and it was insufficient to support conclusions due to methodological limitations, unknown consistency and imprecision. Types of direct evidence available were:
    - Maternal depression symptomatology
        - One small observational study with high risk of bias (n=46) compared mean Center for Epidemiologic Studies Depression Scale (CES-D) scores between depressed pregnant women treated with fluoxetine and untreated depressed pregnant women.
        - One small RCT with high risk of bias (n=109) compared response and remission rates between sertraline and nortriptyline in postpartum women with depression.
        - Two small, medium risk of bias RCTs and one small, high risk of bias observational study (n=150) compared the effects of combining pharmacologic treatments with nonpharmacological treatments versus nonpharmacological treatments alone on depression symptomatology when used to treat depression in postpartum women.
        - One small, medium risk of bias RCTs and one small, high risk of bias observational study (n=58) compared the effects of combining pharmacologic treatments with nonpharmacological treatments versus pharmacological treatments alone on depression symptomatology when used to treat depression in postpartum women.
    - Maternal functional capacity:
        - One small observational study with medium risk of bias (n=62) compared mean Medical Outcomes Survey 12-Item Short Form (SF-12) mental component scores between depressed pregnant women treated with SSRIs and untreated depressed pregnant women.
    - Breastfeeding
        - One small observational study with medium risk of bias compared the effects of SSRI treatment during pregnancy on the proportions of women breastfeeding 6 weeks after birth.
        - One small RCT with high risk of bias (n=70) compared the effects on breastfeeding rates of taking sertraline versus nortriptyline for depression during the postpartum period.
    - Preterm birth
        - Low strength evidence from two medium risk of bias (n=266) studies suggested no difference in risk with use of SSRIs compared with no treatment for depression during pregnancy.
    - Infant/child development
        - One small observational study with medium risk of bias (n=49) compared mean scores on the Brazelton Neonatal Behavioral Assessment Scale between depressed pregnant women treated with SSRIs and untreated depressed pregnant women.
        - One small observational study with medium risk of bias (n=44) compared the effects of SSRIs plus psychotherapy versus psychotherapy alone

during pregnancy on the Bayley Mental Development Index and Psychomotor Development Index and Behavioral Rating Scale.

Detailed Assessment of the Evidence

Key Question 1. What are the comparative benefits of pharmacological and nonpharmacological treatments for women with depression during pregnancy and in the postpartum period?

There were no clinical trials of pharmacologic treatment during pregnancy to inform the question of the comparative benefits of treatment. Evidence was limited to observational studies (cohort and case control designs). Most of these studies provide only indirect evidence, comparing women treated with antidepressants during pregnancy for any reason to pregnant women who were not treated. The diagnosis for treatment in the treated group was most often not reported, or it was reported as a baseline characteristic but with no subgroup analysis based on diagnosis. The rates of depression in the control groups were rarely reported. However, some studies controlled for depression in statistical analyses. We found both RCTs and observational studies of depression treatment in the postpartum period.

The evidence below is organized first by the subquestions of Key Question 1, then by pregnancy status at the time of exposure—during pregnancy or postpartum. Within those categories we present the evidence by pharmacological class with all outcomes for a given class presented together. Direct evidence was the primary focus, with indirect evidence reported only for important outcomes for which evidence in pregnant women with depression did not exist or was sparse, particularly for serious harms for which even such indirect evidence may be useful in guiding clinical decisions. Outcomes for which no evidence was found are not itemized below.

Key Question 1a. How do pharmacological treatments affect maternal and child outcomes when compared with placebo or no active treatment or usual care?

Antidepressant Exposure During Pregnancy

Selective Serotonin Reuptake Inhibitors

Maternal Outcomes
Twenty-five observational studies reported maternal health outcomes for active SSRI treatment (as a class or as an individual drug),[66,69,71,76,77,80,82,99,115,122,129,131,143,145,146,150,152,165,166,169,177,181,184,189] with only three[40,69,177] explicitly including women with depression during pregnancy in both the intervention and control groups (i.e., direct evidence). Two were methodologically weak with high risk of bias, due primarily to potentially biased selection of patients, unclear completeness of data, and lack of appropriate statistical analysis, including failure to control for potential confounding.[145,177]

Depression symptomatology. Associations of treatment effect require study populations that include depressed pregnant women with and without treatment, and ideally the study would include an assessment prior to initiation of treatment in the treated group. Six reports of five observational studies[69,131,145,146,150,177] reported some feature of mood or depression symptoms with SSRI use; only two[69,177] provide direct comparative evidence on depression symptomatology among depressed pregnant women with and without pharmacological treatment. These studies are small, totaling 106 women (59 treated, 31 depressed without pharmacologic treatment, and 16 without depression and no treatment). The smallest, totaling 44 depressed pregnant women,[69] 31 of whom were taking SSRIs, showed no significant difference between treated and untreated in change in symptoms across pregnancy. The larger study of 62 women[177] focused exclusively on fluoxetine treatment and found significant improvement in depression symptoms as measured by CES-D score with treatment; the women's symptoms improved with each trimester. By the third trimester the mean CES-D score for depressed women on fluoxetine was 14.33±12.02 compared with 25.93±4.91 for those not treated with fluoxetine (p=0.0010). However, it is important to note both that these two studies differed in the scales they used to measure depression and that all studies used measures not commonly used in studies of depression in the general population. The four other studies provided only indirect evidence because the untreated group included a mixture of women with and without depression or other mood disorders.

Anxiety symptoms. No direct evidence was found; no studies examined anxiety symptom change in depressed pregnant women with and without treatment or comparing treatments. Indirect evidence comes from two studies with medium[131] and high risk of bias[145] that monitored anxiety and depression symptoms in depressed women taking SSRIs or SNRIs and made comparisons to women with and without mood disorders not taking antidepressants. Both studies used the Hamilton Rating Scale for Anxiety (HAM-A), as well as additional scales to measure anxiety. Anxiety scores were higher among women taking antidepressants compared with women not taking antidepressants. While there was a trend toward declining anxiety scores postpartum, it is unclear whether the declines were statistically significant.

Functional capacity. Only one medium risk of bias study[122,189] provided direct evidence on functional capacity in pregnant women with depression with and without SSRI use. Women who were depressed continually throughout pregnancy and treated with an SSRI continuously throughout pregnancy had better functional capacity as measured by the mental component of the SF-12 compared with those that were depressed throughout pregnancy but untreated (45.2 +/- 13.7 compared with 35.3 +/- 11.4).[189] Women treated with SSRIs for only part of their pregnancy had a mean score of 44.6, and those with depression in only part of their pregnancy but who received no SSRI had a mean score of 40.5 (on a scale of 1 to 100). A control group with no depression and no SSRI treatment had a mean score of 55.7. While the p-value across all groups was statistically significant (p<0.001), pairwise comparisons were not undertaken. Additionally, the specific timing of the SF-12 scores was not clear from the study report.

Pregnancy weight gain. We found no direct evidence on the effect of different treatments for depression on weight gain in pregnant women with depression. In a 1990 report,[195] the Institute of Medicine recommended a maternal weight gain of 25 to 35 pounds for women with normal weight for height. Weight gain is associated both with the use of antidepressant drugs and with some forms of depression, and it can have a significant effect on maternal health; even so, there were only two medium risk of bias studies that addressed these associations. Both studies were indirect evidence because they included women treated with an SSRI for any reason and made comparisons to women who did not receive an SSRI (unknown depression status). Therefore, the strength of evidence was considered insufficient (see Appendix E, Table 2). A study of 5961 women reported mean weight gain during pregnancy, which was 33.4 pounds for non-SSRI users, 34.0 pounds for women who discontinued SSRIs two months before pregnancy, and 37.0 pounds for women who continued SSRIs through the first trimester. Although the group who continued SSRIs through the first trimester is the only group to have a mean weight gain in excess of the 1990 Institute of Medicine guidelines, the statistical significance of this difference is unknown.[181] Another small study found that women in treated with fluoxetine gained an average of 37 +/- 15.4 pounds, which exceeds recommendations, but no data were available for the control group.[71]

Breastfeeding. No direct evidence was found on the effect of SSRIs used during pregnancy on breastfeeding outcomes postpartum.

Indirect evidence consisted of four prospective observational studies ranging in size from 44 to 466 women. These studies reported on breastfeeding rates among women taking SSRIs compared with the rates among women not taking SSRIs (depression status unknown in either group).[66,69,99,115,166] All four studies had medium risk of bias due to potentially biased selection of patients and lack of controlling for potential confounding (e.g., not controlling for parity or prior experience breastfeeding). The best indirect evidence on breastfeeding came from a study of 168 pregnant women enrolled by 20 weeks gestation and assessed for breastfeeding intention, initiation, and breastfeeding up to 12 weeks postpartum.[66] This study assessed depression symptoms at weeks 20, 30 and 36. The analysis controlled for depression symptoms and presence of a diagnosis of major depressive disorder, as well as parity and prior experience breastfeeding (factors known to be strongly associated with future breastfeeding). Intention to exclusively breastfeed was the most significant factor associated with breastfeeding initiation and duration. Neither depression symptoms nor symptom severity was associated with intention to breastfeed; however, there was a significant and negative association between SSRI use (for any reason) and intention to breastfeed compared with no antidepressant use in women with and without depression (relative risk reduction[RRR] 12.31; 95% CI 2.50-60.66) for intention to formula feed). There was also no association between diagnosis of major depressive disorder or depressive symptoms and initiation of breastfeeding. Furthermore, even though SSRI use at 2 weeks postpartum was associated with lower depression symptom scores, women taking SSRIs at 2 weeks postpartum were more likely to stop breastfeeding by 12 weeks (RRR 12.0; 95% CI 1.64-88.3) compared with women not taking SSRIs. This evidence was insufficient strength to draw conclusions for the questions posed in this report.

Infant/Child Outcomes: Birth Parameters
Preterm birth. Direct evidence on the risk of preterm birth was limited to two small observational studies (n=266 total) that provided low strength evidence that SSRIs had no statistically significant effect on rates of preterm birth (Figure 3).[187,192] Both medium risk of bias studies reported preterm birth rates for depressed women treated with an SSRI during pregnancy compared with those who were depressed but did not receive an SSRI. In both studies, preterm birth was defined as delivery prior to the 37th week of gestation, and gestational age was based on ultrasound when available in one (proportion with ultrasound validation available not reported)[192] and no method reported in the other study.[187,189] Pooled analysis resulted in an odds ratio of 1.87 (95% CI 0.89 to 3.89, Cochran Q = 0.089 p=0.77). The larger study (n=77 with depression) attempted to assess early preterm birth (delivery prior to 34 weeks gestation), but no

births met this criterion for the group of women with depression and treated with an SSRI.[192]

Figure 3. Risk of preterm birth (< 37 weeks gestation) with selective serotonin reuptake inhibitors compared with nonexposure

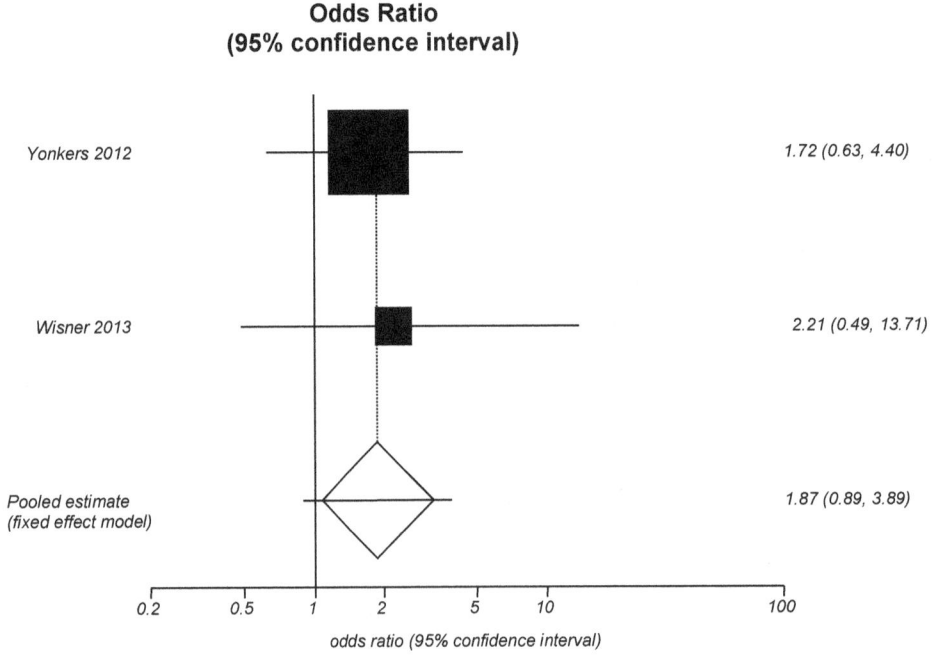

There was a large volume of indirect evidence on the risk of preterm birth. Based on 11 observational studies, there was evidence of an increased risk of preterm birth (< 37 weeks gestation) birth with use of SSRIs during pregnancy in women with unknown depression status.[81,95,100,107,117,118,138,167,180,184,189,192] The magnitude of risk may have varied by timing of exposure, but evidence was inadequate to establish reliable estimates. The most relevant of these studies was a medium risk of bias study that reported a statistically significant increased risk of preterm birth with SSRI use during pregnancy for any reason, compared with pregnant women with a documented psychiatric illness who did not receive an SSRI (or other antidepressant or antipsychotic drug) during pregnancy (adjusted odds ratio [OR] 2.68; 95% CI 1.83 to 3.93).[100] While this study did not limit the diagnoses to depression, gestational age was determined by ultrasound. This study adjusted for several key factors, including history of prior preterm birth, but it did not adjust for severity or type of psychiatric illness.

Four studies provided some information on the effect of timing of exposure to an SSRI during pregnancy.[100,117,118,138] These studies performed ultrasound verification of gestational age, defined preterm birth as delivery at less than 37 weeks gestation, and found an increased risk of preterm birth. A single study found the risk with early exposure to be extremely increased (adjusted OR 11.7; 95% CI 2.20 to 60.70); a second study found increased risk with late exposure (adjusted OR 2.48; 95% CI 1.75 to 3.50). Pooling the two studies reporting exposure at any time during pregnancy also resulted in a statistically significant, but lower, increase in risk (pooled adjusted OR 1.24; 95% CI 1.12 to1.38).

Evidence on the risk of preterm birth with individual SSRIs was very limited, with few studies for each drug. None of these studies made comparisons of pregnant women with depression and therefore only provide indirect evidence for the risk in such women. The estimate of risk was highest with citalopram and escitalopram,[76,111,172,173] with non-statistically significant increase in risk with fluoxetine,[71,76,84,153] sertraline[76,172] and paroxetine[71,76,84,107,111,153,172,173] but all of the estimates are likely to shift with additional studies, particularly those that control for potential confounders.

Growth for gestational age. Evidence on the risk for an infant to be small for gestational age at birth following maternal treatment for depression with an SSRI during pregnancy was insufficient because there was no direct evidence available. To determine whether SSRIs influence infant growth, it is necessary to understand whether depression in pregnancy itself influences infant growth parameters.

The best indirect evidence came from two of the five studies using ultrasound confirmation of gestational age.[93,100] A study from Denmark identified three groups of women, those with depressive symptoms but who received no pharmacological treatment, women who took SSRIs (indication for the SSRI not recorded), and a control group of pregnant women not depressed and not taking an SSRI.[93,100] This study did not report the outcome of small for gestational age for the group with depression, but it did report the outcome of head circumference at birth. This study found no statistically significant difference in head circumference between the depressed, untreated group and controls, but it did find a difference when comparing the group taking an SSRI for any reason with controls (−5.88 millimeters; 95% CI −11.45 to −0.30). A study that included women with a psychiatric illness who did not receive an antidepressant or an antipsychotic treatment during pregnancy compared with a group of similar women who were taking an SSRI did not find an increased risk with use of SSRIs late in pregnancy (adjusted OR 1.13; 95% CI 0.65 to 1.94). This study did not adjust for severity or type of mental illness.

Eleven other medium and high risk of bias observational studies reported on infants small for gestational age; these studies compared women taking an SSRI during pregnancy for unknown reasons with pregnant women not taking an SSRI (depression status unknown)[93,95,100,107,110,118,142,145,162,181,193]. Only five of these studies used ultrasound to determine gestational age,[93,95,100,110,118] and four reported odds ratios adjusted for confounding factors.[93,95,100,110,118] These studies did not find an increased risk of an infant being small for gestational age (adjusted pooled OR of 1.04; 95% CI 0.64 to 1.69; I^2=30%) with SSRI use during pregnancy.

Infant/Child Development
Bayley development assessments. Direct evidence from a very small (n=44) medium risk of bias study of children of women who were depressed during pregnancy and were treated with an SSRI or taking no antidepressant provided insufficient evidence on neonatal development. Both groups received "supportive psychotherapy" (no further details reported), and Beck Depression Inventory maximum scores were 24.0 in the untreated group and 21.3 in the treated group (on a scale of 0 to 63), p=0.58 at baseline.[69,178] At 6–40 months of age, Bayley Scales for Infant Development, 2nd Edition, scores were not statistically significantly different between groups on the mental development index (MDI) or the behavioral rating scale (BRS) portions of the Bayley after adjusting for APGAR scores. Ratings on the psychomotor development index (PDI) portion of the Bayley indicated lower scores in the SSRI-exposed group compared with the group whose mothers were depressed but not treated with an SSRI (90.0 versus 98.2, p=0.02). Examining the

BRS factor scales found the motor quality factor to be lower in the SSRI-exposed group (68.6 versus 88.8, p=0.05).

We found indirect evidence from a small medium risk of bias study (n=84) of children at 10 months of age who had been exposed to SSRIs compared with those who were not exposed in-utero; this study reported that after adjusting for depression, scores on the gross motor, social-emotional and adaptive behavior subscales were significantly lower in the exposed children.[102] The absolute differences were small and clinical relevance was not clear (e.g. gross motor scores 9.5 versus 8.3). Depression scores in the women who did not receive antidepressants were significantly lower than scores in the treated group. The study also analyzed outcomes for children whose mothers were depressed compared with those who were not and found no difference between groups. In contrast, two other studies found no difference between groups, but they did not control for depression among mothers during or after pregnancy.[62Reebye, 2002 #3454164] Another study assessed development of children born preterm (< 37 weeks), using the Bayley scale at 36 months of age; the study compared those exposed to SSRIs during pregnancy to children whose mothers did not take an SSRI (depression status unknown).[62] This medium risk of bias study (n=38) did not find differences between groups on the MDI or PDI. The other study was a small medium risk of bias study (n=61) of children, 24 of whom were exposed to SSRIs prenatally compared with 23 children born to mothers with unknown depression status who did not receive an SSRI during pregnancy and 14 whose mothers took an SSRI plus another psychoactive drug.[166] This study found no difference in the MDI or PDI scores across groups.

Brazelton Neonatal Behavioral Assessment Scale (BNBAS) assessments. Direct evidence from a single small study of neurobehavioral outcomes in infants was insufficient to draw conclusions. Using the Brazelton Neonatal Behavioral Assessment Scale (BNBAS), neurobehavioral assessments for young infants exposed to SSRIs during at least second and third trimester (n=33) were recorded at 1 week and again at 6-8 weeks by blinded trained raters.[178] Differences were not seen in children exposed to SSRIs compared with children of depressed mothers without antidepressant exposure (no antidepressants, discontinued antidepressants in first trimester, or <10 days, n=16).

Language development. The best indirect evidence on language development came from a medium risk of bias study in which children 15–71 months who were exposed prenatally to TCAs (n=45) or fluoxetine (n=38) were compared with children of nondepressed women (n=34), using the Reynell Verbal and Expressive Language Scales.[141] Scores for all three groups were within the normal range, but children in the TCA group scored higher than those in the fluoxetine or nonexposed group on Reynell Developmental Language Scales. This study measured McCarthy cognitive development scores but missing data made this outcome high risk of bias.

Developmental milestones. The best indirect evidence on achievement of developmental milestones at 6 months was available from a medium risk of bias study that compared children exposed in utero to antidepressants (n=415; 81%=SSRIs, 3%=TCAs) with children of mothers with untreated depression during pregnancy (n=489) and children of women not receiving an antidepressant during pregnancy and not identified as being depressed by study methods.[158] This study used maternal interviews at 6 months and 19 months after delivery to obtain assessments of milestone achievement, and information about depression was obtained from two prenatal interviews. At 6 months, children with antidepressant exposure at any time during pregnancy had greater risk of not achieving milestones compared with children of mothers with untreated depression during pregnancy (OR 1.5; 95% CI 1.1-2.0)]. A similar increase in risk was found for those with exposure in the second or second and third trimesters compared with untreated depression (OR 2.6; 95% CI 1.2-5.8)], while exposure only in the first trimester was not statistically significant (OR 1.1; 95% CI 0.6-2.1). At 19 months, there was no difference between the groups in the risk of not meeting one or more milestones. Analysis of the effect of specific types of antidepressants found no differences at 6 months, but on retrospective recall at 19 months, the group exposed to SSRIs in utero was found to have longer days to sitting or walking unassisted; however, the reported days to sit and/or walk for all groups were within the normal range of development.

Motor and speech delays. In a medium risk of bias retrospective study, motor and speech delays in children exposed to antidepressants in utero were compared with children of women who did not take antidepressants during pregnancy (depression status of mothers in either group unknown).[171] Delays were identified by blinded chart review and required physician diagnosis confirmed by a formal developmental evaluation in the course of routine clinical care. No statistically significant differences were found in motor delays or speech delays and SSRI exposure (OR 3.07; 95% CI 0.61-15.40 and OR 1.0; 95% CI 0.14-7.18), respectively). Another study providing indirect evidence examined neonates neurological functioning by assessing the quality of an infant's general movements (Precht method), finding more "abnormal movements" in the SSRI group at 1 week of age (3.0; 95% CI 1.3 to 6.9) after controlling for maternal depression. Depression scores in the third trimester were significantly lower in the non-SSRI group. It does not appear that outcome assessment was conducted with blinding to SSRI exposure.

Early childhood behavioral outcomes. In a medium risk of bias follow-up study of a cohort of children exposed to antidepressants during gestation (n=127) and children whose mothers had depression during pregnancy but no antidepressant exposure (n=98), the Strengths and Difficulties Questionnaire (SDQ) was used to assess behavior at age 4 to 5 years.[157] No difference was found on the overall scores between treated and untreated groups, (any antidepressant compared with untreated depression OR 1.3; 95% CI 0.3 to 6.0). Results are reported to be similar for SSRIs, odds ratio not reported.

Autism spectrum disorders. No direct evidence on the risk of different treatments for depression during pregnancy on development of autism spectrum disorders in the child was found.

We found indirect evidence in two large case-control studies (n=1,805; n=47,656, respectively), which reported the risk of ASD in offspring of mothers who used SSRIs during pregnancy.[79,161] Both used health system databases, one in the United States[79] and the other in Sweden.[161] The Swedish study[161] was rated low risk of bias and the U.S. study[79] was rated moderate risk of bias. Both studies adjusted for maternal age and mental health disorders and the Swedish study additionally adjusted for paternal age.[161] Only the U.S. study adjusted for child's sex.[79] Neither adjusted for family history of ASD or prematurity, both factors known to be strongly associated with ASD. These studies find that maternal SSRI use at any time during pregnancy is statistically significantly associated with an increased risk of autism spectrum disorder in offspring (pooled adjusted OR 1.82; 95% CI 1.14 to 2.91). The U.S. study additionally evaluated whether risk of ASD varied based on exposure period and found that the risk only reached statistical significance during the first trimester (adjusted OR 3.5; 95% CI 1.5 to 7.9), and not during the preconception period (adjusted OR 1.9; 95% CI 0.9 to 4.2), the second trimester (adjusted OR 1.5; 95% CI 0.5 to 5.0) or the third trimester (adjusted OR 2.2; 95% CI 0.7 to 6.9).[79]

In one of these studies, results of subgroup analyses suggested that depression itself may contribute to ASD diagnosis. Compared with the risk for ASD in children of pregnant women without depression or antidepressant use, the risk for ASD in the children of pregnant women with depression and antidepressant use was statistically significantly elevated (OR 3.34; 95% CI 1.50 to 7.47). In contrast, the risk in pregnant women taking an antidepressant for another indication was lower than the risk in children of pregnant women without depression or antidepressant use and not statistically significant (OR 1.61; 95% CI 0.85 to 3.06).

Education and Learning

We found no evidence on school performance or educational outcomes. Observational studies were found comparing maternal antidepressant exposure compared with nonexposure and risk of lowered intelligence testing results in their children. Indirect evidence on SSRIs and intelligence testing is based on two observational studies that assessed childhood intelligence by performance on standardized testing and compared exposure to antidepressants compared with nonexposure.[139,146] Both were high risk of bias observational studies.

Illness Outcomes

We did not find evidence on the risk of stress related chronic disease in children associated with maternal SSRI use during pregnancy. We found evidence on the risk of developing ADHD or having internalizing or externalizing behaviors, reported below.

Attention deficit hyperactivity disorder (ADHD). No direct evidence on the risk of different treatments for depression during pregnancy on development of ADHD in the child was found. One retrospective cohort study with medium risk of bias assessed ADHD diagnoses by age 5 years using a large national claims-based dataset from self-insured employers,[96] providing indirect evidence as a mental health diagnosis was identified in only 33 percent of women, including 10 percent with a depressive disorder and 5 percent with an anxiety disorder. After multiple logistic regression analysis, risk of diagnosis with ADHD in children born to women who used bupropion, SSRIs, or any other antidepressant during or after pregnancy was compared with women not exposed during pregnancy. SSRI use at any time during pregnancy was not associated with increased risk of ADHD in offspring (OR 0.91; 95% CI 0.51 to 1.60), but use after pregnancy (up to four years post-delivery) was associated with increased risk of ADHD diagnosis (OR 2.04; 95% CI 1.43 to 2.91). No breastfeeding data were provided to determine whether direct exposure may have occurred. Children of mothers with depressive disorders had statistically significantly higher risk of ADHD at age 5 than those without (OR 2.58; 95% CI 2.02 to 3.29).

We identified two additional high risk of bias studies that reported on ADHD symptoms.[139,146] Neither study found an association between exposure to SSRIs in utero (n=22) and ADHD symptoms in offspring compared with nonexposed, presumed nondepressed groups.

Internalizing behaviors. No direct evidence on the risk of internalizing behaviors in the child with different treatments for depression during pregnancy was found. Internalizing behaviors are described as behaviors directed internally or "within the self". They include emotional reactivity, depression, anxiety, irritability and withdrawal.

Three observational studies provide indirect evidence. One of medium risk of bias[133] and two of high risk of bias[139,145] reported on outcomes of children exposed to SSRIs and venlafaxine in utero. Levels of internalizing behaviors were assessed by maternal and teacher/caregiver reports in 36 children aged 4 to 5 years exposed to SSRIs and/or clonazepam prenatally.[133] Mothers rated their children on the Child Behavior Checklist (CBCL) and teachers/caregivers rated children using the Child-Teacher Report Form (C-TRF). Maternal mood and anxiety was assessed by the Hamilton Rating Scale for Depression (HAM-D) and HAM-A. No statistically significant differences in internalizing behaviors were found in maternal or caregiver/teacher ratings of children at 4-5 years exposed to SSRIs during pregnancy compared with nonexposed controls [OR (95% CI) HAM-D 1.53 (0.24-9.85);HAM-A 2.89 (0.29-28.90)]. This remained true when controlled for maternal depression [OR (95% CI) HAM-D 0.99 (0.13-7.88); HAM-A 2.85 (0.26-31.20)]. However, increased maternal but not teacher reports of internalizing behaviors were associated with maternal depression ($p<0.05$) and anxiety ($p<0.05$).

Both high risk of bias studies found increased risk of internalizing behaviors associated with SSRI use during pregnancy compared with general nonexposed populations, but both also found that the increase was correlated with maternal depression.[139,145]

Externalizing behaviors. We found no direct evidence on the risk of externalizing behaviors in the child with different treatments for depression during pregnancy. Externalizing behaviors (noncompliance, verbal/physical aggression, disruptive acts, and emotional outbursts) are described as behaviors which are "directed outward". The presence of these behaviors may herald a diagnosis of externalizing disorders such as ADHD, oppositional defiant disorder (ODD) and/or conduct disorder (CD). Indirect evidence comes from three observational studies, but all are high risk of bias, and are not described further.[139,145,146]

Health Care Utilization

We found no direct evidence on health care utilization among children born to mothers with depression during pregnancy, comparing those treated with antidepressants to those not treated, or comparing antidepressants. Indirect evidence, based on one medium risk of bias observational study (n=38,602), suggests that antidepressant use (primarily SSRIs, 71%) is associated with increased health care utilization among children born to women who were prescribed SSRIs during pregnancy compared with nonexposed children (Table 3).[182] The depression status of mothers was not reported. For continuous SSRIs exposure during pregnancy the risk was increased for several markers of resource utilization both during the first two weeks and the first year of life, including a two-fold increase in the utilization of physiotherapy. Intermittent use of SSRIs during pregnancy was also associated with increased risk for some measures, primarily in the first year of life and the risk for those who discontinued an antidepressant during pregnancy; only risks for increased risk during the first two weeks of life were statistically significant.

Table 3. Association between antidepressant use during pregnancy and general practitioner visits and hospital admissions; unadjusted relative risk (95% confidence interval)[182]*

N = 38,602	First 2 Weeks After Birth			First Year After Birth	
Antidepressant Use	Continuous	Intermittent	Discontinued	Continuous	Irregular
≥ 1 GP visits	NS	NS	**1.3 (1.2 to 1.5)**	--	--
>2 GP visits	--	--	--	**1.5 (1.3 to 1.8)**	**1.2 (1.1 to 1.4)**
1 hospital admission	NS	NS	**1.3 (1.1 to 1.7)**	NS	NS
≥ 2 Hospitalizations	**2.4 (1.8 to 3.1)**	**1.4 (1.1 to 1.8)**	**1.4 (1.1 to 1.9)**	NS	**1.5 (1.1 to 2.1)**
1 specialist visit	**1.3 (1.1 to 1.5)**	1.2 (1.0 to 1.3)		**1.4 (1.1 to 1.8)**	NS
>2 specialist visits	**2.4 (1.7 to 3.3)**	NS	**1.2 (1.1 to 1.4)**	**1.5 (1.2 to 1.9)**	**1.4 (1.2 to 1.6)**
1 specialist procedure	**1.5 (1.2 to 1.8)**	1.1 (1.0 to 1.3)		**1.6 (1.3 to 2.0)**	NS
>2 specialist procedures	**1.7 (1.1 to 2.6)**	NS		NS	**1.3 (1.1 to 1.5)**
2 diagnostic tests	**1.9 (1.4 to 2.5)**	NS		NS	NS
Physiotherapy	--	--	--	**2.0 (1.5 to 2.6)**	**1.3 (1.1 to 1.7)**

GP = general practitioner; NS = not significant
*Results are in bold type where they are statistically significant

Tricyclic Antidepressants

Maternal Outcomes
We found no evidence for maternal outcomes with the use of TCAs during pregnancy.

Infant/Child Outcomes
Preterm birth. No direct evidence on the effect of different treatments for depression on preterm birth in women with depression during pregnancy was found.

Indirect evidence based on two observational studies indicates an increased risk of preterm birth with exposure to TCAs during pregnancy for any reason, compared with pregnant women who were not treated with TCAs (depression status unknown for both groups).[81,167]

Growth for gestational age. We found no direct evidence on the effect of different treatments for depression on fetal growth in women with depression during pregnancy.

Indirect evidence indicated no increased risk for the infant to be small for gestational age at birth with exposure to TCAs for any reason compared with pregnant women who were not treated with TCAs (depression status unknown for both groups), based on two medium risk of bias studies.[107,162] The pooled adjusted OR for exposure at any time point during pregnancy is 0.97 (95% CI 0.64 to 1.46), with no statistical heterogeneity. One of the studies reported the rates of a depression diagnosis in the treated and untreated group (46% and 36%, respectively). This study also evaluated the result by timing of exposure (first, second or third trimester) and found no statistically significant increase in risk for any of these time points.

Child Development
We found no direct evidence on the effect of maternal treatment with TCAs for depression during pregnancy on infant and child development. Indirect evidence was limited to three observational studies reporting on comparisons of children whose mothers took TCAs during

pregnancy for any reason, compared with children whose mothers did not take TCAs; depression status was unknown for both groups.[141,158,171]

The best indirect evidence on developmental milestones came from a medium risk of bias study (described above regarding SSRI use).[158] Adjusted odds ratios (days) were calculated for maternal report of sitting without support (at 6 months interview) for TCA exposure at any point during pregnancy. No statistically significant differences were found for exposure to TCAs (OR 2.9; 95% CI 0.89-9.51) at any point in pregnancy, nor were there differences with 1st or 2nd/3rd trimester exposure. On retrospective recall at 19 months, statistically significant delays with TCA exposure were also not found. The best evidence on motor and speech delays comes from a medium risk of bias retrospective study of children exposed to antidepressants in utero who were compared with children of women who did not take antidepressants during pregnancy (depression status of mothers in either group unknown).[171] Delays were identified by blinded chart review and required physician diagnosis confirmed by a formal developmental evaluation in the course of routine clinical care. No statistically significant differences were found with motor or speech delays and TCA exposure (OR 1.0; 95% CI 0.14-7.17) Another study of language development used the Reynell Verbal and Expressive Language Scales.[141] Scores for children 15-71 months exposed prenatally to TCAs (n=45) or fluoxetine (n=38) were compared with children of nondepressed comparison women (n=34). All three groups scored within the normal range. Children in the TCA group scored higher than those in the fluoxetine or nonexposed group on Reynell Developmental Language Scales.

Autism spectrum disorder. We found no direct evidence on the risk of different treatments for depression during pregnancy on development of autism spectrum disorders in the child.

Indirect evidence was found in two large case-control studies (n=1,805; n=47,656, respectively) reported the risk of ASD in offspring of mothers who used antidepressants, including TCAs, described in detail in the section on SSRIs, above.[79,161] These studies included subgroups of women exposed to either TCAs or TCAs/SNRIs (as a group). In the study examining TCAs as a group (n=6 cases, n=20 controls), there is indirect evidence that maternal use of TCAs during pregnancy is statistically significantly associated with an increased risk of autism spectrum disorder in offspring (adjusted OR 2.69; 95% CI 1.04 to 6.96).[161] This study was rated low risk of bias and adjusted for any maternal psychiatric disorder, maternal age, paternal age, parental income, education, occupation, maternal country of birth, and birth parity. It did not adjust for family history of ASD or prematurity, both factors known to be strongly associated with ASD.

The other study included SNRIs with their analysis of TCAs (n=5 cases, n=16 controls).[79] Adding SNRIs to the group resulted in a nonstatistically significant associated increase in risk of ASD (adjusted OR 1.6; 95% CI 0.5 to 4.5). This study was rated moderate risk of bias and provides indirect evidence for this outcome, adjusting for maternal age, race/ethnicity, maternal education, birth weight, sex, birth year of child and birth facility, but not family history of ASD or prematurity, both factors known to be strongly associated with ASD.

Selective Norepinephrine Reuptake Inhibitors and Norepinephrine Reuptake Inhibitors

Maternal Outcomes

We found no evidence for maternal outcomes with the use of SNRIs/NRIs during pregnancy.

Child Outcomes
Preterm birth. We found no direct evidence on the effect of different treatments for depression on preterm birth in women with depression during pregnancy.

Indirect evidence, based on two medium-risk of bias observational studies, indicates an increased risk of preterm birth associated with use of an SNRI/NRI (including bupropion for one study) during pregnancy for any reason (adjusted OR 1.79, 95% CI 1.46 - 2.19).[118,167] These studies compared birth outcomes of women treated with an SNRI or NRI during pregnancy to pregnant women who were not treated with an SNRI or NRI; depression status of either group was not analyzed.

Growth for gestational age. We found no direct evidence on the effect of SNRIs or NRIs for depression on having an infant that is small for gestational age in women with depression during pregnancy. Indirect evidence was limited to two studies, one of venlafaxine[162] and the other including any SNRI or NRI, both with comparison with infants of mothers not receiving an SNRI or NRI during pregnancy but with no known depression.[118] These studies had results in opposite directions. The reason for the discrepancy may simply be inadequate sample sizes – the larger study, the analysis of SNRI or NRI included only 27 exposures,[118] and the smaller study included only five exposures to venlafaxine.[162]

Education and learning. No direct evidence on the effect of SNRI/NRIs for depression on education or learning outcomes in children of women with depression during pregnancy was found. Indirect evidence regarding prenatal SNRI exposure and subsequent intelligence testing in offspring is limited to one high risk of bias observational study, described in detail above (under SSRIs).[139]

Illness Outcomes
We did not find evidence on the risk of stress related chronic disease in children associated with maternal SNRI use during pregnancy. We found evidence on the risk of developing ADHD, internalizing or externalizing behaviors, or mental illness, reported below.

Internalizing behaviors. No direct evidence on the risk of internalizing behaviors and exposure to an SNRI/NRI during pregnancy was found. Indirect evidence was found to determine an effect of SNRI exposure during pregnancy on internalizing or externalizing behaviors in offspring compared with nonexposed children. Increased internalizing behaviors reported by mothers using the CBCL (n=178) correlated with severity of maternal depression during pregnancy and at time of testing, not maternal venlafaxine treatment in pregnancy. Depression in pregnancy and at time of testing, not exposure to venlafaxine, predicted externalizing behaviors as reported by mothers on the CBCL.[139]

Other Antidepressants: Bupropion

Infant/Child Outcomes
Attention deficit hyperactivity disorder. We found no direct evidence on the effect of bupropion for depression on the risk of children of women with depression during pregnancy developing ADHD. One retrospective cohort study with medium risk of bias provides indirect evidence on the risk of ADHD in children of women exposed to bupropion during pregnancy. This study assessed ADHD diagnoses by age 5 years using a large national claims-based

dataset.[96] A mental health diagnosis was identified in only 33 percent of women, including 10 percent with a depressive disorder. After multiple logistic regression analysis, risk of diagnosis with ADHD in children born to women who used bupropion, SSRIs, or any other antidepressant during or after pregnancy was compared with children of women who did not take any antidepressant during pregnancy. Exposure to bupropion at any time during pregnancy was associated with increased risk of ADHD diagnosis in children (OR 3.63; 95% CI 1.20 to 11.04), in particular for exposure during the second trimester (OR 14.66; 95% CI 3.27 to 65.73), but not first or third trimesters (OR 2.06; 95% CI 0.35 to 12.16; OR=<0.01, <0.01 to >99.9, respectively).

Postpartum Exposure

Selective Serotonin Reuptake Inhibitors

Maternal Outcomes

We found one high risk of bias placebo-controlled RCT of paroxetine in women who were depressed in the postpartum period.[191] The trial was small (70 women enrolled and 31 completed) and short-term (8 weeks). This is the only direct evidence for maternal outcomes of treatment for depression in the postpartum period. Additionally, there was indirect evidence from a medium risk of bias observational study that compared treatment with citalopram during pregnancy and up to 2 months postpartum with pregnant and postpartum women who did not receive an SSRI (depression status unknown).[103]

Danger to self or infant. Evidence on the risk of danger to self or infant while being treated for depression with an SSRI is insufficient. The small, high risk of bias RCT reported zero such events.[191]

Depression symptomatology. Evidence on the effect of SSRIs on depressive symptoms in the postpartum period is insufficient to draw conclusions. Only one RCT with high risk of bias compared depression symptom improvement during the postpartum period, between paroxetine and placebo.[191] Response at week 8 was defined as a Clinical Global Impression-Improvement (CGI-I) of 1 or 2 with 43 percent (n=15/35) of the paroxetine group achieving response as compared with 32 percent (n=11/35) of the placebo group (OR 1.31; 95% CI 0.50 to 3.41). Remission by week 8 as defined as a rating of <8 on the 17 Item Hamilton rating Scale for Depression (HAM-D-17) was significantly improved for women taking paroxetine with 37 percent achieving remission in the paroxetine group and 14 percent in the placebo group (OR 3.54; 95% CI 1.10 to 11.41).

Delivery and Postpartum Parameters
Breastfeeding. Evidence on the effect of SSRI treatment for depression during the postpartum period on breastfeeding outcomes is insufficient as there is no direct evidence available. Indirect evidence from one very small observational study (n=21) comparing women who took citalopram to during pregnancy and in the postpartum period (for any reason) to women who did not (depression status not reported) reported equal numbers of mothers breastfeeding in both groups (n=9) and so there is no significant difference between groups (OR 0.91; 95% CI 0.26 to 3.20).[103]

Key Question 1b. How do pharmacological treatments affect maternal and child outcomes when compared with each other (drug A vs. drug B)?

Pregnancy Exposure

Maternal Outcomes

We found no evidence for maternal outcomes comparing antidepressants to each other for depression during pregnancy.

Child Outcomes

Preterm birth. No direct evidence was available comparing one antidepressant to another in women with depression during pregnancy. Three studies provide indirect evidence for risk of preterm birth in women taking specific SSRIs compared with other SSRIs in women taking the drugs during pregnancy. A single high risk of bias study (n = 809) provides opportunity to compare paroxetine and fluoxetine, where no difference between the drugs was found.[84] Additionally, two studies compared citalopram or escitalopram with "other SSRIs"; the unadjusted pooled estimate from these studies is 1.26 (95% CI 0.54 to 2.96).[172,173] These are small studies, one high risk of bias and one medium.

Growth for gestational age. No direct evidence was available comparing one antidepressant with another in women with depression during pregnancy. Indirect evidence was limited to one medium risk of bias study reporting the risk of having an infant that is small for gestational age at birth for any specific drug compared with other drugs.[107] The risk with paroxetine treatment during pregnancy compared with other SSRIs was an adjusted odds ratio of 0.9 (95% CI 0.09 to 4.34).

Postpartum Exposure

Maternal Outcomes

The evidence comparing one antidepressant with another in women with depression during the postpartum period is insufficient to draw conclusions for maternal outcomes. We found one small RCT (n=109) that compared sertraline with nortriptyline in treating depression in postpartum women.[188] Additionally, there are two publications of post-hoc analyses using data from this trial.[116,121] The study was high risk of bias, due to unclear allocation concealment, dissimilarity of groups at baseline and high levels of overall attrition. See Appendix D for strength of evidence ratings for selected outcomes. There was also no difference between the groups in response or remission rates; by week 8 the proportions with either response or remission were 69 percent in the sertraline group, and 73 percent in the nortriptyline group. In a post-hoc analysis using a subset of the data (n=70), no difference in breastfeeding rates between the sertraline and nortriptyline was found (OR 2.78; 95% CI 0.86-8.94).[116] No information in intention to breastfeed or baseline breastfeeding status is presented.

Key Question 1c. How do pharmacological treatments affect outcomes when compared with active nonpharmacological treatments?

No evidence was found for this question in either pregnant or postpartum women.

Key Question 1d. How does combination therapy affect maternal and child outcomes?

1. Using a Second Drug To Augment the Effects of the Primary Drug and Comparing This Treatment With Monotherapy With a Single Drug

Pregnancy Exposure

Maternal Outcomes

No evidence was found for maternal outcomes for this question.

Child Outcomes

We found no direct comparative evidence on the benefits to children of combination pharmacological treatment for maternal depression during pregnancy. Indirect evidence from observational studies comparing results for children of women taking combination antidepressant therapy during pregnancy for any reason with women who did not take an antidepressant during pregnancy, but with unknown depression status was found.

The best indirect evidence on the risk of preterm birth with combination therapy with an antidepressant during pregnancy comes from a single observational study that reported a non-statistically significant unadjusted odds ratio of 1.3 (95% CI 0.5 to 3.33) for comparison of using two drugs (one SSRI and a second antidepressant from a different class) with use of a single SSRI.[92]

Indirect evidence on combination antidepressant therapy during pregnancy and having an infant that is small for gestational age is limited to a single observational study.[162] Although this study was medium risk of bias, it is important for this outcome that the method used to determine gestational age was not reported. Seventy percent were taking an SSRI in combination with a non-SSRI drug. In women who took two antidepressants in the second trimester, there was an increased risk of having a small for gestational age infant compared with women who did not take an antidepressant during pregnancy (ARR = 3.48; 95% CI 1.56 to 7.75).

2. Combining Pharmacological Treatments With Nonpharmacological Treatments and Comparing Them With Nonpharmacological Treatments Alone

Postpartum Exposure

Maternal Outcomes

Direct evidence on maternal outcomes with combination pharmacological and nonpharmacological treatments for depression during the postpartum period compared with nonpharmacological treatments alone is insufficient to draw conclusions due to limited, inconsistent evidence. We found three small RCTs,[58,65,69] rated medium risk of bias, and one small observational study,[155] rated high risk of bias, that compared combining pharmacologic treatments with nonpharmacological treatments and comparing them with nonpharmacological treatments alone. All of the studies focused on the postpartum period only and reported on depression symptoms. See Appendix D for strength of evidence ratings.

Depression symptomatology. Two RCTs compared a nonpharmacological treatment combined with an SSRI with the nonpharmacological intervention alone. A medium risk of bias RCT (n=40)[65] compared sertraline and brief psychodynamic psychotherapy with psychotherapy alone, finding no statistical differences in the rate of response (>50% reduction in either the Montgomery Asberg Depression Rating Scale [MADRS] or Edinburgh Postnatal Depression Scale [EPDS] scores) over 8 weeks of treatment (70% in the combination group and 50 percent psychotherapy only group, OR 1.91; 95% CI 0.52 to 7.00). Similarly, there was no statistically significant difference in remission (defined as final score on the MADRS of <10 or the EPDS <7) at week 8 (combination group 65T and psychotherapy only group 50%, OR 3.09; 95% CI 0.78 to 12.14). At week 12, the combination group had a remission rate of 94 percent and the psychotherapy only group had a rate of 82 percent (OR 3.64; 95% CI 0.34 to 39.02).

The other small (n=86) trial randomized women with depression six to eight weeks after delivery to fluoxetine plus cognitive behavioral counseling (one or six sessions) compared with counseling alone (one or six sessions).[58] Scores > 12 on the Revised Clinical Interview Scale (CIS-R) and the EPDS were considered clinically important morbidity and 'mild depression' was defined as a score of 8-17 on the HAM-D. Analysis based on study completers, few differences were found between groups with all but the single counseling session reducing symptoms. However, because the drop-out rate was high, 30 percent, the results based on intention to treat analysis are different - only the fluoxetine plus one or six counseling sessions had CIS-R scores less than 12 at week 12. The two counseling alone groups did not have scores less than 12 at any time point. This pattern held true for the analysis of EPDS scores. For the HAM-D at week 12, only the single session of counseling did not have a mean score less than 8.

Breastfeeding. Direct evidence on the effect of different treatments for depression used in combination with nonpharmacological treatments compared with nonpharmacological treatments alone on breastfeeding outcomes in women with depression during pregnancy comes from a single observational study and is insufficient to draw conclusions.[69] In this very small (n=44) medium risk of bias study women with major depressive disorder (based on DSM-IV criteria) were enrolled and two groups were identified: those taking an SSRI during pregnancy and those who were not taking a pharmacologic treatment. Both groups received what is described only as "supportive psychotherapy" with no further details reported. No details on the psychotherapy received were reported. The duration of breastfeeding was two months longer in the untreated group (8.5 months) compared with the group treated with an SSRI (6.4 months, p = 0.4), but the difference was not statistically significant.

A high risk of bias observational study[155] compared sertraline plus interpersonal psychotherapy (IPT) with IPT alone in postpartum women, which also included a third sertraline only group. This was a small observational study (n=23) with high loss to followup and high risk of bias.

3. Comparing Pharmacological Treatments Alone With Pharmacological Treatments Used in Combination With Nonpharmacological Treatments

Postpartum Exposure

Maternal Outcomes

Direct evidence was insufficient to draw conclusions, based only on one small medium risk of bias RCT[132] and one small high risk of bias observational study[155] that compared SSRI treatment (as a class or as an individual drug) with pharmacological treatments used in combination with nonpharmacological treatments. The observational study was high risk of bias due to high overall and differential loss to followup and potentially inadequate handling of confounders.[155] Both of the studies focused on the postpartum period only and both concluded that all treatment groups produced reduction in depression symptomatology compared with baseline. Please see Appendix D for strength of evidence ratings for selected outcomes. The RCT[132] compared 16 postpartum women on paroxetine with 19 on paroxetine plus cognitive behavioral therapy. It was a small study with high loss to followup. There was no difference in response between the two groups on either the HAM-D (OR 1.87; 95% CI 0.29 to 11.84) or on the EPDS (OR 1.71; 95% CI 0.36 to 8.16). The response rate at the last visit on the HAM-D was 87.5 percent in the paroxetine only group verses 78.9 percent in the combination group and on the EPDS it was 50 percent compared with 58.3 percent. With anxiety symptoms, there was no difference in response between the two groups on either the HAM-A (OR 1.12; 95% CI 0.16 to 7.82) or on the YBOCS (OR 0.72; 95% CI 0.19 to 2.77).

The high risk of bias observational study[155] comparing sertraline with sertraline plus interpersonal psychotherapy (IPT) in postpartum women. This was a small observational study (n=23) with high loss to followup and high risk of bias. Those who completed the study experienced significant overall improvement and in an analysis of covariance comparing outcomes on the HAM-D, Beck Depression Inventory, and EPDS, controlling for pretreatment depression, no differences in outcome were identified between the IPT and IPT plus sertraline.

Key Question 2. What are the comparative harms of pharmacological and nonpharmacological treatments for women with depression during pregnancy and in the postpartum period?

Summary

- Direct evidence was sparse on the maternal and infant/child harms associated with pharmacological and nonpharmacological treatment for depression during pregnancy and the postpartum period.
    - Direct evidence provided sufficient data to draw the following low-strength conclusions:
        - Results from one observational study with medium risk of bias (n=107,877) suggest that infants of depressed mothers treated with SSRIs during pregnancy do not have a statistically significantly higher risk of convulsions than those of depressed mothers not treated with medication (0.14% compared with 0.11%; risk difference 0.0005; 95% CI −0.0015 to 0.0025).
        - Consistent results from three medium risk of bias observational studies (n=15,793) suggest that, compared with untreated maternal depression during pregnancy, SSRI treatment is associated with a statistically significant increase in risk of respiratory distress in infants (pooled unadjusted OR 1.91; 95% CI 1.63 to 2.24; $I^2 = 0\%$).
    - Direct evidence provided insufficient data to support conclusions on the following additional harms due to methodological limitations, unknown consistency and imprecision:
        - Major malformations:

- One small medium risk of bias observational study (n=62) compared the effects of SSRIs with no treatment of depression during pregnancy.
- One small medium risk of bias observational study (n=44) compared the effects of SSRIs plus psychotherapy with psychotherapy alone for depression during pregnancy.
- Respiratory distress: One small medium risk of bias observational study (n=21) compared the effects of SSRIs with TCAs when used to treat depression during pregnancy.
- Overall adverse events and withdrawals due to adverse events in babies of breastfeeding mothers:
  - One RCT with high risk of bias (n=109) compared risk between women taking either sertraline or nortriptyline for postpartum depression.
  - One small observational study with high risk of bias (n=23) compared risk between women treated with either sertraline or interpersonal psychotherapy for postpartum depression.

Detailed Assessment of the Evidence

Key Question 2. What are the comparative harms of pharmacological and nonpharmacological treatments for women with depression during pregnancy and in the postpartum period?

There were no RCTs of antidepressant drugs used to treat depression in pregnancy to provide direct evidence on the comparative harms. Direct evidence was limited to 16 observational studies of pharmacological treatments given at unknown dosages. Indirect evidence consists of studies of women taking an antidepressant during pregnancy for any reason compared with women who did not take an antidepressant during pregnancy, with unknown depression status in either group. Both RCTs and observational studies were found for comparative harms of pharmacologic treatment in the postpartum period.

We found no direct evidence on maternal harms of pharmacologic treatments for depression during pregnancy, primarily because for this population there is only observational evidence and the harms outcomes for this report, for example, rates of specific adverse effects (e.g., suicidal ideation, hepatoxicity, and loss of libido) are not reported. The risk of mortality may have been reported sporadically, but most of these retrospective observational studies would have excluded women who died during pregnancy, and the remaining studies did not have explicit methodology to ascertain this and other serious harms.

How do pharmacological treatments affect child outcomes when compared with active nonpharmacological treatments?

Antidepressant Exposure During Pregnancy

Selective Serotonin Reuptake Inhibitors

Infant/Child Outcomes
All-cause mortality. No direct evidence was available assessing comparative harms of pharmacologic treatment for depression during pregnancy.

Indirect evidence for this important outcome is available from one Danish cohort study with low risk of bias[105] and four cohort studies with medium risk of bias.[77,106,118,175] This evidence suggested an increased risk of neonatal/postneonatal death over the first year following maternal use of SSRIs during pregnancy, but not when we examined early and late deaths separately. None accounted for depression in analysis and only one small retrospective cohort study (n=105) reported the proportions of women diagnosed with depression, with 65 percent in the SSRI group and 46 percent in the nonexposed group; there were no neonatal deaths in either group.[106]

The remaining four studies did not have data on treatment indication or proportions of women with depression in groups.[77,105,118,175] A population-based cohort study (n=98,365) found a statistically significant increase in risk of neonatal death at any time during the first year of life for SSRIs as a group, paroxetine, escitalopram, and fluvoxamine, but not for other individual SSRIs (Table 4).[77] The remaining studies separately evaluated early and late death. Based on a study of all Nordic countries, maternal use of SSRIs as a group during pregnancy is not statistically significantly associated with a higher risk of early or late neonatal death (Table 4).[175] A Danish study additionally evaluated individual SSRIs and found that citalopram, but not fluoxetine, escitalopram, paroxetine, or sertraline was associated with a statistically significant increase in risk of early death.

Table 4. Risk of neonatal/postneonatal death for maternal use of a selective serotonin reuptake inhibitor in pregnancy*

Author Year Country Sample Size	Results
First year as a whole	
Colvin 2012[77] Western Australia n=98,325	Adjusted OR for deaths during first year of life (95% CI): **SSRIs grouped: 1.81 (1.26, 2.60)** Citalopram: 1.28 (0.61, 2.72) **Escitalopram: 3.52 (1.30, 9.49)** Fluoxetine: 2.30 (0.85, 6.19) **Fluvoxamine: 4.52 (1.44, 14.24)** **Paroxetine: 2.18 (1.03, 4.61)** Sertraline: 1.40 (0.72, 2.72)
Early death	
Jimenez-Solem 2013[105] Denmark n=920,620	Adjusted OR for death within 28 days of birth (95% CI): Any SSRI: 1.27 (0.82 to 1.99) **Citalopram: 2.49 (1.33 to 4.65)** Escitalopram: 2.07 (0.29 to 14.85) Fluoxetine: 0.63 (0.24 to 1.69) Paroxetine: 1.95 (0.73 to 5.23) Sertraline: 0.26 (0.04 to 1.81)
Stephansson 2013[175] Nordic countries n=1,633,877	Adjusted OR (95% CI) for any SSRI Neonatal death (0-27 days): 1.23 (0.96 to 1.57)
Lennestal 2007[118] Sweden n=860,947	Adjusted RR (95% CI) for any SSRI compared with expected: Early: 0.8 (0.6 to 1.2)
Jordan 2008[106] n=105	No neonatal deaths
Late Death	
Stephansson 2013[175] Nordic countries n=1,633,877	Adjusted OR (95% CI) for any SSRI Postneonatal death (28-364 days): 1.34 (0.97 to 1.86)
Lennestal 2007[118] Sweden n=860,947	Adjusted RR (95% CI) for any SSRI compared with expected: Late: 1.2 (0.7 to 2.0)

CI = confidence interval; OR = odds ratio; RR = relative risk; SSRI = selective serotonin reuptake inhibitor
*Results are in bold type where they are statistically significant

Congenital Anomalies

Major malformations. Only three studies provide direct evidence of the comparative risk of major malformations for the comparison of antidepressant-treated and untreated treated depressed pregnant women.[69,72,189] The studies were small (n=44, n=136, and n=238) and reported one or zero major malformations.

In addition to these studies, indirect evidence was available from 26 other observational studies that report on the risk of major malformations in women taking an antidepressant during pregnancy for any reason compared with women who did not take an antidepressant during pregnancy – with depression status unknown for both groups.[56,60,63,76,78,84,88,95,104,109,111,113-115,123,125-127,130,140,149,153,160,163,173,185,190] Two of these studies reported that all included women in the antidepressant groups were depressed, with control groups of women who did not take an antidepressant during pregnancy but whose depression status was unknown.[88,153] Eight studies reported rates of depression in the exposed group; they reported widely varying numbers, from

26 percent[95] to 77 percent.[127] These studies did not report data in a way that allowed clear analysis of the effect of depression on the outcomes in the exposed or nonexposed groups. Several studies explicitly used a comparison group exposed to drugs known to be nonteratogenic.[72,84,88,115,127,140,153,173]

Selective serotonin reuptake inhibitors as a group. Direct evidence on the risk of major congenital malformations associated with the use of any SSRI or specific SSRIs for depression during pregnancy is limited to only two small, medium risk of bias observational studies.[69,189] These studies were small; one reported no major malformations, and the other study reported one malformation in the group of women who were depressed but did not receive an SSRI.

A substantial amount of indirect evidence was available from 15 cohort studies that reported the incidence of major congenital malformations associated with the use of any SSRI, or specific SSRIs, during pregnancy, compared with the children of women who did not receive an SSRI and were not known to be depressed.[76,80,104,109,113-115,125,126,138,142,159,167,171,184] Two of the studies were methodologically strong, rated low risk of bias,[104,125] and two were methodologically weak, rated high risk of bias, due primarily to potentially biased selection of patients, lack of assessment of comparability of subjects at baseline, and lack of appropriate statistical analysis, including controlling for potential confounding.[114,126] Major malformations are a fairly rare and serious adverse event; therefore, a signal from indirect evidence may be important.

Specific malformations that were classified as major varied across these studies, with most studies using ICD-9 codes[196] to identify infants with malformations and some using additional methods to exclude more minor malformations. Other methods used to identify malformations were the EUROCAT[197] classification system, and the approach identified by Holmes et al.[198,199] This variability in what was categorized as "major" may result in heterogeneity in the data set; based on information presented, we were not able to refine this analysis further. As such, we focus our analysis on the best evidence – six studies that were methodologically stronger (medium or low risk of bias), used a formal system to identify and classify malformations (e.g., EUROCAT, Holmes, ICD), and controlled for at least three of the four types of potential confounders we had identified as critical, a priori (age, race, parity, and other relevant exposures such as smoking and drug use).[104,109,125,138,167,184] None of the studies adjusted for race, and none reported on race characteristics of their study populations. None of these studies were conducted in the United States; all were conducted in Nordic countries. This evidence, based six studies of over 2.4 million pregnancies, suggests no increased risk of major malformations with exposure during pregnancy to SSRIs (as a group) compared with not being exposed (pooled adjusted OR 1.08; 95% CI 0.95 to 1.22) (Table 5). However, the I^2 value of 67 percent suggests the presence of moderate heterogeneity. To explore potential sources of heterogeneity, we conducted exploratory subgroup analyses based on exposure timing, timing of diagnosis, and methods used to identify malformations. Exposure timing in these studies varied from first trimester to "any" time point in the 10 studies that reported adjusted odds ratios; limiting the best evidence analysis to only exposures in the first trimester resulted in a similar estimate (pooled adjusted OR 1.11; 95% CI 0.97 to 1.28). The studies varied in the timing of diagnosis of the malformation in that two allowed diagnosis up to 1 year, one was unclear, and three included malformations diagnosed soon after birth (e.g., within 7 days or during the initial hospitalization). Limiting to these early diagnosis studies resulted in a pooled adjusted odds ratio of 0.99 (95% CI 0.85 to 1.16), again not changing the estimate in a meaningful way. Limiting the analysis to those studies that used ICD coding resulted in an odds ratio of 0.99 (95% CI 0.85 to 1.15) while limiting to studies that used EUROCAT coding resulted in a slightly higher risk estimate, although still not statistically significant (OR 1.19; 95% CI 0.97 to 1.47). None of these sensitivity analyses reduced the heterogeneity to below 30 percent.

Compared with the results of our pooled analysis above the pooled estimate based on unadjusted rates from all studies, regardless of methods, showed a larger and statistically significant increased risk (OR 1.19; 95% CI 1.02 to 1.40). Heterogeneity was even higher in this analysis, with an inconsistency estimate (I^2) of 78 percent.

Table 5. Best evidence estimates of risk for major malformations with use of selective serotonin reuptake inhibitors during pregnancy*

SSRI	Number of Studies Sample Size	Pooled Adjusted OR (95% CI)	Heterogeneity (I^2)
Any SSRI	6 ; 2,421,444	1.08 (0.95 to 1.22)	67%
Any SSRI during pregnancy vs. prior use of an SSRI	8	1.07 (0.78 to 1.47)	Not estimable Cochran Q 0.29, P = 0.59
Citalopram/escitalopram	8; 4,091,225	1.06 (0.97 to 1.16)	0%
Fluoxetine	7; 3,397,479	**1.14 (1.01 to 1.30)**	0%
Paroxetine	11; 4,192,613	**1.17 (1.02 to 1.35)**	0%
Sertraline	7; 4,020,791	0.98 (0.85 to 1.13)	23%
Fluvoxamine	2; 1,492,881	0.76 (0.38 to 1.50)	Not estimable (Cochran Q = 0.17; P = 0.68)

CI = confidence interval; OR = odds ratio; SSRI = selective serotonin reuptake inhibitor
*Results are in bold type where they are statistically significant

Citalopram and/or escitalopram. Twelve studies reported indirect evidence on the risk of malformations with citalopram and/or escitalopram for any reason.[56,76,90,109,111,113,125,138,149,159,167,173] One of the studies was methodologically strong, with low risk of bias,[125] and three were methodologically weak, high risk of bias, due primarily to potentially biased selection of patients, lack of assessment of comparability of subjects at baseline, and lack of appropriate statistical analysis, including controlling for potential confounding.[90,111,173]

Based on eight medium and low risk of bias studies (seven cohort and one case control) reporting adjusted odds ratios, there was evidence that there is no increased risk of major malformations associated with use of either citalopram or escitalopram for any reason compared with women who did not take an antidepressant during pregnancy (depression status unknown) (Table 5). Using unadjusted rates for all 12 studies, regardless of methods, the pooled OR was slightly greater, although not statistically significant (1.12; 95% CI 0.91 to 1.38), but statistical heterogeneity was present (I^2=64%). Because there was no heterogeneity in the adjusted analysis, we did not pursue subgroup analyses.

Fluoxetine. Thirteen observational studies provided indirect evidence on major malformations associated with fluoxetine use during pregnancy for any reason.[56,71,76,84,90,109,113,125,140,149,153,159,167] Of these again one was low risk of bias[125] and five were high risk of bias.[71,84,90,140,153] We focused our analysis on the seven studies that were medium to low risk of bias and that reported adjusted odds ratios.[56,76,109,113,125,159,167] Based on these studies, there was evidence that fluoxetine use during pregnancy for any reason is statistically significantly associated with an increased risk of major malformations compared with women who did not take an antidepressant (depression status unknown) (Table 5). Sensitivity analysis removing the only study that did not use a recognized classification system did not alter these results in a meaningful way (pooled adjusted OR 1.15; 95% CI 1.00 to 1.31; p=0.045).[56,76,109,113,125,159,167]

Paroxetine. Eleven observational studies[56,76,84,90,109,113,125,138,149,159,167] provided indirect evidence on major malformation rates associated with paroxetine use during pregnancy for any reason compared with women who did not take an antidepressant during pregnancy (depression status unknown), of which two were high risk of bias.[84,90] Based on analysis of the eight medium and low risk of bias studies that adjusted for potential confounders and reported odds ratios,[56,76,109,113,125,138,159,167] we found an increased risk of major malformations (Table 5). Sensitivity analysis removing the two studies that did not adjust for at least three of four key confounding factors resulted in a similar estimate (pooled adjusted OR 1.20; 95% CI 1.03 to 1.41).

Sertraline. Nine medium and low risk of bias observational studies provided indirect evidence on rates of major malformations associated with sertraline use during pregnancy for any reason compared with women who were not treated with an antidepressant (depression status unknown).[56,76,90,109,113,125,149,159,167] Analysis based on the seven studies that reported adjusted odds ratios indicates no increased risk for major malformations (Table 5).[56,76,109,113,125,159,167] Sensitivity analysis removing studies that did not adjust for at least three of the four key confounding factors identified for this review left four studies and resulted in a more precise estimate (pooled adjusted OR 0.92; 95% CI 0.80 to 1.05).[56,109,125,167]

Fluvoxamine. Three medium and low risk of bias observational studies provided indirect evidence of the risk of major malformations with fluvoxamine use during pregnancy for any reason compared with women who did not use an antidepressant (depression status unknown), although the numbers of women using this SSRI were smaller than the others above.[109,125,149] The pooled estimate from two studies reporting adjusted odds ratios indicated no increased risk (Table 5),[109,125] nor did the third study that reported adjusted mean differences.[149]

Cardiac malformations. In addition to major malformations, we examined cardiac malformations as a separate category, in part because there is uncertainty in the ascertainment definitions and methods identifying major malformations, but also because although not all cardiac malformations are major, even those that are minor, if diagnosed, result in resource utilization and stress for families. No direct evidence was available on the risk of cardiac malformations following fetal exposure to SSRIs to treat maternal depression during pregnancy.

Ten observational studies provided indirect evidence on the risk of SSRIs as a group for cardiac malformations, compared with nonexposure.[104,109,113,123,125,138,142,159,167,185] Two of the studies were methodologically strong, with low risk of bias,[104,125] and one was methodologically weak, with high risk of bias, due primarily to potentially biased selection of patients, lack of assessment of comparability of subjects at baseline, and lack of appropriate statistical analysis, including controlling for potential confounding.[185] Similar to identification of major malformations, above, we had concerns over the accuracy of ascertainment of serious cardiovascular anomalies in these studies, as they depended on ICD coding to identify a defect, with some studies applying additional criteria to categorize the type of anomaly according to developmental groupings. As a result there may have been heterogeneity in what was recorded as a major cardiac malformation across these studies. Because of this we focused our analysis on the best evidence—five studies that were methodologically stronger (medium or low risk of bias), used a formal system to identify and classify malformations (e.g., EUROCAT), and controlled for at least three of the four types of potential confounders we had identified as critical, a priori (age, race, parity, and other relevant exposures such as smoking and drug use).[104,123,125,138,167] These studies provided evidence that there is no increased risk of cardiac malformations with SSRI use during pregnancy for any reason; however, there was statistically significant heterogeneity present in the analysis. In order to address this heterogeneity, we conducted a sensitivity analysis removing the studies that did not use an additional method to classify the type of cardiovascular defect, leaving three studies with a pooled adjusted odds ratio of 1.07 (95% CI 0.94 to 1.2), with no heterogeneity present.[123,125,167]

Citalopram and/or escitalopram. Eight studies reported indirect evidence on the risk of malformations with citalopram and/or escitalopram.[113,123,125,130,138,149,159,167] One of the studies was methodologically strong, with low risk of bias,[125] and one was methodologically weak, high risk of bias, due primarily to potentially biased selection of patients, uncertain accuracy of outcome ascertainment, and lack of appropriate statistical analysis, including controlling for potential confounding.[130]

Based on six medium and low risk of bias studies reporting adjusted odds ratios,[113,123,125,138,159,167] there was evidence of no increased risk of cardiac malformations associated with use of either citalopram or escitalopram for any reason during pregnancy compared with women who did not take an antidepressant during pregnancy (depression status unknown) (Table 6). Because there was very little heterogeneity in the adjusted analysis, we did not pursue subgroup analyses. Analysis of unadjusted risk of a cardiac malformation in women taking citalopram or escitalopram during pregnancy compared with those who discontinued an SSRI prior to pregnancy resulted in a nonstatistically significant difference (OR 1.86; 95% CI 0.31 to 8.21).[138]

Table 6. Best evidence on risk of cardiac malformations with selective serotonin reuptake inhibitors compared with nonexposure*

SSRI (N = 15, 709)	Pooled Adjusted OR (95% CI)	Heterogeneity (I^2)
Any SSRI	1.29 (0.96 to 1.72)	84%
Sensitivity analysis	1.07 (0.94 to 1.20)	0%
Comparison to Prior SSRI use	Unadjusted OR 1.29 (0.77 to 2.18)	Cochran Q=0.71, p=0.40
Citalopram/escitalopram	1.05 (0.84 to 1.39)	5%
Fluoxetine	**1.31 (1.08 to 1.58)**	0%
Sensitivity analysis	1.2 (0.99 to 1.51)	0%
Paroxetine	**1.49 (1.20 to 1.85)**	0%
Sensitivity analysis	**1.45 (1.13 to 1.85)**	0%
Sertraline	1.08 (0.70 to 1.65)	68%
Sensitivity analysis	0.76 (0.57 to 1.00)	0%

CI = confidence interval; OR = odds ratio; SSRI = selective serotonin reuptake inhibitor
*Results are in bold type where they are statistically significant

Fluoxetine. Eleven observational studies provide indirect evidence on the risk of major malformations associated with fluoxetine use during pregnancy for any reason, compared with women who did not take an antidepressant (depression status unknown).[56,76,84,109,113,125,149,159,167] Of these one was low risk of bias[125] and one was high risk of bias.[84] We focused our analysis on the eight studies that were medium to low risk of bias and that reported adjusted odds ratios.[56,76,109,113,125,159,167] Based on these studies, there was evidence that fluoxetine is associated with an increased risk of cardiac malformations (Table 6), with no statistical heterogeneity. Sensitivity analysis removing the three studies that did not adjust for at least three of four key confounders resulted in a nonstatistically significant finding (pooled adjusted OR 1.2; 95% CI 0.99 to 1.51).[56,109,125,167]

Paroxetine. Ten observational studies provided indirect evidence on the risk of cardiac malformation rates associated with paroxetine use during pregnancy for any reason compared with women who did not use an antidepressant during pregnancy (depression status unknown), of which one was high risk of bias.[56,60,84,109,113,123,125,149,159,167] Based on analysis of the six medium and low risk of bias studies that adjusted for potential confounders and reported odds ratios,[56,60,109,123,125,167] we found an increased risk of cardiac malformations (Table 6). Sensitivity analysis removing one study that did not report additional methods of identifying serious cardiac malformations resulted in a similar estimate (pooled adjusted OR 1.45; 95% CI 1.13 to 1.85). Statistical heterogeneity was not present in any of these analyses.

Sertraline. Eight observational studies, all medium to low risk of bias, provide indirect evidence of the risk of cardiac malformations associated with sertraline use during pregnancy for any reason compared with women who did not use an antidepressant during pregnancy (depression status unknown).[56,109,113,123,125,149,159,167] Pooled analysis of the seven studies that reported adjusted odds ratios resulted in no increased risk of cardiac malformations (Table 6) but with statistical heterogeneity. Sensitivity analysis, first removing two studies that did not adjust for at least three of the four potential confounding factors identified for this review, resulted in a pooled estimate suggesting a reduced risk of cardiac anomalies with sertraline (pooled adjusted OR 0.76; 95% CI 0.59 to 0.97), but further limiting to the four studies that also indicated efforts to identify serious cardiac malformations yielded a pooled estimate of 0.76 (95% CI 0.57 to 1.00; p=0.51).

Fluvoxamine. Three observational studies provide indirect evidence on the risk of cardiac malformations associated with use of fluvoxamine use during pregnancy for any reason compared with women who did not use an antidepressant during pregnancy (depression status unknown),[125,140,149] one being low risk of bias,[125] another being medium,[149] and the last being high risk of bias.[140] Collectively, these studies provided evidence of no increased risk of cardiac malformations with fluvoxamine. None reported adjusted results in a similar way across the studies, preventing a meta-analysis of adjusted odds. The best of these studies, which adjusted for three of four key confounding factors and used both ICD-9 and EUROCAT coding, reported an adjusted odds ratio of 0.56 (95% CI 0.14 to 2.25), and the medium risk of bias study reported am adjusted risk difference of -0.55 (95% CI -1.45 to 0.36). Pooling the crude rates from these studies resulted in an odds ratio of 0.67 (95% CI 0.19 to 2.34).

Other Specific Adverse Events
Withdrawal symptoms (neonatal abstinence symptoms). No direct evidence was available on the risk of withdrawal symptoms following fetal exposure to SSRIs to treat maternal depression during pregnancy. Five small cohort studies with medium risk of bias provide indirect evidence suggesting increased risk of neonatal withdrawal/abstinence syndrome symptoms following maternal use of SSRIs for any reason during pregnancy compared with infants of women who did not take an antidepressant (depression status unknown).[71,95,106,119,165] Signs of neonatal

withdrawal/abstinence syndrome were consistently more frequent in SSRI-exposed newborns (Table 7). In the largest studies that adjusted for multiple potential confounding factors, neonates exposed to fluoxetine during the first trimester had almost a nine-fold greater risk of poor neonatal adaptation[71] and those exposed to an SSRI or venlafaxine in late pregnancy had three-fold higher odds of neonatal behavioral signs.[95]

Table 7. Risk of neonatal withdrawal/abstinence syndrome for maternal use of a selective serotonin reuptake inhibitor in pregnancy

Author Year Country Sample Size	Depression	Comparison	Results
SSRIs grouped			
Jordan 2008[106] US N = 108	SRI: 65% Control: 46%	SSRI during pregnancy vs. nonexposed	NBS: Any component present: 28% vs. 17%; NSD
Levinson-Castiel, 2006[119] Israel n=120	NR	SSRI during entire pregnancy or at least during the third trimester vs. nonexposed	Finnegan severe score of ≥ 8: 13% vs. 0% Any symptoms: 30% vs. 0% p=NR
Individual SSRIs			
Chambers 1996[71] US n=482	Fluoxetine: 76.9% Control: NR	Fluoxetine during first trimester vs. nonexposed	Poor neonatal adaptation: Adjusted RR, 8.7 (2.9 to 26.6)
SSRIs or SNRIs			
Ferreira 2007[95] USA n=166	Exposed: 41% Control: NR	SSRI or venlafaxine during third trimester or at least two weeks prior to delivery vs. nonexposed	Neonatal behavioral signs: Adjusted OR, 3.1 (1.3–7.1)
Rampono, 2009[165] Australia N=56	NR	SSRI/SNRI during pregnancy vs. nonexposed	Maximum median NAS on day 1: SSRI/SNRI=2 vs. nonexposed=0; P<0.05 No other differences in NAS scores (days 1 to 3) Percent infants with NAS > 12 or 3 scores > 8: SSRI=4% vs. SNRI=9%, NSD

NAS = Finnegan neonatal abstinence scoring system; NBS = neonatal behavioral syndrome; NR = not reported; NSD = no significant difference' OR = odds ratio; RR = risk ratio; SNRI = serotonin norepinephrine reuptake inhibitor; SSRI = selective serotonin reuptake inhibitor

Pulmonary hypertension. No direct evidence was available on the risk of withdrawal symptoms following fetal exposure to SSRIs to treat maternal depression during pregnancy. Indirect evidence indicates an increased risk of persistent pulmonary hypertension is associated with use of SSRIs for any reason during pregnancy compared with women who did not take an antidepressant (depression status unknown), based on eight observational studies.[57,70,106,108,110,167,185,186] All but one of these studies were medium risk of bias, but only four reported odds ratios adjusted for potential confounding factors.[70,108,110,167]

Using a broad "any exposure" category, the pooled adjusted odds ratio is 2.41 (95% CI 1.47 to 3.95), with only 14 percent inconsistency.[70,108,167] Exposure later in pregnancy (generally after week 20, excluding women who used SSRIs both early and late) was associated with a statistically significant increase in risk (pooled adjusted OR 2.72; 95% CI 1.63 to 4.54), based on three studies.[70,110,167] However, this pooled analysis had moderate heterogeneity, I^2=48%. While all three adjusted for multiple confounders, including three of the four key confounders identified for this review, the categorization of exposure timing (early) was described in a way that may not exclude overlap between the groups of early, late, or any exposure. Pooled analysis of "early" exposure, reported in four studies,[70,108,110,167] produced concerning statistical heterogeneity, I^2=69% (pooled adjusted OR 1.45; 95% CI 0.84 to 2.49), with three studies showing an increased risk and one showing a nonsignificant lower risk compared with nonexposure. In both analyses it appears that the earliest study estimates were outliers.[70] This was a prospective study that identified infants with persistent pulmonary hypertension prospectively using patient charts and blinded review by a pediatric cardiologist. The other three studies relied on ICD-9 coding to identify cases. However, the prospective study used mother's recall of medications used to identify exposure, while the other studies used combinations of medical and pharmacy records. Thus, none of the studies is superior to the others and the heterogeneity cannot be fully explained.

Respiratory distress. Direct evidence was available from three medium risk of bias observational studies that directly compared the risk of respiratory distress in infants between SSRI-treatment of maternal depression during pregnancy and untreated maternal depression.[69,147,189] Methods for measuring respiratory distress-related outcomes varied across studies, including use of ICD-9 codes,[147] the Peripartum Events Scale (tachypnea, required oxygen, respiratory distress, acrocyanosis, and cyanosis),[189] and admission to the neonatal intensive care unit due to respiratory distress.[69] Based on these three studies, there is low-strength evidence that, compared with untreated maternal depression during pregnancy, SSRI treatment is associated with a statistically significant increase in risk of respiratory distress in infants (pooled unadjusted OR 1.91; 95% CI 1.63 to 2.24; I^2 = 0%).

Seven observational studies with medium risk of bias provide additional indirect evidence on the risk of respiratory distress among infants following maternal use of SSRIs for any reason during pregnancy compared with women who did not use SSRIs (depression status unknown).[77,81,95,106,107,118,142] Four of the studies used ICD codes to identify infants with respiratory distress and used multivariate regression analyses to control for at least one of key confounders identified for this review (n=748,658).[77,81,107,118] Focusing our analysis on the best evidence from these studies, this indirect evidence supports the direct evidence that maternal exposure to SSRIs primarily in late pregnancy is associated with a statistically significant increased risk of respiratory distress in infants exposed to SSRIs during pregnancy compared with infants of nonexposed pregnant women (pooled adjusted OR 1.79; 95% CI 1.64 to 1.97; I^2 = 0%).[77,81,107,118]

A medium risk of bias study of pharmacy dispensing data from the Netherlands suggested a small increase in risk of a child whose mother had taken an SSRI during pregnancy being prescribed a drug for a respiratory condition (incidence risk ratio 1.17; 95 % CI 1.16–1.18).[179] Because ascertainment of exposure was not ideal, and control for confounding possibly not adequate (e.g., did not control for smoking status of mother), these findings should be interpreted with caution.

Neonatal convulsions. Eight observational studies with low to moderate risk of bias reported risk of neonatal convulsions/seizures following maternal use of SSRIs during pregnancy.[80,95,106,107,115,119,147,171] Only one study (n=107,877) provides direct evidence by comparing outcomes from infants of depressed mothers treated with SSRIs with infants of depressed mothers not treated with medication and nondepressed mothers.[147] Infants of depressed mothers treated with SSRIs (incidence 0.14%) did not have a statistically significantly higher risk of convulsions than those of depressed mothers not treated with medication (incidence=0.09%) or nondepressed mothers (incidence =0.11%; risk difference 0.0005; 95% CI −0.0015 to 0.0025).

Indirect evidence from the remaining studies suggests that maternal use of SSRIs during pregnancy for any indication is associated with a statistically significantly increased risk of convulsions compared with infants of nonexposed pregnant women (pooled unadjusted OR 4.11; 95% CI 1.78 to 9.48). These findings are in conflict with the direct evidence.

Tricyclic Antidepressants

Infant/Child Outcomes

Congenital anomalies. No direct evidence was available on the risk of congenital anomalies following fetal exposure to TCAs to treat maternal depression during pregnancy. We identified indirect evidence form five observational studies that reported rates of congenital malformations following exposure to TCAs for any indication during pregnancy compared with women not taking an antidepressant during pregnancy, who were not known to be depressed.[68,140,153,167,171] Of these, one was methodologically strong, low risk of bias,[171] one was medium,[167] and three were methodologically weak, high risk of bias.[68,140,153] These studies had less clear methods for obtaining an unbiased sample and ascertaining exposures and outcomes.

Major malformations. Limiting our analysis to two low and medium risk of bias studies,[167,171] both of which adjusted for at least three of four key confounding factors, we found indirect evidence of an increased risk of major malformations associated with TCAs as a group compared with non-use (pooled adjusted OR 1.31; 95% CI 1.04 to 1.65). Evidence was not reported in a way that allowed investigation of specific drugs in this class.

Cardiac malformations. Based on two low and medium risk of bias studies,[167,171] both of which adjusted for at least three of four key confounding factors, indirect evidence indicated a statistically significant increased risk of cardiovascular malformations associated with use of TCAs as a group for any indication during pregnancy compared with nonuse (pooled adjusted OR 1.58; 95% CI 1.10 to 2.29). Evidence was not reported in a way that allowed investigation of specific drugs in this class.

Other specific adverse events.
Respiratory distress. No direct evidence was available on the risk of neonatal respiratory distress following fetal exposure to TCAs to treat maternal depression during pregnancy. Indirect evidence from two large observational studies with medium risk of bias reported risk of respiratory distress among infants exposed to TCAs during late pregnancy.[81,107] The first evaluated 16,299 cases and 566,497 controls using data from the Swedish Medical Birth Registry.[107] The second was a cohort study of 76,093 women from five health maintenance organizations (HMOs) participating in the HMO Research Network's Center for Education and Research on Therapeutics project.[81] Neither study matched groups based on maternal depression and do not allow direct comparison of the risks of TCA-treated depression to untreated depression. Based on the results of these studies, there is evidence that exposure to TCAs during

late pregnancy leads to a statistically significant increased risk of respiratory distress (pooled adjusted OR 2.11; 95% CI 1.57 to 2.83; Cochran Q=0.08, df=1, p=0.78).

Neonatal convulsions. We found no direct evidence on the risk of neonatal convulsions following fetal exposure to TCAs to treat maternal depression during pregnancy. Indirect evidence indicates a statistically significant increase in risk of convulsions in infants of mothers exposed to TCAs during pregnancy. Two observational studies with moderate risk of bias evaluated risk of neonatal convulsions/seizures following maternal use of TCAs during pregnancy.[107,171] Neither accounted for depression exposure. The best evidence comes from the large Swedish population-based case-control study (cases n=1009; controls n=581,787) that provided indirect evidence that infants exposed to TCAs during pregnancy have almost a seven-fold higher risk of convulsions (adjusted RR 6.8; 95% CI 2.2 to 16.0).[107] A much smaller study (n=418) using data from a health plan also found that more infants of mothers treated with TCAs during pregnancy (1.9%) had seizure disorder than nonexposed infants (0.0%).[171] This study did not provide an adjusted odds ratio. When we combined data from both studies, the unadjusted pooled odds ratio indicated an even higher risk of convulsions/seizures than in the Swedish study alone (7.82; 95% CI 2.81 to 21.76).

Selective Norepinephrine Reuptake Inhibitors and Norepinephrine Reuptake Inhibitors

Infant/Child Outcomes

All-cause mortality. There was no direct evidence to draw conclusions about the risk for infant death associated with use of SNRIs or NRIs during pregnancy to treat depression. One Swedish cohort study with medium risk of bias reported neonatal/postneonatal deaths following maternal use of SNRIs or NRIs during pregnancy.[118] There was no statistically significant increased risk of either early (RR 1.3; 95% CI 0.5 to 2.8) or late (RR 0.0; 95% CI 0.0 to 4.4) neonatal death with SNRIs or NRIs as a group.

Congenital anomalies. There was no direct evidence to draw conclusions about the risk for congenital anomalies associated with use of SNRIs or NRIs during pregnancy to treat depression. Indirect evidence on the risk of congenital malformations with an SNRI indicated no statically significant increase in risk compared with pregnant women who did not use an antidepressant and were not known to be depressed. Two studies reported on malformations with venlafaxine.[90,149] One was medium risk of bias and adjusted for depression and other diseases among other confounders, but did not control for the four key confounders identified for this review.[149] The other was high risk of bias and presented unadjusted rates.[90] There was no increased risk compared with a nonexposed group based on the adjusted risk difference presented in the medium risk of bias study (-1.18; 95% CI -3.20 to 0.84) or the pooled unadjusted rates from both studies (OR 0.68; 95% CI 0.33 to 1.38). Evidence for NRIs (nefazodone or trazodone) was limited to two small, high risk of bias studies.[88,90]

Other Specific Adverse Events
Respiratory distress. There was no direct evidence to draw conclusions about the risk for neonatal respiratory distress associated with use of SNRIs or NRIs during pregnancy to treat depression. Indirect evidence was limited with one very small cohort study with medium risk of

bias reported risk of respiratory distress among infants exposed to SNRIs or NRIs during pregnancy.[118]

Other Antidepressants: Bupropion

Infant Outcomes

Congenital malformations. Two observational studies reported on the risk of congenital malformations associated with use of bupropion during pregnancy.[55,72] One was high risk of bias, but it was the only study provided direct evidence on major malformations.[72] There were few malformations in any group and the p value for comparison across the groups was 0.51. The second, medium risk of bias study[55] was a case control study (n=12,749) designed to examine the risk of cardiac malformations provides only indirect evidence. Compared with nonexposed controls, the adjusted odds ratio for any cardiac malformation was 1.4 (95% CI 0.8 to 2.5).

Postpartum Exposure

Selective Serotonin Reuptake Inhibitors

Child Outcomes

Overall adverse events. One observational study with high risk of bias provided direct evidence on the comparative risk of overall adverse events in babies of 20 women taking an SSRI or venlafaxine for postpartum depression compared with 68 babies of breastfeeding mothers not treated with any medication and of unspecified depression status.[64] Total adverse event symptom score was 5.9 in the treatment group and 7.6 in the control group (p not reported). The proportion of withdrawals from study drug due to adverse events was not reported. Due to high methodological limitations, unknown consistency and imprecision, however, this observational study provides insufficient evidence to draw strong conclusions about comparative risk of overall adverse events in babies.

How do pharmacological treatments affect maternal outcomes when compared with each other (drug A compared with drug B)?

Antidepressant Exposure During Pregnancy

We found no direct evidence comparing antidepressants to each other in pregnant women with depression.

Class Compared With Class: Selective Serotonin Reuptake Inhibitors Compared With Tricyclic Antidepressants

Infant/Child Outcomes

Congenital malformations. Indirect evidence from two medium risk of bias studies reported major malformations and cardiac malformations associated with specific classes of antidepressant drugs.[167,171] Both studies adjusted for at least three of four key confounding factors. Both studies provide adjusted odds ratios for TCAs and SSRIs (and one includes SNRIs) compared with pregnant women who did not receive antidepressants during pregnancy but were not known to be depressed. These studies do not make direct comparisons across classes. The adjusted odds ratios are presented in Table 8. Findings from these studies differ in that a statistically significant increase in risk of major and cardiac malformations was found with TCAs, but not SSRIs in the larger study that used ICD-9 codes to identify malformations,[167] while the other smaller study that used an unblinded pediatric specialist review of patient records to identify malformations found a nonstatistically significant lower risk with TCAs, and a nonsignificant increase in risk with SSRIs.[171] Pooling the unadjusted rates from these two studies, we find SSRIs to have a statistically significantly lower risk of major or cardiac malformations compared with TCAs (Table 8). The comparison of SSRIs and SNRIs comes from a single medium risk of bias study (Table 8), where similar odds were found for both classes and neither was statistically significant.

Table 8. Class compared with class: Risk of congenital malformations

Study	SSRIs (Adjusted OR [95% CI] Compared With Nonexposure)	TCAs (Adjusted OR [95% CI] Compared With Nonexposure)	SNRIs (Adjusted OR [95% CI] Compared With Nonexposure)	SSRIs vs. TCAs (Unadjusted Pooled Odds Ratio [Fixed Effect Model])
Major malformations				
Reis 2010 Sweden n=17,425 exposed	1.08 (0.97 to 1.21)	1.39 (1.07 to 1.72)	1.00 (0.73 to 1.37)	
Simon 2002 US n=385 exposed	1.36 (0.56 to 3.30)	0.82 (0.35 to 1.95)	--	
				0.77 (0.60 to 0.98)
Cardiac malformations				
Reis 2010 Sweden n=14, 821 exposed	0.99 (0.82 to 1.20)	1.63 (1.12 to 2.36)	1.33 (0.84 to 2.09)	
Simon 2002 US n=385 exposed	Non-estimable (0 events in control group)	0.5 (0.05 to 5.53)	--	
				0.66 (0.44 to 0.99)

OR = odds ratio; SNRI = serotonin norepinephrine reuptake inhibitor; SSRI = selective serotonin reuptake inhibitor; TCA = tricyclic antidepressant

Other Specific Adverse Events

Withdrawal symptoms (neonatal abstinence symptoms). Indirect evidence comparing the risk of neonatal abstinence symptoms in infants of women treated for depression with SSRIs compared with SNRIs during pregnancy comes from only one small (n=56) prospective cohort study with medium risk of bias evaluated the comparative risks of neonatal abstinence syndrome between maternal use of SSRIs as a group and SNRIs as a group during pregnancy.[165] Depression status of the women was not reported. Only one cohort study with medium risk of bias include both classes and made any comparison between them, finding no difference in the proportion of infants with neonatal abstinence symptoms scores greater than 12 (on the Finnegan scale, range of 0 to 21) or with 3 days of scores greater than 8 (SSRI=4%, SNRI=9%, p = NR).

Respiratory distress: SSRI compared with TCA. Indirect evidence comparing the risk of neonatal respiratory distress in infants of women treated for depression with SSRIs compared with TCAs during pregnancy comes from only one small study with medium risk of bias

compared the risk of respiratory distress among infants between treatment of maternal depression during pregnancy with different SSRIs or nortriptyline.[172] The study included 21 women from the Women's Behavioral HealthCARE Program at the University of Pittsburgh Medical Center's Western Psychiatric Institute and Clinic. Results from this study suggest that SSRIs and nortriptyline are associated with similar risks of respiratory distress in infants (10% vs. 0%; p=NR).

Bupropion Compared With Other Antidepressants

Infant/Child Outcomes
Congenital malformations. One high risk of bias, observational study reported no increase in risk of congenital malformations associated with the use of bupropion during pregnancy compared with other antidepressants as a group in women with depression during pregnancy.[72] Indirect evidence came from a larger (n=7005), medium risk of bias study that also reported no statistically significant increase in risk with bupropion compared with other antidepressants and reported an adjusted odds ratio of 0.95 (95% CI 0.62 to 1.45).[74] Depression status of women in either group was not known in this study.

Within Class Comparisons: Selective Serotonin Reuptake Inhibitors Compared With Selective Serotonin Reuptake Inhibitors

Congenital Anomalies
Indirect evidence based on nine observational studies[76,84,90,109,125,138,149,159,167] suggested that that there is no difference in risk of major (unadjusted pooled OR 1.14; 95% CI 0.95 to 1.37) or cardiac (unadjusted pooled OR 1.10; 95% CI 0.85 to 1.43) malformations between paroxetine and fluoxetine used for any indication during pregnancy. The evidence was limited by a lack of adjusted analyses directly comparing the two drugs (these findings are based on unadjusted rates), and the methodological limitations of individual studies (range from high to low risk of bias), but is strengthened by the strong consistency across estimates.

Based on eight observational studies,[76,90,109,125,138,149,159,167] we compared the risk of citalopram or escitalopram with that of fluoxetine or paroxetine. Using unadjusted rates, we found that the pooled odds of a major malformations is 0.94 (95% CI 0.82 to 1.07; I^2=0%), suggesting no statistically significant difference between the drugs. Similarly, analysis of the unadjusted risk for cardiac malformations did not result in a statistically significant difference (OR 0.94; 95% CI 0.60 to 1.47). This analysis resulted in significant statistical heterogeneity (I^2 = 49%), sensitivity analyses based on risk of bias did not reduce this heterogeneity. These findings compare to adjusted analyses reported for the individual drugs (above) where the confidence intervals overlap considerably.

These same eight studies indicated a lower risk of major malformations with sertraline compared with fluoxetine or paroxetine (pooled unadjusted OR 0.59; 95% CI 0.38 to 0.90; I^2 = 0%). The risk for cardiac malformations is also lower, based on pooled unadjusted rates (OR 0.59; 95% CI 0.38 to 0.93) but statistically significant heterogeneity (I^2 = 42%) suggested caution in interpreting these results. Sensitivity analysis removing a high risk of bias study did not alter these results.

Other Specific Adverse Events
Persistent pulmonary hypertension. Of the eight observational studies reporting persistent pulmonary hypertension rates with SSRIs, only one conducted an analysis by drug.[110] Based on this medium risk of bias study, there was indirect evidence that only escitalopram did not have statistically significant increased risk when exposure occurs after 20 weeks gestation (Table 9). For early exposure (up to 8 weeks gestation), only citalopram was associated with a statistically significant increase in risk, while escitalopram had the lowest risk. No direct statistical comparisons across the drugs were made. While increased odds are similar for late exposure across the four drugs (citalopram, fluoxetine, paroxetine and sertraline), they are less similar for the early exposure comparison, and a study designed to directly compare the drugs may result in differences being found.

Table 9. Risk of persistent pulmonary hypertension with individual selective serotonin reuptake inhibitors[110]*

N exposed = 30,115 N control = 1 588 140	Adjusted OR	Lower Bound (95% CI)	Upper Bound (95% CI)
Late exposure (20 weeks or after)			
Fluoxetine	**2.0**	**1.0**	**3.8**
Citalopram	**2.3**	**1.2**	**4.1**
Paroxetine	**2.8**	**1.2**	**6.7**
Sertraline	**2.3**	**1.3**	**4.4**
Escitalopram	1.3	0.2	9.5
Early exposure (up to 8 weeks)			
Fluoxetine	1.3	0.6	2.8
Citalopram	**1.8**	**1.1**	**3.0**
Paroxetine	1.3	0.5	3.5
Sertraline	1.9	1	3.6
Escitalopram	0.3	0	2.2

CI = confidence interval, OR = odds ratio
*Results are in bold type where they are statistically significant

Respiratory distress. Indirect evidence comparing the risk of neonatal abstinence symptoms in infants of women treated for depression with SSRIs compared with each other during pregnancy comes from only one small study (n=20) with medium risk of bias that compared the risk of respiratory distress among infants between treatments of maternal depression during pregnancy with different SSRIs.[172] Results from this study suggest that sertraline is not associated with a statistically significant increase in risk of respiratory distress compared with other SSRIs (22% vs. 0%; p=NR).

Postpartum Exposure

Class Compared With Class: Selective Serotonin Reuptake Inhibitors Compared With Tricyclic Antidepressants

Child Outcomes
Overall adverse events and withdrawals due to adverse events. One RCT with high risk of bias provided direct evidence on the comparative risk of overall adverse events in babies of 109 women taking either sertraline or nortriptyline for postpartum depression.[188] There were no adverse events or withdrawals due to adverse events in the babies of the breastfeeding mothers.

Due to high methodological limitations, unknown consistency and imprecision, however, this trial provided insufficient evidence to draw strong conclusions about comparative risk of overall adverse events in babies.

How do pharmacological treatments affect child outcomes when compared with active nonpharmacological treatments?

Antidepressant Exposure During Pregnancy

We found no evidence on the risk of serious adverse outcomes in the infant (e.g., mortality, malformations, and pulmonary hypertension) when comparing pharmacologic and nonpharmacologic treatments.

Postpartum Exposure: Selective Serotonin Reuptake Inhibitors

Overall Adverse Events and Withdrawals Due To Adverse Events

One observational study with high risk of bias provided evidence on the comparative risk of overall adverse events and withdrawal due to adverse events in babies of 23 women treated with either sertraline or interpersonal psychotherapy for postpartum depression.[155] Breastfeeding women reported no adverse events in their babies and none withdrew from the study due to adverse events. Due to high methodological limitations, unknown consistency and imprecision, however, this study provides insufficient evidence to draw strong conclusions about comparative risk of overall adverse events in babies.

How does combination therapy affect maternal and child outcomes?

Using a Second Drug To Augment the Effects of the Primary Drug and Comparing This Treatment With Single Drug Monotherapy

Congenital Anomalies

We found no direct evidence on the risk of congenital anomalies with multiple antidepressants taken during pregnancy for depression compared with monotherapy. Indirect evidence comes from only two small studies specifically addressed this question.[92,159] Both studies reported nonstatistically significant risks with wide confidence intervals for the comparison of multiple antidepressants to nonexposure, but the direction of the estimates were opposite. A medium risk of bias study that adjusted for age, calendar year, income, marriage and smoking status presented an adjusted odds ratio of 1.62 (95% CI 0.83 to 3.16),[159] while a high risk of bias study that matched patients for age, smoking status, and alcohol use reported an odds ratio of 0.68 (95% CI 0.11 to 4.16).[92] This study also reported the comparison to monotherapy, finding an odds ratio of 1.03 (95% CI 0.14 to 7.48). Pooling these data results in an odds ratio of 1.58 (95% CI 0.86 to 2.93), still an imprecise result.

A statistically significant increase in risk of cardiac malformations was found in the one study reporting this outcome, compared with nonexposure; adjusted odds ratio of 3.42 (95% CI 1.40 to 8.34) compared with nonexposure. Because the use of multiple antidepressants may indicate more severe or resistant depression, and since this study did not control for depression or severity of depression, we cannot determine the role of the antidepressants compared with the role of the disease in these findings.

Combining Pharmacological Treatments With Nonpharmacological Treatments and Comparing Them With Nonpharmacological Treatments Alone

Antidepressant Exposure During Pregnancy

We found no evidence on the risk of serious adverse outcomes in the infant (e.g., mortality, malformations, pulmonary hypertension) when comparing combination pharmacologic treatments with nonpharmacologic treatments.

Postpartum Exposure

Overall Adverse Events or Withdrawal Due to Adverse Events

One RCT with high risk of bias provided direct evidence on the comparative risk of overall adverse events in babies of 23 women treated with either sertraline plus interpersonal psychotherapy or sertraline alone for postpartum depression.[155] Breastfeeding women reported no adverse events or withdrew from the study due to adverse events in their babies. Due to high methodological limitations, unknown consistency and imprecision, however, this trial provides insufficient evidence to draw strong conclusions about comparative risk of overall adverse events in babies.

Comparing Pharmacological Treatments Alone With Pharmacological Treatments Used in Combination With Nonpharmacological Treatments

Antidepressant Exposure During Pregnancy

No evidence on the risk of serious adverse outcomes in the infant (e.g., mortality, malformations, pulmonary hypertension) was found comparing pharmacologic treatments used alone with pharmacologic treatments combined with nonpharmacologic treatments.

Key Question 2e. In babies born to women who become pregnant while taking medications to treat depression, what is the comparative risk of teratogenicity?

The evidence on the risk of exposure to an antidepressant drug during the conception period in women with depression was extremely limited, and it was insufficient to draw conclusions. The studies included in the sections above reporting on the risk of congenital malformations comprised the best evidence to answer this question, but even among those that specified exposure in the first trimester, there were few that specified exposure during conception and none that made direct comparisons with a control group of untreated depression. For example, of the studies that reported specifically on first trimester exposure to SSRIs, and met our criteria for risk of bias (controlled for three of four of our key confounders and used a recognized categorization system to identify malformations), only one reported exposure timeframes that required exposure in the conception period.[104] Compared with the other three studies reporting major malformations following exposure in the first trimester, but without necessarily including the conception period, this study reported the highest odds (Figure 4). All of these studies made comparisons with nonexposed pregnant women, with unknown proportions in either group with depression, but the Jiminez-Salem study also reported on a small group of women who had taken an SSRI in the year prior to pregnancy but had discontinued it prior to conception. The risk in this group was similar to the exposed group, (OR 1.27; 95% CI 0.91 to 0.78) but not statistically significant. This study also examined the effect of dose, with the risk associated with low dose SSRIs (e.g., $\leq$ 20 mg fluoxetine daily) having an odds ratio of 1.26 (95% CI 1.05 to 1.51) compared with 1.44 (95% CI 1.15 to 1.79) for high doses. While the high dose risk was slightly higher, analysis comparing the odds ratios indicated no statistically significant difference, indicating no clear dose-response relationship. Because this was a single observational study using a control group of presumably mainly nondepressed women, with unknown consistency in findings and imprecise results, this evidence was insufficient to draw firm conclusions.

Based on this single study, the risk of a cardiovascular malformation was also found to be significantly increased in exposed women compared with nonexposed pregnant women, (adjusted OR 2.01; 95% CI 1.60 to 2.53). In this case, the risk in women who stopped taking an SSRI prior to conception was also statistically significantly elevated, (adjusted OR 1.85; 95% CI 1.07 to 3.20). Dose again showed a small increase in risk with greater dose, but comparison of the odds ratios resulted in a p value of 0.41, indicating no clear dose-response relationship. Analysis of other specific malformations did not result in any statistically significant increased risk estimates.

While there were a few other studies that reported the risk of malformations after exposure during the conception period for individual or grouped SSRIs, SNRIs, and individual drugs,[73,74,149,184] none controlled for more than two of the key confounders, and all suffered from inferior methods for ascertainment of exposure or outcomes.

Insufficient evidence was available to reliably assess the risk of autism spectrum disorder in children of women taking an antidepressant at the time of conception. A single observational study examined this group and found no statistically significant increase in risk compared with nonexposed pregnant women.[79]

Figure 4. Risk of major malformations with selective serotonin reuptake inhibitors compared with nonexposure

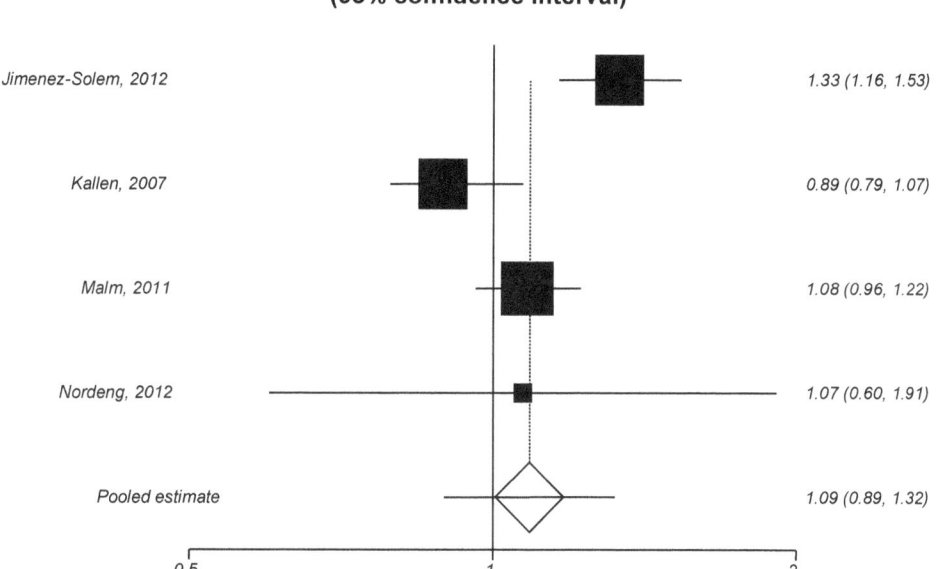

Key Question 3. Is there evidence that the comparative effectiveness of pharmacological and nonpharmacological treatments for women with depression during pregnancy and in the postpartum period varies based on characteristics such as interventions, populations, and providers?

Summary

- Evidence in subgroups based on characteristics such as interventions, populations, and providers was insufficient to draw conclusions. Direct evidence was limited.

Exposure During Pregnancy

Duration of Treatment

- Compared with partial SSRI exposure during pregnancy, there was not a statistically significantly greater risk of preterm birth (< 37 weeks) associated with continuous exposure (unadjusted pooled OR 3.23; 95% CI 0.74 to 14.17).
- Evidence on the influence of antidepressant dose on adverse effects was insufficient.

Postpartum Exposure

Depression Severity Level
- In women with postpartum depression, symptom response to brief dynamic psychotherapy, with or without sertraline, did not vary based on depression severity level.

Duration of Treatment
- In women with postpartum depression, symptom improvement did not differ when fluoxetine was used in combination with either one or six sessions of cognitive-behavioral counseling.

Depression History
- Evidence was insufficient to allow analysis of the impact of history of major depressive disorder prior to pregnancy versus those with a first episode during pregnancy or the postpartum period.

Other
- Studies with definite depression in all comparison groups and that had medium to low risk of bias provided only insufficient evidence to draw conclusions about variation in treatment effects based on all other patient characteristics and comorbidities, intervention characteristics, co-administration of other drugs, medical provide characteristics, medical care environments, and characteristics of diagnosis.

Detailed Assessment of the Evidence

There were six medium to low risk of bias observational studies of the comparative effectiveness of pharmacological and nonpharmacological treatments in women with depression during pregnancy[69,147,152,172,189,192] and three RCTs of treatment during the postpartum period that met this best evidence criteria.[58,65,132] Among those, only one RCT of women with postpartum depression evaluated the effects of depression severity[65] and four studies evaluated the effects of treatment duration.[58,152,189,192]

Exposure During Pregnancy

Duration of Treatment
Preterm birth. Two prospective cohort studies conducted in the United States (n=95) provided evidence that, compared with partial SSRI exposure, there was not a statistically significantly greater risk of preterm birth (< 37 weeks) associated with continuous exposure (unadjusted pooled OR 3.23; 95% CI 0.74 to 14.17).[189,192]

Postpartum Exposure

Severity of Symptoms
One RCT of 40 women treated for postpartum depression for 8 weeks with brief dynamic psychotherapy, with or without sertraline add-on, evaluated the effects of baseline depression severity (above and below the median MADRS scores).[65] The main analysis of all patients

provided evidence of no statistically significant difference between add-on sertraline (70%) and placebo (55%) in response rates (>50% reduction in either the MADRS or EPDS scores). The post-hoc analysis of the high depression severity subgroup also found no statistically significant difference in response rate (p=0.31).

Duration of Treatment

One 12-week RCT of 87 women treated for postpartum depression with fluoxetine, cognitive-behavioral counseling or their combination evaluated the effects of treatment duration.[58] Treatment groups that received fluoxetine plus either one or six session(s) had similar mean changes on the Edinburgh postnatal depression scale (-67% compared with -69%; p=not reported) and on the Hamilton Depression Scale (-78% compared with -79%; p=not reported).

Discussion

Key Findings and Strength of Evidence

The results of our review highlight important concerns over the state of the evidence on benefits and harms of treating depression during and after pregnancy. The majority of the comparative evidence applies to selective serotonin reuptake inhibitors (SSRIs) taken during pregnancy, with little evidence for other types of antidepressant drugs or nonpharmacological interventions. Additionally, the majority of the evidence for this report was indirect, in that studies made comparisons of outcomes for women who took an antidepressant during pregnancy for any reason, with women who did not take an antidepressant during pregnancy; proportions of women with depression in either group were rarely reported and never analyzed. The applicability of indirect evidence of findings from studies of pregnant women with unknown depression status is unclear. We are left with a small body of direct evidence: studies that were designed to directly compare the benefits and harms of pharmacological treatments for depression in pregnant or postpartum women.

The overarching findings for Key Question 1 on comparative benefits are that there is little direct evidence on the maternal benefits of antidepressants used to treat depression in pregnancy, including important health outcomes such as functional status. Our questions were intended to compare a broad range of benefits with antidepressants compared with each other, with nonpharmacological treatments, and with 'usual care' or no treatment. The evidence was divided into treatment during pregnancy and treatment during the postpartum period. With exposure during pregnancy, the evidence we found was limited initially by the population comparisons made (the control groups) and also by the way outcomes were measured. In addition, the evidence was limited to observational studies, and these studies were generally not designed to measure health outcomes when women are treated during pregnancy. We were left with spotty evidence that did not allow comparisons among the specific classes or individual drugs. For example, while anxiety is a common feature of depression during pregnancy, direct evidence on the impact of treatment on this symptom was lacking. Where we did have evidence (Table 9), it was based on one or two small studies, with some methodological problems (none were low risk of bias), imprecise estimates of effect, and inconsistency when more than one study was found. These factors led to strength of evidence ratings of insufficient for the benefit of SSRI treatment on depressive symptoms during pregnancy and no evidence for other drug classes or other possible benefits. Similarly, the evidence on the effects of SSRI treatment during pregnancy on breastfeeding outcomes was insufficient to draw conclusions, as it was limited to a single study reporting the duration of breastfeeding. While the duration was two months longer in the group that received psychotherapy alone (8.5 months) compared with the group treated with an SSRI plus psychotherapy (6.4 months, p = 0.4), the difference was not statistically significant and the study was very small (n = 44). In contrast, women treated for depression with an SSRI throughout pregnancy were found to have better functional capacity than those with depression but not treated in a single small study. Again, this evidence was insufficient to draw conclusions for the reasons noted above. Evidence for benefits in mothers was insufficient for other antidepressant drugs or for nonpharmacologic therapy, and for all other maternal benefit outcomes we studied.

The potential benefits we evaluated in children included outcomes related to parameters at birth, child development, diagnosis of chronic diseases, and health care utilization. Here evidence was again very limited, with only the effect of SSRI treatment for depression compared with no treatment on preterm birth and some child development scales studied in direct comparisons of these populations. Although no differences were found between groups on rates of preterm birth (defined as less than 37 weeks gestation), and most child development scales (SSRI-exposed infants may have lower scores on the Bayley Psychomotor Development Index), this evidence was insufficient to draw conclusions.

While we identified randomized controlled trials (RCTs) on treatment of postpartum depression, they were small and included limited comparisons and outcomes. For benefits to mothers, this direct evidence was insufficient to draw conclusions on the benefits of drug therapy compared with placebo or to other drug therapies, and we found no evidence comparing drug therapy to nondrug therapy. Evidence for other outcomes or comparisons either for exposure during pregnancy or in the postpartum period was either not found or insufficient.

Indirect evidence was available for several other benefits outcomes, including the risk of autism spectrum disorder or attention deficit/hyperactivity disorder (ADHD). Diagnosis of ADHD in the children by the age of 5 was found to be associated with use of bupropion use (OR 3.63; $p < 0.02$), particularly in the second trimester. In contrast, a diagnosis of ADHD was not associated with use of SSRIs or other antidepressants during pregnancy. Filling a prescription for an SSRI after pregnancy (timing not reported) was statistically significantly associated with increased risk of ADHD diagnosis by age five in the child (OR 2.04, $p<0.001$). These analyses controlled for parental mental health diagnoses and found that a diagnosis of depression in the mother was statistically significantly associated with the diagnosis of ADHD in the child (OR 2.58; $p<0.001$).

Two studies suggested that maternal use of SSRIs is statistically significantly associated with diagnosis of autism spectrum disorder (ASD) in the child (OR 1.82; 95% CI 1.14 to 2.91). Both studies examined other antidepressant drugs but grouped them differently, one finding an increased risk with TCAs and the other finding no increased risk with TCAs combined with SNRIs or NRIs. Although these results were controlled for depression, the comparison groups were women who did not receive an antidepressant during pregnancy, rather than women with untreated depression. The role of depression was examined in one study through subgroup analyses. Analysis of women with depression who received an SSRI compared with a population of pregnant women who did not receive an SSRI (depression status unknown) found the risk for ASD was statistically significantly elevated with a greater odds ratio than the overall analysis (OR 3.34, 95% CI 1.50 to 7.47), while the risk in women taking an SSRI for another indication was lower and not statistically significant (OR 1.61; 95% CI 0.85 to 3.06).

Evidence on Key Question 2, comparative harms of pharmacological and nonpharmacological treatments for women with depression during pregnancy and in the postpartum period, was also limited by the comparison groups selected by most studies (pregnant women taking an antidepressant for any reason). The overarching findings for harms associated with exposure during pregnancy are that there is limited direct evidence about serious infant harms, with suggestion of increased risk of respiratory distress associated with exposure to SSRIs. The only outcomes for which we had direct evidence are major malformations, convulsions and respiratory distress in the neonate after exposure to SSRIs in utero (Table 10). This evidence is insufficient to draw conclusions for major malformations due to the limitations of the few small studies found. Low strength evidence suggests that there is no increased risk of neonatal convulsions, but a statistically significant increase in risk of neonatal respiratory distress with use of SSRIs. The increase in risk for respiratory distress is a pooled unadjusted odds ratio of 1.91 (95% CI 1.63 to 2.24). Because this is low strength evidence, the findings are likely to be altered by future studies.

Indirect evidence was available for several other harms outcomes. In cases where there is a signal of a serious harm, this evidence may be useful both clinically and to direct future research. An increased risk of infant death in the first year of life was found with exposure to SSRIs (as a group and individually) during pregnancy, compared with nonexposed children (SSRIs OR 1.81; 95% CI 1.26 to 2.60). While exposure to SSRIs as a group did not result in increased risk of major malformations in infants, evidence indicated a small but statistically significant risk with exposure to fluoxetine (OR 1.14, 95% CI 1.01 to 1.30) or paroxetine (OR 1.17, 95% CI 1.02 to 1.35), but not the other SSRIs individually. Timing of exposure was primarily in the first trimester, although sensitivity analyses removing studies that may have included exposures at other time points did not alter the results. Similar results were found for cardiac malformations, except that limiting our analysis to the highest quality studies of fluoxetine resulted in a nonsignificant increase in risk. The increased risk with paroxetine was 1.49 (95% CI 1.20 to 1.85). TCAs were also associated with increased risk for major (OR 1.31; 95% CI 1.04 to 1.65) and cardiac malformations (OR 1.58; 95% CI 1.10 to 2.29). Evidence for other antidepressants was insufficient.

Persistent pulmonary hypertension was statistically significantly associated with maternal SSRI use during late pregnancy (OR 2.72; 95% CI 1.63 to 4.54). Indirect evidence suggested that neonatal withdrawal symptoms were more common with fluoxetine use during the first trimester (RR 8.7; 95% CI 2.9 to 26.6), and with SSRIs or venlafaxine (grouped) in late pregnancy, but suggested no difference in risk between SSRIs and SNRIs. The risk of respiratory distress in the neonate was statistically significantly elevated for SSRIs and TCAs, but not with SNRIs. The pooled odds ratio was 2.11 (95% CI 1.57 to 2.83), comparing TCA exposure to nonexposed pregnant women. A single study indicated no difference in the risk of respiratory depression in the infant with maternal exposure to SSRIs compared with nortriptyline.

Only a few well-designed studies examined the risk for teratogenicity with exposure to antidepressants during the conception period, and even fewer studies specifically isolated exposure during this period; the evidence was insufficient.

In Key Question 3, we attempted to examine a wide range of subgroups defined by patient and intervention characteristics. Given the difficulty we had in identifying direct evidence for the first two Key Questions with appropriate control and intervention groups, it is not surprising that we found very little evidence to address these questions. Based on the best evidence, with comparisons between pregnant women with depression who did and did not take an antidepressant during pregnancy, and with data stratified to continuous use and use during only one trimester, the duration of treatment did not appear to influence the risk of preterm birth. In the postpartum period, we found that multiple sessions of cognitive behavioral therapy were not superior to a single session, when both were combined with fluoxetine. Depressive symptom response to dynamic psychotherapy, with or without sertraline, did not vary based on depression severity level. For all other subgroups (including co-administration of other drugs, medical provider characteristics, medical care environments, and characteristics of diagnosis) the evidence was limited. For example, co-administration of antidepressants and benzodiazepines in pregnant women may modify or confound adverse outcomes in neonates, but most studies did not report on this exposure. This may have been due to decreasing prevalence of benzodiazepine use, but we were not able to draw conclusions. Studies with definite diagnosis of depression in all comparison groups and that had medium or low risk of bias provided only insufficient evidence to draw conclusions about variation in treatment effects.

Table 10 highlights the findings from studies of depression in pregnant or postpartum women; these studies were designed to compare directly the benefits or the harms of pharmacological treatments with other pharmacological treatments, nonpharmacological treatment, and/or no treatment. As noted, we regarded these investigations as direct evidence (all comparison groups comprised participants with depression). We believe that this is the best evidence for the Key Questions posed for this review, as it is unclear how untreated or nonpharmacologically treated depression in control groups, or indications other than depression in the treatment groups, may have affected outcomes in the remainder of the evidence. (Table 10 does not show outcomes for which we only had indirect evidence.)

Table 10. Key findings and strength of evidence of directly comparative evidence for depression during pregnancy

Intervention	Comparison	Outcome	Strength of Evidence Conclusions
Pregnancy			
Potential benefits			
SSRIs+psychotherapy	Psychotherapy alone	Depressive symptoms	Insufficient; no conclusions drawn
SSRIs: Fluoxetine	No treatment	Depressive symptoms	Insufficient; no conclusions drawn
SSRIs	No treatment	Functional capacity	Insufficient; no conclusions drawn
SSRIs+psychotherapy	Psychotherapy alone	Breastfeeding	Insufficient; no conclusions drawn
SSRIs	No treatment	Preterm birth	Low; Risk not increased
SSRIs+psychotherapy	Psychotherapy alone	Infant and child development: Bayley Scales	Insufficient; no conclusions drawn
SSRIs	No treatment	Infant and child development: Brazelton Neonatal Behavioral Assessment Scale	Insufficient; no conclusions drawn
Potential harms			
SSRIs	No treatment	Major malformations	Insufficient; no conclusions drawn
SSRIs+psychotherapy	Psychotherapy alone	Major malformations	Insufficient; no conclusions drawn
SSRIs	No treatment	Neonatal convulsions	Low; Risk not increased
SSRIs	No treatment	Neonatal respiratory distress	Low; Risk higher with SSRIs
SSRIs	TCA (nortriptyline)	Neonatal respiratory distress	Insufficient; no conclusions drawn

Table 11. Key findings and strength of evidence of directly comparative evidence for depression during pregnancy (continued)

Intervention	Comparison	Outcome	Strength of Evidence Conclusions
Postpartum			
Potential benefits			
Sertraline+brief dynamic psychotherapy	brief dynamic psychotherapy	Depressive symptoms.	Low No difference in response or remission
Sertraline	Sertraline+interpersonal psychotherapy	Depressive symptoms	Insufficient; no conclusions drawn
Paroxetine	Paroxetine+cognitive behavioral therapy	Depressive symptoms.	Low No difference in response or remission
Potential harms			
Sertraline+brief dynamic psychotherapy	brief psychodynamic	Adverse events	Insufficient; no conclusions drawn
Sertraline	Sertraline+interpersonal psychotherapy	Adverse events	Insufficient; no conclusions drawn
Fluoxetine+cognitive behavioral therapy	cognitive behavioral therapy	Adverse events	Insufficient; no conclusions drawn

SSRI = selective serotonin reuptake inhibitor; TCA = tricyclic antidepressant

Findings in Relationship to What Is Already Known

Putting these findings into the context of prior comparative effectiveness evidence reviews was difficult; we did not identify any other studies with as broad a scope as ours or other reviews that applied comparable methodologies. For example, a review by Bromley, et al.,[31] assessed fetal and child outcomes and SSRIs only, but those authors did not limit their comparison group to women with depression, so our results are quite different from theirs. Additionally, we formally assessed the risk of bias in individual studies and graded the strength of evidence for the body of evidence for each key outcome, which other reviews did not.[29-41]

Applicability

The comparative evidence on pharmacological treatment during pregnancy was limited to observational studies that generally met criteria for effectiveness studies. The evidence on treatment for postpartum depression came almost entirely from RCTs that met criteria for efficacy studies. These studies were limited by the exclusion of patients with common comorbidities, such as drug and alcohol misuse/abuse, other Axis I disorders, and suicidal ideation, the lack of health outcomes and comprehensive assessment of adverse events, short study durations, and small sample sizes.

The majority of studies were indirect in terms of population, comparing women using antidepressants during pregnancy for any reason to nonexposed pregnant women, with rates of depression not reported for either group. As maternal depression is widely recognized as a risk factor for poorer pregnancy outcomes, the findings from all the studies that do not account for maternal depression likely have very low applicability to our target population of pregnant women with depression. The mean maternal age ranged from 26 years to 34 years. Few studies reported race or socioeconomic status. In the studies that reported race, the populations were predominantly White. When reported, a medium socioeconomic status level was most common, and applicability to lower U.S. socioeconomic groups, including lesser availability of resources (e.g., insurance, family support) and access to mental health care was certainly not clear. The data sources for these studies typically did not include access to information about depressive symptom severity, co-existing anxiety diagnoses and other mental health or medical conditions, family history of depressive/mood disorders, prior use of antidepressive drugs, situation at home, unplanned pregnancy, marital/partner status, etc.; therefore, we know very little about these important patient characteristics.

There was very little evidence available to assess the benefits and harms of nonpharmacological treatment modalities, and what we found was limited to treatment during the postpartum period. The clinical relevance of the nonpharmacological treatment modalities was difficult to assess because of the general lack of detail about the characteristics of these interventions. Likewise, the clinical relevance of the pharmacological treatment regimens was also difficult to assess, due to a general lack of information about dose, duration, and co-interventions.

Only approximately 30 percent of included studies were conducted in the United States. Canada and Nordic countries each accounted for additional thirds of the studies, respectively. Findings from many of the studies conducted in the United States and Canada may not be reflective of the general population in North America, due to their reliance on highly selected samples with participants who voluntarily called teratogen information services, had specific health plan membership, or who attended specific community prenatal clinics. As they primarily relied on birth registry data, the studies from the Nordic countries are likely the most representative of the broad general populations. It is unclear how the differences in the health care systems and demographic characteristics between the United States and the various Nordic countries impact the applicability of the findings from the Nordic country studies to the U.S. context. Provider characteristics were generally not reported.

We were looking for evidence on women with a new episode (not necessarily the first) of depression during pregnancy or postpartum, rather than a continuing episode. The studies were unclear on this point and most simply identified women taking an antidepressant during pregnancy, with few identifying proportions of women with a history of depression, and even fewer reporting the number with a continuing episode. None analyzed results based on these characteristics. We believe that the evidence base applies to a mixed group, and does not reflect clearly one or the other.

Overall, the applicability of this evidence to programs such as the federal Children's Health Insurance Program (CHIP) is somewhat limited because of the issues noted above. The large number of studies conducted in health care settings outside the United States and in samples of women with medium socioeconomic status likely limits how well this evidence applies to children served by the CHIP program.

Implications for Clinical and Policy Decisionmaking

Depression during pregnancy and postpartum can have adverse consequences for both mother and child. Knowing the best course of action when a woman is diagnosed with depression during these times is extremely important. For multiple reasons, the evidence base at present is extremely limited in the specific guidance it can provide. Our overall findings were based on insufficient or low strength of evidence. This means that future studies are very likely to alter the findings in a meaningful way. The implications for decisionmaking for women with depression during pregnancy are unclear. Without better evidence specific to this population, the balance of benefit and harm are uncertain. Shared decisionmaking based on the best evidence available and a woman's particular characteristics and circumstances is the best use for a comparative effectiveness review such as this.

Based on the best evidence available today, the benefits to mothers are unclear. For pregnant women, treatment with drugs may offer benefits, although the specific benefits, particularly in terms of tangible benefits (health outcomes), and how benefits compare across potential treatments are still very unclear. Although we believe that treating depressed women with SSRIs is likely to improve some symptoms based on indirect evidence from studies of nonpregnant patients, direct evidence comparing the interventions of interest in the population of interest is currently insufficient. Similarly, the evidence on functional outcomes for the mother is unfortunately insufficient, although it leans towards better outcomes in women treated with an SSRI compared with untreated pregnant women

Women taking antidepressants may be less likely to breastfeed or to breastfeed for shorter durations than women who are not taking an antidepressant in the postpartum period. We did not find evidence of harm to the infant of breastfeeding while the mother was taking an antidepressant, although evidence was insufficient to draw specific conclusions. Clinicians can know in advance that, for women treated with antidepressants, decisions about breastfeeding can be problematic; thus, early discussion and support for maternal intention to breastfeed is warranted. Women who receive antenatal education and professional encouragement, or who report that their health care provider encouraged them to breastfeed are more likely to initiate and sustain breastfeeding.[200-202] Antidepressants are widely used in postpartum women. For most antidepressants, no or only negligible amounts are passed from mother to baby through breast milk (fluoxetine and citalopram may be exceptions, but the amount varies with dose and frequency of dosing).[21-23]

Evidence on the comparative benefits of treating depression during pregnancy (compared with not treating) is expected to include benefits in developmental achievement in the child. Our evidence indicates that SSRIs result in no differences on most measures, but may result in slightly worse motor development than no treatment at all, but again this evidence is insufficient to guide clinical decisions. When making direct comparisons, while the evidence does not indicate higher rates of preterm birth with use of SSRIs during pregnancy (unadjusted OR 1.73; 95% CI 0.63 to 4.42), it is insufficient to guide clinical decisions.

Numerous potentially serious harms have been suggested to be associated with use of antidepressants during pregnancy. However, in the comparison of treated and untreated depressed women, we found only the risk for respiratory distress to be associated with SSRIs (as a drug class). The fact that different conclusions may be drawn for some outcomes based on a large body of evidence that we consider indirect for our questions highlights the importance of making clinically relevant comparisons.

An example is the risk of ASD in children of women treated for depression during pregnancy. The increasing prevalence of ASD diagnosis, likely in part attributable to increased detection, temporally parallels an increasing tendency to prescribe antidepressants in pregnancy. Based on indirect evidence, whether ASD in the child is associated with maternal depression during pregnancy, treatment with antidepressants, or a combination of the two, remains unclear. Although we found that ASD was associated with maternal exposure to antidepressants, particularly SSRIs, compared with the maternal nonexposure (depression status unknown), we did not find clear evidence on the risk when untreated depressed women were the comparison group. Any suggestion of increased risk for ASD is very concerning. In studies comparing with maternal nonexposure, although researchers controlled for depression, the relationship between depression, antidepressant use, and risk of ASD remains unclear. The small, but statistically significant risk of ASD diagnosis with antidepressant use or depression or both is important to understand better, because treatment could mitigate this risk if severe depression underlies the association with ASD. One study examined the risk of having depression during pregnancy and a diagnosis of ASD in the child, finding statistically significant increased odds in depressed mothers (with and without known treatment), and a nonsignificant increase in mothers without depression. An interaction between depression and antidepressant treatment is possible, but has not been fully elucidated. Nevertheless, women should be informed about the risk of ASD in their offspring if antidepressants are found more conclusively to increase this risk. Because the fraction of cases of ASD that could potentially be attributed to antidepressants in these studies is exceedingly small (0.6 to 2.5 percent of the study populations), prenatal antidepressant use is not a major risk factor for ASD and does not explain the increasing prevalence of autism.

Evidence on the benefits or harms of treatment of depression in the postpartum is insufficient to draw conclusions. Women and clinicians are currently left with only evidence in nonpregnant populations and evidence on intermediate outcomes (e.g., which drugs are passed into breast milk) to guide treatment choices.

Limitations of the Review Process

Methodological limitations of the review within the defined scope included the exclusion of studies published in languages other than English and lack of a specific search for unpublished studies. The review process and results could have benefited from further refinement of the scope to limit inclusion of studies of pregnant or postpartum women with depression, both in the intervention and control groups.

Gaps in the Research

A major caveat to interpreting the findings of the majority of observational studies of exposure during pregnancy is the potential confounding role of depression itself and its severity.[152] Most of the studies identified women taking an antidepressant for any reason, with few reporting the proportions with depression and even fewer using this information in their analyses. Studies of women who were taking an antidepressant during or after pregnancy but not known to be depressed are problematic; a major drawback is that we do not know what the differential baseline risk of various outcomes are for the various indications for which antidepressants can be used. We do know, however, that some baseline risks are associated with depression during pregnancy; this fact underscores the importance of limiting the treated group to women with depression.[7,8] In this report we were interested in women who became depressed during pregnancy, with or without prior episodes, but the studies do not report on the timing of diagnosis in most cases. Equally problematic is the control groups used in most of the studies, which were general populations of nonexposed pregnant women. These groups could have included a proportion of women with depression, but in general this characteristic is not reported. When it was reported, the range of depression in the control groups was large (from 6% to 36%). For much of the evidence, then, the comparison is mostly depressed-treated women compared with nondepressed, untreated women. This comparison is problematic because of known effects of untreated depression on both mother and child. A small number of studies set out to examine these questions by comparing to untreated, depressed, pregnant women, but these did not measure both benefits and harms (in both mother and baby) simultaneously.

Some clinicians or investigators may still hesitate to conduct RCTs in pregnant women.[203] Nevertheless, the assumption that the comparative effectiveness of interventions in nonpregnant populations is directly applicable to pregnant women may not be valid for various reasons (e.g., changes in pharmacokinetics of the drugs); moreover, trials in nonpregnant populations do not measure outcomes specific to pregnant or postpartum women. Various groups do advocate for RCTs in pregnant women;[204,205] furthermore, the U.S. Department for Health and Human Services outlines detailed rules[206] on protecting pregnant women research subjects, their fetuses, and fathers. Because clinicians already prescribe antidepressants on a regular basis to pregnant women, RCTs comparing treatments and adequately measuring appropriate outcomes, with measurement of depression severity at baseline and during followup among such populations do not necessarily increase risk to either the women or their fetuses. Comparisons of specific treatments in pregnancy are badly needed to better uncover variation in risk across drugs, even within a class. Ascertainment of exposure, including both timing and dose, must be done in a way that insures accuracy and reliability. Outcomes should be determined by blinded evaluators, which is possible for nearly all outcomes considered here. Randomization would be the best approach to minimize potential confounding, but observational studies could also be done in a way that addresses the gaps in the research. For example, studies could identify women being treated for depression as the study population and make comparisons across treatments (including no treatment). These studies should adjust for important prognostic factors such as pre-existing illness, depression history, depression severity, age, race, parity, socioeconomic status, and other exposures (e.g., alcohol, smoking, and other potential teratogens).

Nonpharmacological treatments are generally thought to have fewer risks than antidepressants. Nonetheless, evidence is almost entirely lacking on this point or on the question of the effectiveness of combinations of drug and nondrug treatments. Newer approaches to nonpharmacological interventions using technology such as Internet-based therapies, web-camera counseling, and mobile phone applications are emerging. These may offer pregnant and postpartum women alternatives to more established treatments, particularly in lower-income or rural populations.[207-209]

Studies of women in the postpartum period are both small and methodologically weak. These limitations leave a large gap in knowledge about treatments for a group of patients in whom RCTs could be undertaken. In addition to comparative efficacy (e.g., effects on symptoms) little is known about the benefits of treatments on important outcomes such as improving the mother-infant dyad, enhancing breastfeeding outcomes or reducing domestic violence. The need for specifically-designed research that addresses these problems is substantial.

Conclusion

The current evidence base is insufficient to fully support clinical decisionmaking, which requires knowing both benefits and harms and being able to determine the tradeoffs that individual patients might make. For example, if a medication has a lower adverse event profile but is also less effective for a given condition, it would not make sense to prescribe that for a patient who needs treatment for that particular condition, just because of a lower adverse event profile. We know that depression during pregnancy and the postpartum period can lead to serious adverse outcomes for both mother and child, such that treatment is important. There is a real need for research in this area to simultaneously measure both benefits and harms so that better evidence can inform the tradeoffs that women and clinicians need to weigh in making their health care decisions.

References

1. Blazer DG, Kessler RC, McGonagle KA, et al. The prevalence and distribution of major depression in a national community sample: the National Comorbidity Survey. Am J Psychiatry. 1994 Jul;151(7):979-86. PMID: 8010383.

2. Le Strat Y, Dubertret C, Le Foll B. Prevalence and correlates of major depressive episode in pregnant and postpartum women in the United States. J Affect Disord. 2011 Dec;135(1-3):128-38. PMID: 21802737.

3. Dietz PM, Williams SB, Callaghan WM, et al. Clinically identified maternal depression before, during, and after pregnancies ending in live births. Am J Psychiatry. 2007 Oct;164(10):1515-20. PMID: 17898342.

4. Halbreich U, Karkun S. Cross-cultural and social diversity of prevalence of postpartum depression and depressive symptoms. J Affect Disord. 2006 Apr;91(2-3):97-111. PMID: 16466664.

5. Le Strat Y, Dubertret C, Le Foll B. Prevalence and correlates of major depressive episode in pregnant and postpartum women in the United States. J Affect Disord. 2011 Dec;135(1-3):128-38. PMID: 21802737.

6. Norwitz ER, Lye SJ. Chapter 5: Biology of parturition. In: Creasy RK, Resnick R, Iams JD, eds. Creasy and Resnik's maternal-fetal medicine : principles and practice. 6th ed. Philadelphia, PA: Saunders/Elsevier; 2009. Pages 69-86.

7. Hallberg P, Sjoblom V. The use of selective serotonin reuptake inhibitors during pregnancy and breast-feeding: a review and clinical aspects. J Clin Psychopharmacol. 2005 Feb;25(1):59-73. PMID: 15643101.

8. Nonacs R, Cohen LS. Assessment and treatment of depression during pregnancy: an update. Psychiatr Clin North Am. 2003 Sep;26(3):547-62. PMID: 14563097.

9. Alder J, Fink N, Bitzer J, et al. Depression and anxiety during pregnancy: a risk factor for obstetric, fetal and neonatal outcome? A critical review of the literature. J Matern Fetal Neonatal Med. 2007 Mar;20(3):189-209. PMID: 17437220.

10. Henry AL, Beach AJ, Stowe ZN, et al. The fetus and maternal depression: implications for antenatal treatment guidelines. Clin Obstet Gynecol. 2004 Sep;47(3):535-46. PMID: 15326416.

11. Grote NK, Bridge JA, Gavin AR, et al. A meta-analysis of depression during pregnancy and the risk of preterm birth, low birth weight, and intrauterine growth restriction. Arch Gen Psychiatry. 2010 Oct;67(10):1012-24. PMID: 20921117.

12. Murray L, Cooper PJ. Postpartum depression and child development. Psychol Med. 1997 Mar;27(2):253-60. PMID: 9089818.

13. Ludermir AB, Lewis G, Valongueiro SA, et al. Violence against women by their intimate partner during pregnancy and postnatal depression: a prospective cohort study. Lancet. 2010 Sep 11;376(9744):903-10. PMID: 20822809.

14. Doucet S, Jones I, Letourneau N, et al. Interventions for the prevention and treatment of postpartum psychosis: a systematic review. Arch Womens Ment Health. 2011 Apr;14(2):89-98. PMID: 21128087.

15. Halbreich U. Prevalence of mood symptoms and depressions during pregnancy: implications for clinical practice and research. CNS Spectr. 2004 Mar;9(3):177-84. PMID: 14999158.

16. Myers E, Aubuchon-Endsley N, Bastian L, et al. Efficacy and Safety of Screening for Postpartum Depression. Comparative Effectiveness Review 106. (Prepared by the Duke Evidence-based Practice Center under Contract No. 290-2007-10066-I.) AHRQ Publication No. 13-EHC064-EF. Rockville, MD: Agency for Healthcare Research and Quality; 2013. Available from www.effectivehealthcare.ahrq.gov/reports/final.cfm.

17. Hayes RM, Wu P, Shelton RC, et al. Maternal antidepressant use and adverse outcomes: a cohort study of 228,876 pregnancies. Am J Obstet Gynecol. 2012 Jul;207(1):49 e1-9. PMID: 22727349.

18. Diagnostic and statistical manual of mental disorders: DSM-IV-TR. 4th ed., text revision ed. Washington DC: American Psychiatric Association; 2000.

19. Gartlehner G, Hansen, RA, Morgan, LC, et al. Second-Generation Antidepressants in the Pharmacologic Treatment of Adult Depression: An Update of the 2007 Comparative Effectiveness Review. (Prepared by the RTI International–University of North Carolina Evidence-based Practice Center, Contract No. 290-2007-10056-I.) AHRQ Publication No. 12-EHC012-EF. Rockville, MD: Agency for Healthcare Research and Quality; 2011. Available from www.effectivehealthcare.ahrq.gov/reports/final.cfm.

20. Gartlehner G, Hansen RA, Morgan LC, et al. Comparative benefits and harms of second-generation antidepressants for treating major depressive disorder: an updated meta-analysis. Ann Intern Med. 2011 Dec 6;155(11):772-85. PMID: 22147715.

21. Hale TW. Medication and Mother's Milk 2012: A Manual of Lactational Pharmacology. 15th ed. Amarillo, TX: Hale Publishing LP; 2012.

22. Lanza di Scalea T, Wisner KL. Antidepressant medication use during breastfeeding. Clin Obstet Gynecol. 2009 Sep;52(3):483-97. PMID: 19661763.

23. Lawrence RA, Lawrence RM. Breastfeeding: A Guide for the Medical Profession. 7th ed. St. Louis, MO: Saunders; 2011.

24. Freeman MP, Fava M, Lake J, et al. Complementary and alternative medicine in major depressive disorder: the American Psychiatric Association Task Force report. J Clin Psychiatry. 2010 Jun;71(6):669-81. PMID: 20573326.

25. Kayser S, Bewernick BH, Grubert C, et al. Antidepressant effects, of magnetic seizure therapy and electroconvulsive therapy, in treatment-resistant depression. J Psychiatr Res. 2011 May;45(5):569-76. PMID: 20951997.

26. Cuijpers P, Geraedts AS, van Oppen P, et al. Interpersonal psychotherapy for depression: a meta-analysis. Am J Psychiatry. 2011 Jun;168(6):581-92. PMID: 21362740.

27. Ishak WW, Ha K, Kapitanski N, et al. The impact of psychotherapy, pharmacotherapy, and their combination on quality of life in depression. Harv Rev Psychiatry. 2011 Dec;19(6):277-89. PMID: 22098324.

28. Nieuwsma JA, Trivedi RB, McDuffie J, et al. Brief psychotherapy for depression: a systematic review and meta-analysis. Int J Psychiatry Med. 2012;43(2):129-51. PMID: 22849036.

29. Ross EL, Grigoriadis S, Mamisashvili L. Selected pregnancy and delivery outcomes after exposure to antidepressant medication: A systematic review and meta-analysis. JAMA Psychiatry. 2013:1-8. PMID: 23446732.

30. 't Jong GW, Einarson T, Koren G, et al. Antidepressant use in pregnancy and persistent pulmonary hypertension of the newborn (PPHN): A systematic review. Reprod Toxicol. 2012;34(3):293-7. PMID: 22564982.

31. Bromley RL, Wieck A, Makarova D, et al. Fetal effects of selective serotonin reuptake inhibitor treatment during pregnancy: Immediate and longer term child outcomes. Fetal Matern Med Rev. 2012;23(3-4):230-75.

32. Sockol LE, Epperson CN, Barber JP. A meta-analysis of treatments for perinatal depression. Clin Psychol Rev. 2011 Jul;31(5):839-49. PMID: 21545782.

33. Gentile S. Neonatal withdrawal reactions following late in utero exposure to antidepressant medications. Curr Womens Health Rev. 2011;7(1):18-27.

34. Wurst KE, Poole C, Ephross SA, et al. First trimester paroxetine use and the prevalence of congenital, specifically cardiac, defects: a meta-analysis of epidemiological studies. Birth Defects Res Part A Clin Mol Teratol. 2010 Mar;88(3):159-70. PMID: 19739149.

35. Ng RC, Hirata CK, Yeung W, et al. Pharmacologic treatment for postpartum depression: a systematic review. Pharmacotherapy. 2010 Sep;30(9):928-41. PMID: 20795848.

36. Kendall-Tackett K, Hale TW. The use of antidepressants in pregnant and breastfeeding women: a review of recent studies. J Hum Lact. 2010 May;26(2):187-95. PMID: 19652194.

37. Santone G, Ricchi G, Rocchetti D, et al. Is the exposure to antidepressant drugs in early pregnancy a risk factor for spontaneous abortion? A review of available evidences. Epidemiol Psichiatr Soc. 2009;18(3):240-7. PMID: 20034202.

38. Myles N, Newall H, Ward H, et al. Systematic meta-analysis of individual selective serotonin reuptake inhibitor medications and congenital malformations. Aust N Z J Psychiatry; 2013. p. 1002-12. doi: Epub 2013 Jun 12.

39. Grigoriadis S, VonderPorten EH, Mamisashvili L. Antidepressant exposure during pregnancy and congenital malformations: is there an association? A systematic review and meta-analysis of the best evidence. J Clin Psychiatry. 2013 April;74(4):e293-e308. PMID: 23656855.

40. Grigoriadis S, VonderPorten EH, Mamisashvili L. The effect of prenatal antidepressant exposure on neonatal adaptation: a systematic review and meta-analysis. J Clin Psychiatry. 2013 April;74(4):e309-e20. PMID: 23656856.

41. Painuly N, Heun R, Painuly R, et al. Risk of cardiovascular malformations after exposure to paroxetine in pregnancy: meta-analysis. Psychiatrist. 2013 June 1, 2013;37(6):198-203.

42. Methods Guide for Effectiveness and Comparative Effectiveness Reviews. AHRQ publication no. 10(12)-EHC063-EF. Rockville, MD: Agency for Healthcare Research and Quality; April 2012. Chapters available at: www.effectivehealthcare.ahrq.gov.

43. Moher D, Liberati A, Tetzlaff J, et al. Preferred reporting items for systematic reviews and meta-analyses: the PRISMA statement. PLoS medicine. 2009;6(7). PMID: 1000097.

44. McDonagh MS, Jonas DE, Gartlehner G, et al. Methods for the Drug Effectiveness Review Project. BMC Med Res Methodol. 2012;12(140). PMID: 22970848.

45. Whitlock EP, Lin JS, Chou R, et al. Using existing systematic reviews in complex systematic reviews. Ann Intern Med. 2008 May 20;148(10):776-82. PMID: 18490690.

46. Center for Reviews and Dissemination. Undertaking Systematic Reviews of Research on Effectiveness: CRD's Guidance for Those Carrying Out or Commissioning Reviews. CRD Report Number 4 (2nd edition). York, UK: NHS Centre for Reviews and Dissemination, York University; 2001.

47. Harris RP, Helfand M, Woolf SH, et al. Current methods of the third U.S. Preventive Services Task Force. Am J Prev Med. 2001;20(3Suppl):21-35. PMID: 11306229.

48. Fu R, Gartlehner G, Grant M, et al. Conducting Quantitative Synthesis When Comparing Medical Interventions: AHRQ and the Effective Health Care Program. J Clin Epidemiol 2011;64(11):1187-97. PMID: 21477993.

49. Guyatt GH, Norris SL, Schulman S, et al. Methodology for the development of antithrombotic therapy and prevention of thrombosis guidelines. Chest. 2012 February 1, 2012;141(2 suppl):53S-70S. PMID: 22315256

50. Sutton AJ, Abrams KR, Jones DR, et al. Methods for Meta-Analysis in Medical Research. Chichester, UK: John Wiley & Sons, Inc.; 2000.

51. Higgins JP, Thompson SG, Deeks JJ, et al. Measuring inconsistency in meta-analyses. BMJ. 2003;327(7414):557-60. PMID: 12958120.

52. Higgins JPT, Thompson SG. Quantifying heterogeneity in a meta-analysis. Stat Med. 2002;21(11):1539-58. PMID: 12111919.

53. Owens D, Lohr K, Atkins D, et al. Chapter 10. Grading the Strength of a Body of Evidence When Comparing Medical Interventions. Methods Guide for Effectiveness and Comparative Effectiveness Reviews [Prepublication Draft Copy]. AHRQ Publication No. 10(12)-EHC063-EF. Rockville, MD: Agency for Healthcare Research and Quality; April 2012.

54. Owens DK, Lohr KN, Atkins D, et al. AHRQ series paper 5: Grading the strength of a body of evidence when comparing medical interventions—Agency for Healthcare Research and Quality and the Effective Health Care Program. J Clin Epidemiol. 2010 May;63(5):513-23. PMID: 19595577.

55. Alwan S, Reefhuis J, Botto LD, et al. Maternal use of bupropion and risk for congenital heart defects. Am J Obstet Gynecol. 2010 Jul;203(1):52.e1-6. PMID: 20417496.

56. Alwan S, Reefhuis J, Rasmussen SA, et al. Use of selective serotonin-reuptake inhibitors in pregnancy and the risk of birth defects. N Engl J Med. 2007 Jun 28;356(26):2684-92. PMID: 17596602.

57. Andrade SE, McPhillips H, Loren D, et al. Antidepressant medication use and risk of persistent pulmonary hypertension of the newborn. Pharmacoepidemiol Drug Saf. 2009 Mar;18(3):246-52. PMID: 19148882.

58. Appleby L, Warner R, Whitton A, et al. A controlled study of fluoxetine and cognitive-behavioural counselling in the treatment of postnatal depression. BMJ. 1997 Mar 29;314(7085):932-6. PMID: 9099116.

59. Bakker MK, De Walle HEK, Wilffert B, et al. Fluoxetine and infantile hypertrophic pylorus stenosis: a signal from a birth defects-drug exposure surveillance study. Pharmacoepidemiol Drug Saf. 2010 Aug;19(8):808-13. PMID: 20572024.

60. Bakker MK, Kerstjens-Frederikse WS, Buys CHCM, et al. First-trimester use of paroxetine and congenital heart defects: a population-based case-control study. Birth Defects Res Part A Clin Mol Teratol. 2010 Feb;88(2):94-100. PMID: 19937603.

61. Ban L, Tata LJ, West J, et al. Live and non-live pregnancy outcomes among women with depression and anxiety: A population-based study. PLoS ONE. 2012;7(8):e43462. PMID: 22937052.

62. Batton B, Batton E, Weigler K, et al. In utero antidepressant exposure and neurodevelopment in preterm infants. Am J Perinatol. 2013;30(4):297-301. PMID: 22893558.

63. Bérard A, Ramos É, Rey É, et al. First trimester exposure to paroxetine and risk of cardiac malformations in infants: The importance of dosage. Birth Defects Res B Dev Reprod Toxicol. 2007;80(1):18-27. PMID: 17187388.

64. Berle JO, Steen VM, Aamo TO, et al. Breastfeeding during maternal antidepressant treatment with serotonin reuptake inhibitors: infant exposure, clinical symptoms, and cytochrome p450 genotypes. J Clin Psychiatry. 2004 Sep;65(9):1228-34. PMID: 15367050.

65. Bloch M, Meiboom H, Lorberblatt M, et al. The effect of sertraline add-on to brief dynamic psychotherapy for the treatment of postpartum depression: a randomized, double-blind, placebo-controlled study. J Clin Psychiatry. 2012 Feb;73(2):235-41. PMID: 22401479.

66. Bogen DL, Hanusa BH, Moses-Kolko E, et al. Are maternal depression or symptom severity associated with breastfeeding intention or outcomes? J Clin Psychiatry. 2010 Aug;71(8):1069-78. PMID: 20584521.

67. Boucher N, Bairam A, Beaulac-Baillargeon L. A new look at the neonate's clinical presentation after in utero exposure to antidepressants in late pregnancy. J Clin Psychopharmacol. 2008 Jun;28(3):334-9. PMID: 18480693.

68. Bracken MB, Holford TR. Exposure to prescribed drugs in pregnancy and association with congenital malformations. Obstet Gynecol. 1981;58(3):336-44. PMID: 7266953.

69. Casper RC, Fleisher BE, Lee-Ancajas JC, et al. Follow-up of children of depressed mothers exposed or not exposed to antidepressant drugs during pregnancy. J Pediatr. 2003 Apr;142(4):402-8. PMID: 12712058.

70. Chambers CD, Hernandez-Diaz S, Van Marter LJ, et al. Selective serotonin-reuptake inhibitors and risk of persistent pulmonary hypertension of the newborn. N Engl J Med. 2006 Feb 9;354(6):579-87. PMID: 16467545.

71. Chambers CD, Johnson KA, Dick LM, et al. Birth outcomes in pregnant women taking fluoxetine. N Engl J Med. 1996 Oct 3;335(14):1010-5. PMID: 8793924.

72. Chun-Fai-Chan B, Koren G, Fayez I, et al. Pregnancy outcome of women exposed to bupropion during pregnancy: a prospective comparative study. Am J Obstet Gynecol. 2005 Mar;192(3):932-6. PMID: 15746694.

73. Cole JA, Ephross SA, Cosmatos IS, et al. Paroxetine in the first trimester and the prevalence of congenital malformations. Pharmacoepidemiol Drug Saf. 2007 Oct;16(10):1075-85. PMID: 17729379.

74. Cole JA, Modell JG, Haight BR, et al. Bupropion in pregnancy and the prevalence of congenital malformations. Pharmacoepidemiol Drug Saf. 2007 May;16(5):474-84. PMID: 16897811.

75. Colvin L, Slack-Smith L, Stanley FJ, et al. Linking a pharmaceutical claims database with a birth defects registry to investigate birth defect rates of suspected teratogens. Pharmacoepidemiol Drug Saf. 2010;19(11):1137-50. PMID: 20602344.

76. Colvin L, Slack-Smith L, Stanley FJ, et al. Dispensing patterns and pregnancy outcomes for women dispensed selective serotonin reuptake inhibitors in pregnancy.[Erratum appears in Birth Defects Res A Clin Mol Teratol. 2011 Apr;91(4):268]. Birth Defects Res Part A Clin Mol Teratol. 2011 Mar;91(3):142-52. PMID: 21381184.

77. Colvin L, Slack-Smith L, Stanley FJ, et al. Early morbidity and mortality following in utero exposure to selective serotonin reuptake inhibitors: a population-based study in Western Australia. CNS Drugs. 2012;26(7):e1-e14. PMID: 22712699.

78. Costei AM, Kozer E, Ho T, et al. Perinatal outcome following third trimester exposure to paroxetine. Arch Pediatr Adolesc Med. 2002 Nov;156(11):1129-32. PMID: 12413342.

79. Croen LA, Grether JK, Yoshida CK, et al. Antidepressant use during pregnancy and childhood autism spectrum disorders. Arch Gen Psychiatry. 2011 Nov;68(11):1104-12. PMID: 21727247.

80. Davidson S, Prokonov D, Taler M, et al. Effect of exposure to selective serotonin reuptake inhibitors in utero on fetal growth: potential role for the IGF-I and HPA axes. Pediatr Res. 2009 Feb;65(2):236-41. PMID: 19262294.

81. Davis RL, Rubanowice D, McPhillips H, et al. Risks of congenital malformations and perinatal events among infants exposed to antidepressant medications during pregnancy. Pharmacoepidemiol Drug Saf. 2007 Oct;16(10):1086-94. PMID: 17729378.

82. De Vera MA, Bérard A. Antidepressant use during pregnancy and the risk of pregnancy-induced hypertension. Br J Clin Pharmacol. 2012;74(2):362-9. PMID: 22435711.

83. de Vries NKS, van der Veere CN, Reijneveld SA, et al. Early Neurological Outcome of Young Infants Exposed to Selective Serotonin Reuptake Inhibitors during Pregnancy: Results from the Observational SMOK Study. PLoS ONE. 2013;8(5):e64654. PMID: 23785389.

84. Diav-Citrin O, Shechtman S, Weinbaum D, et al. Paroxetine and fluoxetine in pregnancy: a prospective, multicentre, controlled, observational study. Br J Clin Pharmacol. 2008 Nov;66(5):695-705. PMID: 18754846.

85. Djulus J, Koren G, Einarson TR, et al. Exposure to mirtazapine during pregnancy: a prospective, comparative study of birth outcomes. J Clin Psychiatry. 2006 Aug;67(8):1280-4. PMID: 16965209.

86. Dubnov-Raz G, Hemila H, Vurembrand Y, et al. Maternal use of selective serotonin reuptake inhibitors during pregnancy and neonatal bone density. Early Hum Dev. 2012 Mar;88(3):191-4. PMID: 21890289.

87. Dubnov-Raz G, Juurlink DN, Fogelman R, et al. Antenatal use of selective serotonin-reuptake inhibitors and QT interval prolongation in newborns. Pediatrics. 2008 Sep;122(3):e710-5. PMID: 18762507.

88. Einarson A, Bonari L, Voyer-Lavigne S, et al. A multicentre prospective controlled study to determine the safety of trazodone and nefazodone use during pregnancy. Can J Psychiatry. 2003;48(2):106-10. PMID: 12655908.

89. Einarson A, Choi J, Einarson TR, et al. Rates of spontaneous and therapeutic abortions following use of antidepressants in pregnancy: results from a large prospective database. J Obstet Gynaecol Can. 2009;31(5):452-6. PMID: 19604427.

90. Einarson A, Choi J, Einarson TR, et al. Incidence of major malformations in infants following antidepressant exposure in pregnancy: results of a large prospective cohort study. Can J Psychiatry. 2009 Apr;54(4):242-6. PMID: 19321030.

91. Einarson A, Choi J, Einarson TR, et al. Adverse effects of antidepressant use in pregnancy: an evaluation of fetal growth and preterm birth. Depress Anxiety. 2010;27(1):35-8. PMID: 19691030.

92. Einarson A, Choi J, Koren G, et al. Outcomes of infants exposed to multiple antidepressants during pregnancy: results of a cohort study. J Popul Ther Clin Pharmacol. 2011;18(2):e390-6. PMID: 22071601.

93. El Marroun H, Jaddoe VWV, Hudziak JJ, et al. Maternal use of selective serotonin reuptake inhibitors, fetal growth, and risk of adverse birth outcomes. Arch Gen Psychiatry. 2012 Jul;69(7):706-14. PMID: 22393202.

94. Ericson A, Kallen B, Wiholm B. Delivery outcome after the use of antidepressants in early pregnancy. Eur J Clin Pharmacol. 1999 Sep;55(7):503-8. PMID: 10501819.

95. Ferreira E, Carceller AM, Agogue C, et al. Effects of selective serotonin reuptake inhibitors and venlafaxine during pregnancy in term and preterm neonates. Pediatrics. 2007 Jan;119(1):52-9. PMID: 17200271.

96. Figueroa R. Use of antidepressants during pregnancy and risk of attention-deficit/hyperactivity disorder in the offspring. J Dev Behav Pediatr. 2010 Oct;31(8):641-8. PMID: 20613624.

97. Galbally M, Lewis AJ, Buist A. Developmental outcomes of children exposed to antidepressants in pregnancy. Aust N Z J Psychiatry. 2011 May;45(5):393-9. PMID: 21314237.

98. Galbally M, Lewis AJ, Lum J, et al. Serotonin discontinuation syndrome following in utero exposure to antidepressant medication: prospective controlled study. Aust N Z J Psychiatry. 2009 Sep;43(9):846-54. PMID: 19670058.

99. Gorman JR, Kao K, Chambers CD. Breastfeeding among women exposed to antidepressants during pregnancy. J Hum Lact. 2012;28(2):181-8. PMID: 22344850.

100. Grzeskowiak LE, Gilbert AL, Morrison JL. Neonatal outcomes after late-gestation exposure to selective serotonin reuptake inhibitors. J Clin Psychopharmacol. 2012;32(5):615-21. PMID: 22926594.

101. Hale TW, Kendall-Tackett K, Cong Z, et al. Discontinuation syndrome in newborns whose mothers took antidepressants while pregnant or breastfeeding. Breastfeed Med. 2010 Dec;5(4):283-8. PMID: 20807106.

102. Hanley GE, Brain U, Oberlander TF. Infant developmental outcomes following prenatal exposure to antidepressants, and maternal depressed mood and positive affect. Early Hum Dev. 2013;89(8):519-24. PMID: 23384962.

103. Heikkinen T, Ekblad U, Kero P, et al. Citalopram in pregnancy and lactation. Clin Pharmacol Ther. 2002 Aug;72(2):184-91. PMID: 12189365.

104. Jimenez-Solem E, Andersen JT, Petersen M, et al. Exposure to selective serotonin reuptake inhibitors and the risk of congenital malformations: A nationwide cohort study. BMJ Open. 2012;2(3):e001148. PMID: 22710132.

105. Jimenez-Solem E, Andersen JT, Petersen M, et al. SSRI Use During Pregnancy and Risk of Stillbirth and Neonatal Mortality. Am J Psychiatry. 2013 Mar 1;170(3):299-304 PMID: 23361562.

106. Jordan AE, Jackson GL, Deardorff D, et al. Serotonin reuptake inhibitor use in pregnancy and the neonatal behavioral syndrome. J Matern Fetal Neonatal Med. 2008 Oct;21(10):745-51. PMID: 19012191.

107. Kallen B. Neonate characteristics after maternal use of antidepressants in late pregnancy. Arch Pediatr Adolesc Med. 2004 Apr;158(4):312-6. PMID: 15066868.

108. Kallen B, Olausson PO. Maternal use of selective serotonin re-uptake inhibitors and persistent pulmonary hypertension of the newborn. Pharmacoepidemiol Drug Saf. 2008 Aug;17(8):801-6. PMID: 18314924.

109. Kallen BAJ, Otterblad Olausson P. Maternal use of selective serotonin re-uptake inhibitors in early pregnancy and infant congenital malformations. Birth Defects Res Part A Clin Mol Teratol. 2007 Apr;79(4):301-8. PMID: 17216624.

110. Kieler H, Artama M, Engeland A, et al. Selective serotonin reuptake inhibitors during pregnancy and risk of persistent pulmonary hypertension in the newborn: population based cohort study from the five Nordic countries. BMJ. 2012;344:d8012. PMID: 22240235.

111. Klieger-Grossmann C, Weitzner B, Panchaud A, et al. Pregnancy outcomes following use of escitalopram: a prospective comparative cohort study. J Clin Pharmacol. 2012 May;52(5):766-70. PMID: 22075232.

112. Klinger G, Frankenthal D, Merlob P, et al. Long-term outcome following selective serotonin reuptake inhibitor induced neonatal abstinence syndrome. J Perinatol. 2011 Sep;31(9):615-20. PMID: 21311497.

113. Kornum JB. Use of selective serotonin-reuptake inhibitors during early pregnancy and risk of congenital malformations: updated analysis. Clin Epidemiol. 2010 Aug 9;2:29-36. PMID: 20865100.

114. Kulin NA, Pastuszak A, Sage SR, et al. Pregnancy outcome following maternal use of the new selective serotonin reuptake inhibitors: a prospective controlled multicenter study. JAMA. 1998 Feb 25;279(8):609-10. PMID: 9486756.

115. Laine K, Heikkinen T, Ekblad U, et al. Effects of exposure to selective serotonin reuptake inhibitors during pregnancy on serotonergic symptoms in newborns and cord blood monoamine and prolactin concentrations. Arch Gen Psychiatry. 2003 Jul;60(7):720-6. PMID: 12860776.

116. Lanza di Scalea T, Hanusa BH, Wisner KL. Sexual function in postpartum women treated for depression: results from a randomized trial of nortriptyline versus sertraline. J Clin Psychiatry. 2009 Mar;70(3):423-8. PMID: 19284932.

117. Latendresse G, Ruiz RJ. Maternal corticotropin-releasing hormone and the use of selective serotonin reuptake inhibitors independently predict the occurrence of preterm birth. J Midwifery Womens Health. 2011 Mar-Apr;56(2):118-26. PMID: 21429075.

118. Lennestal R, Kallen B. Delivery outcome in relation to maternal use of some recently introduced antidepressants. J Clin Psychopharmacol. 2007 Dec;27(6):607-13. PMID: 18004128.

119. Levinson-Castiel R, Merlob P, Linder N, et al. Neonatal abstinence syndrome after in utero exposure to selective serotonin reuptake inhibitors in term infants. Arch Pediatr Adolesc Med. 2006 Feb;160(2):173-6. PMID: 16461873.

120. Lewis AJ, Galbally M, Opie G, et al. Neonatal growth outcomes at birth and one month postpartum following in utero exposure to antidepressant medication. Aust N Z J Psychiatry. 2010 May;44(5):482-7. PMID: 20397792.

121. Logsdon MC, Wisner K, Hanusa BH. Does maternal role functioning improve with antidepressant treatment in women with postpartum depression? J Womens Health (Larchmt). 2009 Jan-Feb;18(1):85-90. PMID: 19132881.

122. Logsdon MC, Wisner K, Sit D, et al. Depression treatment and maternal functioning. Depress Anxiety. 2011 Nov;28(11):1020-6. PMID: 21898714.

123. Louik C, Lin AE, Werler MM, et al. First-trimester use of selective serotonin-reuptake inhibitors and the risk of birth defects. N Engl J Med. 2007 Jun 28;356(26):2675-83. PMID: 17596601.

124. Lund N, Pedersen LH, Henriksen TB. Selective serotonin reuptake inhibitor exposure in utero and pregnancy outcomes.[Erratum appears in Arch Pediatr Adolesc Med. 2009 Dec;163(12):1143]. Arch Pediatr Adolesc Med. 2009 Oct;163(10):949-54. PMID: 19805715.

125. Malm H, Artama M, Gissler M, et al. Selective serotonin reuptake inhibitors and risk for major congenital anomalies. Obstet Gynecol. 2011 Jul;118(1):111-20. PMID: 21646927.

126. Manakova E, Hubickova L. Antidepressant drug exposure during pregnancy. CZTIS small prospective study. Neuroendocrinol Lett. 2011;32 Suppl 1:53-6. PMID: 22167208.

127. Maschi S, Clavenna A, Campi R, et al. Neonatal outcome following pregnancy exposure to antidepressants: a prospective controlled cohort study. BJOG. 2008 Jan;115(2):283-9. PMID: 17903222.

128. McElhatton PR, Garbis HM, Elefant E, et al. The outcome of pregnancy in 689 women exposed to therapeutic doses of antidepressants. A collaborative study of the European Network of Teratology Information Services (ENTIS). Reprod Toxicol. 1996 Jul-Aug;10(4):285-94. PMID: 8829251.

129. McFarland J, Salisbury AL, Battle CL, et al. Major depressive disorder during pregnancy and emotional attachment to the fetus. Arch Womens Ment Health. 2011;14(5):425-34. PMID: 21938509.

130. Merlob P, Birk E, Sirota L, et al. Are selective serotonin reuptake inhibitors cardiac teratogens? Echocardiographic screening of newborns with persistent heart murmur. Birth Defects Res Part A Clin Mol Teratol. 2009 Oct;85(10):837-41. PMID: 19691085.

131. Misri S, Kendrick K, Oberlander TF, et al. Antenatal depression and anxiety affect postpartum parenting stress: a longitudinal, prospective study. Can J Psychiatry. 2010 Apr;55(4):222-8. PMID: 20416145.

132. Misri S, Reebye P, Corral M, et al. The use of paroxetine and cognitive-behavioral therapy in postpartum depression and anxiety: a randomized controlled trial. J Clin Psychiatry. 2004 Sep;65(9):1236-41. PMID: 15367052.

133. Misri S, Reebye P, Kendrick K, et al. Internalizing behaviors in 4-year-old children exposed in utero to psychotropic medications. Am J Psychiatry. 2006 Jun;163(6):1026-32. PMID: 16741203.

134. Misri S, Sivertz K. Tricyclic drugs in pregnancy and lactation: a preliminary report. Int J Psychiatry Med. 1991;21(2):157-71. PMID: 1894455.

135. Mulder EJ, Ververs FF, de Heus R, et al. Selective serotonin reuptake inhibitors affect neurobehavioral development in the human fetus. Neuropsychopharmacology. 2011 Sep;36(10):1961-71. PMID: 21525859.

136. Nakhai-Pour HR, Broy P, Berard A. Use of antidepressants during pregnancy and the risk of spontaneous abortion. CMAJ. 2010 Jul 13;182(10):1031-7. PMID: 20513781.

137. Nijenhuis CM, ter Horst PGJ, van Rein N, et al. Disturbed development of the enteric nervous system after in utero exposure of selective serotonin re-uptake inhibitors and tricyclic antidepressants. Part 2: Testing the hypotheses. Br J Clin Pharmacol. 2012 Jan;73(1):126-34. PMID: 21848990.

138. Nordeng H, van Gelder MMHJ, Spigset O, et al. Pregnancy outcome after exposure to antidepressants and the role of maternal depression: results from the Norwegian Mother and Child Cohort Study. J Clin Psychopharmacol. 2012 Apr;32(2):186-94. PMID: 22367660.

139. Nulman I, Koren G, Rovet J, et al. Neurodevelopment of children following prenatal exposure to venlafaxine, selective serotonin reuptake inhibitors, or untreated maternal depression. Am J Psychiatry. 2012 Nov 1;169(11):1165-74. PMID: 23128923.

140. Nulman I, Rovet J, Stewart DE, et al. Neurodevelopment of children exposed in utero to antidepressant drugs. N Engl J Med. 1997 Jan 23;336(4):258-62. PMID: 8995088.

141. Nulman I, Rovet J, Stewart DE, et al. Child development following exposure to tricyclic antidepressants or fluoxetine throughout fetal life: a prospective, controlled study. Am J Psychiatry. 2002 Nov;159(11):1889-95. PMID: 12411224.

142. Oberlander TF, Bonaguro RJ, Misri S, et al. Infant serotonin transporter (SLC6A4) promoter genotype is associated with adverse neonatal outcomes after prenatal exposure to serotonin reuptake inhibitor medications. Mol Psychiatry. 2008 Jan;13(1):65-73. PMID: 17519929.

143. Oberlander TF, Eckstein Grunau R, Fitzgerald C, et al. Prolonged prenatal psychotropic medication exposure alters neonatal acute pain response. Pediatr Res. 2002 Apr;51(4):443-53. PMID: 11919328.

144. Oberlander TF, Misri S, Fitzgerald CE, et al. Pharmacologic factors associated with transient neonatal symptoms following prenatal psychotropic medication exposure. J Clin Psychiatry. 2004 Feb;65(2):230-7. PMID: 15003078.

145. Oberlander TF, Papsdorf M, Brain UM, et al. Prenatal effects of selective serotonin reuptake inhibitor antidepressants, serotonin transporter promoter genotype (SLC6A4), and maternal mood on child behavior at 3 years of age. Arch Pediatr Adolesc Med. 2010 May;164(5):444-51. PMID: 20439795.

146. Oberlander TF, Reebye P, Misri S, et al. Externalizing and attentional behaviors in children of depressed mothers treated with a selective serotonin reuptake inhibitor antidepressant during pregnancy. Arch Pediatr Adolesc Med. 2007 Jan;161(1):22-9. PMID: 17199063.

147. Oberlander TF, Warburton W, Misri S, et al. Neonatal outcomes after prenatal exposure to selective serotonin reuptake inhibitor antidepressants and maternal depression using population-based linked health data. Arch Gen Psychiatry. 2006 Aug;63(8):898-906. PMID: 16894066.

148. Oberlander TF, Warburton W, Misri S, et al. Effects of timing and duration of gestational exposure to serotonin reuptake inhibitor antidepressants: population-based study. Br J Psychiatry. 2008 May;192(5):338-43. PMID: 18450656.

149. Oberlander TF, Warburton W, Misri S, et al. Major congenital malformations following prenatal exposure to serotonin reuptake inhibitors and benzodiazepines using population-based health data. Birth Defects Res Part B Dev Reprod Toxicol. 2008 Feb;83(1):68-76. PMID: 18293409.

150. Okun ML, Kiewra K, Luther JF, et al. Sleep disturbances in depressed and nondepressed pregnant women. Depress Anxiety. 2011 Aug;28(8):676-85. PMID: 21608086.

151. Okun ML, Luther JF, Wisniewski SR, et al. Disturbed sleep, a novel risk factor for preterm birth? J Womens Health (Larchmt). 2012 Jan;21(1):54-60. PMID: 21967121.

152. Palmsten K, Setoguchi S, Margulis AV, et al. Elevated risk of preeclampsia in pregnant women with depression: depression or antidepressants? Am J Epidemiol. 2012 May 15;175(10):988-97. PMID: 22442287.

153. Pastuszak A, Schick-Boschetto B, Zuber C, et al. Pregnancy outcome following first-trimester exposure to fluoxetine (Prozac). JAMA. 1993;269(17):2246-8. PMID: 8474204.

154. Pawluski JL, Galea LAM, Brain U, et al. Neonatal S100B protein levels after prenatal exposure to selective serotonin reuptake inhibitors. Pediatrics. 2009 Oct;124(4):e662-70. PMID: 19786426.

155. Pearlstein TB, Zlotnick C, Battle CL, et al. Patient choice of treatment for postpartum depression: a pilot study. Arch Women Ment Health. 2006 Nov;9(6):303-8. PMID: 16932988.

156. Pearson KH, Nonacs RM, Viguera AC, et al. Birth outcomes following prenatal exposure to antidepressants. J Clin Psychiatry. 2007 Aug;68(8):1284-9. PMID: 17854255.

157. Pedersen L, Henriksen T, Bech B, et al. Prenatal antidepressant exposure and behavioral problems in early childhood - A cohort study. Acta Psychiatr Scand. 2013 Feb;127(2):126-35. PMID: 23126521.

158. Pedersen LH, Henriksen TB, Olsen J. Fetal exposure to antidepressants and normal milestone development at 6 and 19 months of age. Pediatrics. 2010 Mar;125(3):e600-8. PMID: 20176667.

159. Pedersen LH, Henriksen TB, Vestergaard M, et al. Selective serotonin reuptake inhibitors in pregnancy and congenital malformations: population based cohort study. BMJ. 2009;339:b3569. PMID: 19776103.

160. Polen KND, Rasmussen SA, Riehle-Colarusso T, et al. Association between reported venlafaxine use in early pregnancy and birth defects, national birth defects prevention study, 1997-2007. Birth Defects Res A Clin Mol Teratol. 2013;97(1):28-35. PMID: 23281074.

161. Rai D, Lee BK, Dalman C, et al. Parental depression, maternal antidepressant use during pregnancy, and risk of autism spectrum disorders: population based case-control study. BMJ. 2013 2013-04-19 12:14:20;346PMID: 23604083.

162. Ramos E, St-Andre M, Berard A. Association between antidepressant use during pregnancy and infants born small for gestational age. Can J Psychiatry. 2010 Oct;55(10):643-52. PMID: 20964943.

163. Ramos E, St-Andre M, Rey E, et al. Duration of antidepressant use during pregnancy and risk of major congenital malformations. Br J Psychiatry. 2008 May;192(5):344-50. PMID: 18450657.

164. Rampono J, Proud S, Hackett LP, et al. A pilot study of newer antidepressant concentrations in cord and maternal serum and possible effects in the neonate. Int J Neuropsychopharmcol. 2004 Sep;7(3):329-34. PMID: 15035694.

165. Rampono J, Simmer K, Ilett KF, et al. Placental transfer of SSRI and SNRI antidepressants and effects on the neonate. Pharmacopsychiatry. 2009 May;42(3):95-100. PMID: 19452377.

166. Reebye P, Morison SJ, Panikkar H, et al. Affect expression in prenatally psychotropic exposed and nonexposed mother-infant dyads. Infant Ment Health J. 2002 Jul;23(4):403-16.

167. Reis M, Kallen B. Delivery outcome after maternal use of antidepressant drugs in pregnancy: an update using Swedish data. Psychol Med. 2010 Oct;40(10):1723-33. PMID: 20047705.

168. Salisbury AL, Wisner KL, Pearlstein T, et al. Newborn neurobehavioral patterns are differentially related to prenatal maternal major depressive disorder and serotonin reuptake inhibitor treatment. Depress Anxiety. 2011 Nov;28(11):1008-19. PMID: 21898709.

169. Salkeld E, Ferris LE, Juurlink DN. The risk of postpartum hemorrhage with selective serotonin reuptake inhibitors and other antidepressants. J Clin Psychopharmacol. 2008 Apr;28(2):230-4. PMID: 18344737.

170. Sharp DJ, Chew-Graham C, Tylee A, et al. A pragmatic randomised controlled trial to compare antidepressants with a community-based psychosocial intervention for the treatment of women with postnatal depression: the RESPOND trial. Health Technol Assess. 2010;14(43):iii-iv, ix-xi, 1-153. PMID: 20860888.

171. Simon GE, Cunningham ML, Davis RL. Outcomes of prenatal antidepressant exposure. Am J Psychiatry. 2002 Dec;159(12):2055-61. PMID: 12450956.

172. Sit D, Perel JM, Wisniewski SR, et al. Mother-infant antidepressant concentrations, maternal depression, and perinatal events. J Clin Psychiatry. 2011 Jul;72(7):994-1001. PMID: 21824458.

173. Sivojelezova A, Shuhaiber S, Sarkissian L, et al. Citalopram use in pregnancy: prospective comparative evaluation of pregnancy and fetal outcome. Am J Obstet Gynecol. 2005 Dec;193(6):2004-9. PMID: 16325604.

174. Smith MV, Sung A, Shah B, et al. Neurobehavioral assessment of infants born at term and in utero exposure to serotonin reuptake inhibitors. Early Hum Dev. 2013;89(2):81-6. PMID: 22999988.

175. Stephansson O, Kieler H, Haglund B, et al. Selective serotonin reuptake inhibitors during pregnancy and risk of stillbirth and infant mortality. JAMA. 2013;309(1):48-54. PMID: 23280224.

176. Suri R, Altshuler L, Hellemann G, et al. Effects of antenatal depression and antidepressant treatment on gestational age at birth and risk of preterm birth. Am J Psychiatry. 2007 Aug;164(8):1206-13. PMID: 17671283.

177. Suri R, Altshuler L, Hendrick V, et al. The impact of depression and fluoxetine treatment on obstetrical outcome. Arch Women Ment Health. 2004 Jul;7(3):193-200. PMID: 15241665.

178. Suri R, Hellemann G, Stowe ZN, et al. A prospective, naturalistic, blinded study of early neurobehavioral outcomes for infants following prenatal antidepressant exposure. J Clin Psychiatry. 2011 Jul;72(7):1002-7. PMID: 21672498.

179. Ter Horst PGJ, Bos HJ, De Jong-Van De Berg LTW, et al. In utero exposure to antidepressants and the use of drugs for pulmonary diseases in children. Eur J Clin Pharmacol. 2013;69(3):541-7. PMID: 22815049.

180. Toh S, Mitchell AA, Louik C, et al. Antidepressant use during pregnancy and the risk of preterm delivery and fetal growth restriction. J Clin Psychopharmacol. 2009 Dec;29(6):555-60. PMID: 19910720.

181. Toh S, Mitchell AA, Louik C, et al. Selective serotonin reuptake inhibitor use and risk of gestational hypertension. Am J Psychiatry. 2009 Mar;166(3):320-8. PMID: 19122006.

182. Ververs TF, van Wensen K, Freund MW, et al. Association between antidepressant drug use during pregnancy and child healthcare utilisation. BJOG. 2009 Nov;116(12):1568-77. PMID: 19681852.

183. Wan MW, Sharp DJ, Howard LM, et al. Attitudes and adjustment to the parental role in mothers following treatment for postnatal depression. J Affect Disord. 2011 Jun;131(1-3):284-92. PMID: 21349585.

184. Wen SW, Yang Q, Garner P, et al. Selective serotonin reuptake inhibitors and adverse pregnancy outcomes. Am J Obstet Gynecol. 2006 Apr;194(4):961-6. PMID: 16580283.

185. Wichman CL, Moore KM, Lang TR, et al. Congenital heart disease associated with selective serotonin reuptake inhibitor use during pregnancy. Mayo Clin Proc. 2009;84(1):23-7. PMID: 19121250.

186. Wilson KL, Zelig CM, Harvey JP, et al. Persistent pulmonary hypertension of the newborn is associated with mode of delivery and not with maternal use of selective serotonin reuptake inhibitors. Am J Perinatol. 2011 Jan;28(1):19-24. PMID: 20607643.

187. Wisner KL, Bogen DL, Sit D, et al. Does fetal exposure to SSRIs or maternal depression impact infant growth? Am J Psychiatry. 2013 May 1;170(5):485-93. PMID: 23511234.

188. Wisner KL, Hanusa BH, Perel JM, et al. Postpartum depression: a randomized trial of sertraline versus nortriptyline. J Clin Psychopharmacol. 2006 Aug;26(4):353-60. PMID: 16855451.

189. Wisner KL, Sit DKY, Hanusa BH, et al. Major depression and antidepressant treatment: impact on pregnancy and neonatal outcomes. Am J Psychiatry. 2009 May;166(5):557-66. PMID: 19289451.

190. Wogelius P, Norgaard M, Gislum M, et al. Maternal use of selective serotonin reuptake inhibitors and risk of congenital malformations. Epidemiology. 2006 Nov;17(6):701-4. PMID: 17028507.

191. Yonkers KA, Lin H, Howell HB, et al. Pharmacologic treatment of postpartum women with new-onset major depressive disorder: a randomized controlled trial with paroxetine. J Clin Psychiatry. 2008 Apr;69(4):659-65. PMID: 18363420.

192. Yonkers KA, Norwitz ER, Smith MV, et al. Depression and serotonin reuptake inhibitor treatment as risk factors for preterm birth. Epidemiology. 2012;23(5):677-85. PMID: 22627901.

193. Zeskind PS, Stephens LE. Maternal selective serotonin reuptake inhibitor use during pregnancy and newborn neurobehavior. Pediatrics. 2004 Feb;113(2):368-75. PMID: 14754951.

194. Liberati A, Altman DG, Tetzlaff J, et al. The PRISMA statement for reporting systematic reviews and meta-analyses of studies that evaluate healthcare interventions: explanation and elaboration. BMJ. 2009;339:b2700. PMID: 19622552.

195. Institute of Medicine. Nutrition During Lactation: Subcommittee on Nutritional Status and Weight Gain during Pregnancy. Washington D.C.: The National Academy Press; 1990.

196. International Classification of Diseases (ICD). Geneva, Switzerland: World Health Organization. http://www.who.int/classifications/icd/en/. Accessed on February 2, 2014.

197. EUROCAT: European Surveillance of Congenital Anomalies. http://www.eurocat-network.eu/. Accessed on February 2, 2014.

198. Holmes LB, Westgate M-N. Inclusion and exclusion criteria for malformations in newborn infants exposed to potential teratogens. Birth Defects Res A Clin Mol Teratol. 2011;91(9):807-12. PMID: 21800414.

199. Holmes LB, Westgate M-N. Using ICD-9 codes to establish prevalence of malformations in newborn infants. Birth Defects Res A Clin Mol Teratol. 2012;94(4):208-14. PMID: 22451461.

200. Lu M, Lange L, Slusser W, et al. Provider encouragement of breast-feeding: Evidence from a National Survey. Obstet Gynecol. 2001;97(2):290-5. PMID:11165597.

201. Philipp BL, Malone KL, Cimo S, et al. Sustained breastfeeding rates at a US baby-friendly hospital. Pediatrics. 2003 Sep;112(3 Pt 1):e234-6. PMID: 12949318.

202. Su LL, Chong YS, Chan YH, et al. Antenatal education and postnatal support strategies for improving rates of exclusive breast feeding: randomised controlled trial. BMJ. 2007 Sep 22;335(7620):596. PMID: 17670909.

203. Howland RH. Update on St. John's wort. J Psychosoc Nurs Ment Health Serv. 2010 Nov;48(11):20-4. PMID: 21053786.

204. Moyer M. Why Pregnant Women Deserve Drug Trials. Body Politic [Blog]. January 6, 2011. http://blogs.plos.org/bodypolitic/2011/01/06/why-pregnant-women-deserve-drug-trials/. Accessed on February 2, 2014.

205. The Second Wave Initiative. Toward the Responsible Inclusion of Pregnant Women in Research. http://www.secondwaveinitiative.org/. Accessed on February 2, 2014.

206. Research involving pregnant women or fetuses [45 CFR Part 46B Section 204]. In Code of Federal Regulations. Title 45: Public Welfare. Part 46: Protection of Human Subjects. Subpart B: Additional Protections for Pregnant Women, Human Fetuses and Neonates Involved in Research. Washington, DC: U.S. Department of Health & Human Services; Revised January 15, 2009; Effective July 14, 2009. http://www.hhs.gov/ohrp/humansubjects/guidance/45cfr46.html#46.204. Accessed on February 2, 2014.

207. Aguilera A, Munoz RF. Text messaging as an adjunct to CBT in low-income populations: A usability and feasibility pilot study. Professional Psychology Research & Practice 2011;42(6):472-8.

208. Boschen MJ, Casey LM. The use of mobile telephones as adjuncts to cognitive behavioral psychotherapy. Professional Psychology Research & Practice 2008;39(5):546-52.

209. Moritz S, Schilling L, Hauschildt M, et al. A randomized controlled trial of internet-based therapy in depression. Behaviour Research and Therapy. 2012;50(7–8):513-21. PMID: 22677231.

Abbreviations and Acronyms

ADHD	Attention deficit hyperactivity disorder
AHRQ	Agency for Healthcare Research and Quality
ASD	Autism spectrum disorder
BNBAS	Brazelton Neonatal Behavioral Assessment Scale
CCRCT	Cochrane Central Register of Controlled Trials
CES-D	Center for Epidemiologic Studies Depression Scale
CDSR	Cochrane Database of Systematic Reviews
CGI–I	Clinical Global Impressions Improvement Scale
CHIP	Children's Health Insurance Program
CI	Confidence interval
CINAHL	Cumulative Index to Nursing and Allied Health Literature
CIS-R	Clinical Interview Schedule–Revised
DSM-IV	Diagnostic and Statistical Manual of Mental Disorders, Fourth Edition
EPC	Evidence-based Practice Center
EPDS	Edinburgh Postnatal Depression Scale
FDA	U.S. Food and Drug Administration
GP	General practitioner
HAM-A	Hamilton Rating Scale for Anxiety
HAM-D	Hamilton Rating Scale for Depression
HMO	Health maintenance organization
ICD	International Classification of Diseases
ICD-9	International Classification of Diseases, Ninth Revision
KQ	Key Question
MADRS	Montgomery Asberg Depression Rating Scale
MDI	Mental Development Index
NR	Not reported
NRI	Norepinephrine reuptake inhibitor
NS	Not significant
NSD	No significant difference
OR	Odds ratio
RCT	Randomized controlled trial
RR	Relative risk
RRR	Relative risk reduction
SD	Standard deviation
SF-12	Medical Outcomes Survey 12-Item Short Form
SF-36	Medical Outcomes Survey 36-Item Short Form
SNRI	Serotonin norepinephrine reuptake inhibitor
SSNRI	Selective serotonin norepinephrine reuptake inhibitor
SSRI	Selective serotonin reuptake inhibitor
TCA	Tricyclic antidepressant
Zung SDS	Zung Self-Rating Depression Scale

Appendix A. Search Strategies

CINAHL Plus With Full Text 1941–July 2013
S1 MH Pregnancy+
S2 "pregnan*"
S3 MH Postnatal Period+
S4 (MH "Affective Disorders+")
S5 MH Seasonal Affective Disorder
S6 MH Depression+ OR MH Depression, Postpartum
S7 MH Serotonin Uptake Inhibitors+
S8 "selective serotonin reuptake inhibitor"
S9 "ssri"
S10 MH Citalopram OR citalopram
S11 "escitalopram"
S12 MH Fluoxetine OR fluoxetine OR MH Olanzapine-Fluoxetine
S13 MH Fluvoxamine Maleate OR fluvoxamine
S14 MH Sertraline Hydrochloride OR sertraline
S15 MH Paroxetine OR paroxetine
S16 "celexa"
S17 "lexapro"
S18 "prozac"
S19 "luvox"
S20 "zoloft"
S21 "paxil"
S22 MH Desvenlafaxine Succinate OR desvenlafaxine
S23 MH Mirtazapine OR mirtazapine
S24 "pristiq"
S25 MH Venlafaxine OR effexor
S26 "noradrenergic and specific serotonergic reuptake inhibitor"
S27 (MH "Duloxetine Hydrochloride") OR "duloxetine"
S28 "cymbalta"
S29 (MH "Norepinephrine") OR "norepinephrine"
S30 MH Dopamine Uptake Inhibitors OR dopamine reuptake inhibitor
S31 MH Bupropion OR bupropion
S32 "wellbutrin"
S33 MH Nefazodone OR nefazodone
S34 "serzone"
S35 (MH "Antidepressive Agents+") OR (MH "Antidepressive Agents, Tricyclic+")
S36 (MH "Amitriptyline") OR "amitriptyline"
S37 (MH "Imipramine") OR "imipramine"
S38 (MH "Desipramine") OR "desipramine"
S39 (MH "Nortriptyline") OR "nortriptyline"
S40 MH Teratogens OR teratogenicity
S41 S1 OR S2 OR S3
S42 S4 OR S5 OR S6

S43 S7 OR S8 OR S9 OR S10 OR S11 OR S12 OR S13 OR S14 OR S15 OR S16 OR S17 OR S18 OR S19 OR S20 OR S21 OR S22 OR S23 OR S24 OR S25 OR S26 OR S27 OR S28 OR S29 OR S30 OR S31 OR S32 OR S33 OR S34 OR S35 OR S36 OR S37 OR S38 OR S39
S44 S41 AND S42 AND S43
S45 S40 AND S43
S46 S44 OR S45
S47 S44 OR S45

EBM Reviews - Cochrane Central Register of Controlled Trials July 2013
1 exp Pregnancy/
2 pregnan$.mp.
3 Perinatal Care/
4 Postnatal Care/
5 Peripartum Period/
6 exp Postpartum Period/
7 mood disorders/ or depressive disorder/ or depression, postpartum/ or depressive disorder, major/ or depressive disorder, treatment-resistant/ or dysthymic disorder/ or seasonal affective disorder/
8 Depression/
9 (depressi$ or dysthymi$ or "mood disorder$" or "seasonal affective disorder" or sad).mp.
10 or/7-9
11 10 and (de or dh or dt or pc or th).fs.
12 Serotonin Uptake Inhibitors/
13 (selective serotonin reuptake inhibitor$ or ssri).mp.
14 (citalopram or escitalopram or fluoxetine or fluvoxamine or sertraline or paroxetine).mp.
15 (celexa or lexapro or prozac or luvox or zoloft or paxil).mp.
16 serotonin norepinephrine reuptake inhibitor.mp.
17 (desvenlafaxine or mirtazapine).mp.
18 (pristiq or effexor).mp.
19 (noradrenergic and specific serotonergic reuptake inhibitor).mp.
20 remeron.mp.
21 (selective serotonin and norepinephrine reuptake inhibitor).mp.
22 ssnri.mp.
23 (duloxetine or cymbalta).mp.
24 (norepinephrine and dopamine reuptake inhibitor).mp.
25 ndri.mp.
26 (bupropion or wellbutrin).mp.
27 (nefazodone or serzone).mp.
28 (olanzapine adj1 fluoxetine).mp.
29 exp Antidepressive Agents/
30 Antidepressive Agents, Tricyclic/
31 (amitriptyline or imipramine).mp.
32 desipramine.mp. or Desipramine/
33 nortriptyline.mp. or Nortriptyline/
34 or/12-33
35 exp Prenatal Injuries/

36 exp Maternal Exposure/
37 exp Pregnancy Complications/
38 exp Pregnancy Outcome/
39 exp Fetal Development/
40 or/35-39
41 exp Infant/
42 exp Infant Mortality/
43 exp child/ or exp child, preschool/
44 (infant$ or child$ or pediatri$).mp.
45 or/41-44
46 exp Prenatal Care/
47 exp Preconception Care/
48 Abnormalities, Drug-Induced/ or Prenatal Exposure Delayed Effects/
49 teratogen$.mp.
50 or/1-6
51 (pregnan$ or perinatal or postpartum).mp.
52 50 or 51
53 46 or 47 or 52
54 48 or 49
55 11 and 34 and 53
56 34 and 40
57 34 and 54
58 34 and 45 and 52
59 or/55-58

EBM Reviews - Cochrane Database of Systematic Reviews 2005 to July 2013

1. (depressi$ or bipolar$ or dysthymi$ or cyclotymi$ or "mood disorder$" or "seasonal affective disorder" or sad).mp.
2. (selective serotonin reuptake inhibitor$ or ssri).mp.
3. (citalopram or escitalopram or fluoxetine or fluvoxamine or sertraline or paroxetine).mp.
4. (celexa or lexapro or prozac or luvox or zoloft or paxil).mp.
5. serotonin norepinephrine reuptake inhibitor.mp.
6. (desvenlafaxine or mirtazapine).mp.
7. (pristiq or effexor).mp.
8. (noradrenergic and specific serotonergic reuptake inhibitor).mp.
9. mirtazapine.mp.
10. remeron.mp.
11. (selective serotonin and norepinephrine reuptake inhibitor).mp.
12. ssnri.mp.
13. (duloxetine or cymbalta).mp.
14. (norepinephrine and dopamine reuptake inhibitor).mp.
15. ndri.mp.
16. (bupropion or wellbutrin).mp.
17. (nefazodone or serzone).mp.
18. (olanzapine adj1 fluoxetine).mp.

19. antidepressant$.mp.
20. (amitriptyline or imipramine or desipramine or nortriptyline).mp.
21. (pregnan$ or prenatal$ or postnatal$ or peripartum or postpartum).mp.
22. or/2-20
23. 1 and 21 and 22
24. limit 23 to full systematic reviews

Ovid MEDLINE and Ovid OLDMEDLINE 1946 to July 2013

1. exp Pregnancy/
2. pregnan$.mp.
3. Perinatal Care/
4. Postnatal Care/
5. Peripartum Period/
6. exp Postpartum Period/
7. mood disorders/ or depressive disorder/ or depression, postpartum/ or depressive disorder, major/ or depressive disorder, treatment-resistant/ or dysthymic disorder/ or seasonal affective disorder/
8. Depression/
9. (depressi$ or dysthymi$ or "mood disorder$" or "seasonal affective disorder" or sad).mp.
10. or/7-9
11. 10 and (de or dh or dt or pc or th).fs.
12. Serotonin Uptake Inhibitors/
13. (selective serotonin reuptake inhibitor$ or ssri).mp.
14. (citalopram or escitalopram or fluoxetine or fluvoxamine or sertraline or paroxetine).mp.
15. (celexa or lexapro or prozac or luvox or zoloft or paxil).mp.
16. serotonin norepinephrine reuptake inhibitor.mp.
17. (desvenlafaxine or mirtazapine).mp.
18. (pristiq or effexor).mp.
19. (noradrenergic and specific serotonergic reuptake inhibitor).mp.
20. remeron.mp.
21. (selective serotonin and norepinephrine reuptake inhibitor).mp.
22. ssnri.mp.
23. (duloxetine or cymbalta).mp.
24. (norepinephrine and dopamine reuptake inhibitor).mp.
25. ndri.mp.
26. (bupropion or wellbutrin).mp.
27. (nefazodone or serzone).mp.
28. (olanzapine adj1 fluoxetine).mp.
29. exp Antidepressive Agents/
30. Antidepressive Agents, Tricyclic/
31. (amitriptyline or imipramine).mp.
32. desipramine.mp. or Desipramine/
33. nortriptyline.mp. or Nortriptyline/
34. or/12-33
35. exp Prenatal Injuries/
36. exp Maternal Exposure/

37. exp Pregnancy Complications/
38. exp Pregnancy Outcome/
39. exp Fetal Development/
40. or/35-39
41. exp Infant/
42. exp Infant Mortality/
43. exp child/ or exp child, preschool/
44. (infant$ or child$ or pediatri$).mp.
45. or/41-44
46. exp Prenatal Care/
47. exp Preconception Care/
48. Abnormalities, Drug-Induced/ or Prenatal Exposure Delayed Effects/
49. teratogen$.mp.
50. or/1-6
51. (pregnan$ or perinatal or postpartum).mp.
52. 50 or 51
53. 46 or 47 or 52
54. 48 or 49
55. 11 and 34 and 53
56. 34 and 40
57. 34 and 54
58. 34 and 45 and 52
59. or/55-58
60. limit 59 to humans
61. limit 60 to english language
62. limit 60 to abstracts
63. 61 or 62

PsychInfo 1806 to July 2013

1. exp Pregnancy/
2. pregnan$.mp.
3. mood disorders/ or depressive disorder/ or depression, postpartum/ or depressive disorder, major/ or depressive disorder, treatment-resistant/ or dysthymic disorder/ or seasonal affective disorder/
4. Depression/
5. (depressi$ or dysthymi$ or "mood disorder$" or "seasonal affective disorder" or sad).mp.
6. (selective serotonin reuptake inhibitor$ or ssri).mp.
7. (citalopram or escitalopram or fluoxetine or fluvoxamine or sertraline or paroxetine).mp.
8. (celexa or lexapro or prozac or luvox or zoloft or paxil).mp.
9. serotonin norepinephrine reuptake inhibitor.mp.
10. (desvenlafaxine or mirtazapine).mp.
11. (pristiq or effexor).mp.
12. (noradrenergic and specific serotonergic reuptake inhibitor).mp.
13. mirtazapine.mp.
14. remeron.mp.

15. (selective serotonin and norepinephrine reuptake inhibitor).mp.
16. ssnri.mp.
17. (duloxetine or cymbalta).mp.
18. (norepinephrine and dopamine reuptake inhibitor).mp.
19. ndri.mp.
20. (bupropion or wellbutrin).mp.
21. (nefazodone or serzone).mp.
22. (olanzapine adj1 fluoxetine).mp.
23. (amitriptyline or imipramine or desipramine or nortriptyline).mp. [mp=title, abstract, heading word, table of contents, key concepts, original title, tests & measures]
24. exp Tricyclic Antidepressant Drugs/ or exp Antidepressant Drugs/
25. exp Pregnancy Outcome/
26. (infant$ or child$ or pediatri$).mp.
27. 1 or 2
28. or/3-5
29. or/6-24
30. 25 and 26
31. 27 and 28 and 29
32. 29 and 30
33. 31 or 32

Sciverse Scopus 1974 to July 2013

(TITLE-ABS-KEY((pregnan*) AND ("mood disorder*" OR "affective disorder*" OR "depressive disorder" OR depression OR "seasonal affective disorder" OR "dysthymic disorder")) OR (TITLE-ABS-KEY(teratogen*)) AND ((TITLE-ABS-KEY(antidepressant* OR antidepressive agent* OR "selective serotonin reuptake inhibitor*" OR "ssri" OR citalopram OR escitalopram OR fluoxetine OR fluvoxamine OR sertraline OR paroxetine OR celexa OR lexapro OR prozac OR luvox OR zoloft OR paxil OR desvenlafaxine OR mirtazapine OR pristiq OR effexor OR "noradrenergic and specific serotonergic reuptake inhibitor" OR "selective serotonin and norepinephrine reuptake inhibitor" OR "ssnri" OR "norepinephrine and dopamine reuptake inhibitor" OR bupropion OR wellbutrin OR nefazodone OR serzone OR amitriptyline OR imipramine OR desipramine OR nortriptyline OR remeron OR olanzapine))

Appendix B. Included Studies

Observational Studies

1. Alwan S, Reefhuis J, Botto LD, et al. Maternal use of bupropion and risk for congenital heart defects. Am J Obstet Gynecol. 2010 Jul;203(1):52.e1-6. PMID: 20417496.

2. Alwan S, Reefhuis J, Rasmussen SA, et al. Use of selective serotonin-reuptake inhibitors in pregnancy and the risk of birth defects. N Engl J Med. 2007 Jun 28;356(26):2684-92. PMID: 17596602.

3. Andrade SE, McPhillips H, Loren D, et al. Antidepressant medication use and risk of persistent pulmonary hypertension of the newborn. Pharmacoepidemiol Drug Saf. 2009 Mar;18(3):246-52. PMID: 19148882.

4. Bakker MK, De Walle HEK, Wilffert B, et al. Fluoxetine and infantile hypertrophic pylorus stenosis: a signal from a birth defects-drug exposure surveillance study. Pharmacoepidemiol Drug Saf. 2010 Aug;19(8):808-13. PMID: 20572024.

5. Bakker MK, Kerstjens-Frederikse WS, Buys CHCM, et al. First-trimester use of paroxetine and congenital heart defects: a population-based case-control study. Birth Defects Res Part A Clin Mol Teratol. 2010 Feb;88(2):94-100. PMID: 19937603.

6. Ban L, Tata LJ, West J, et al. Live and non-live pregnancy outcomes among women with depression and anxiety: A population-based study. PLoS ONE. 2012;7(8)PMID: 22937052.

7. Batton B, Batton E, Weigler K, et al. In utero antidepressant exposure and neurodevelopment in preterm infants. Am J Perinatol. 2013;30(4):297-301. PMID: 22893558.

8. Bérard A, Ramos É, Rey É, et al. First trimester exposure to paroxetine and risk of cardiac malformations in infants: The importance of dosage. Birth Defects Res B Dev Reprod Toxicol. 2007;80(1):18-27. PMID: 17187388.

9. Berle JO, Steen VM, Aamo TO, et al. Breastfeeding during maternal antidepressant treatment with serotonin reuptake inhibitors: infant exposure, clinical symptoms, and cytochrome p450 genotypes. J Clin Psychiatry. 2004 Sep;65(9):1228-34. PMID: 15367050.

10. Bogen DL, Hanusa BH, Moses-Kolko E, et al. Are maternal depression or symptom severity associated with breastfeeding intention or outcomes? J Clin Psychiatry. 2010 Aug;71(8):1069-78. PMID: 20584521.

11. Boucher N, Bairam A, Beaulac-Baillargeon L. A new look at the neonate's clinical presentation after in utero exposure to antidepressants in late pregnancy. J Clin Psychopharmacol. 2008 Jun;28(3):334-9. PMID: 18480693.

12. Bracken MB, Holford TR. Exposure to prescribed drugs in pregnancy and association with congenital malformations. Obstet Gynecol. 1981;58(3):336-44. PMID: 7266953.

13. Casper RC, Fleisher BE, Lee-Ancajas JC, et al. Follow-up of children of depressed mothers exposed or not exposed to antidepressant drugs during pregnancy. J Pediatr. 2003 Apr;142(4):402-8. PMID: 12712058.

14. Chambers CD, Hernandez-Diaz S, Van Marter LJ, et al. Selective serotonin-reuptake inhibitors and risk of persistent pulmonary hypertension of the newborn. N Engl J Med. 2006 Feb 9;354(6):579-87. PMID: 16467545.

15. Chambers CD, Johnson KA, Dick LM, et al. Birth outcomes in pregnant women taking fluoxetine. N Engl J Med. 1996 Oct 3;335(14):1010-5. PMID: 8793924.

16. Chun-Fai-Chan B, Koren G, Fayez I, et al. Pregnancy outcome of women exposed to bupropion during pregnancy: a prospective comparative study. Am J Obstet Gynecol. 2005 Mar;192(3):932-6. PMID: 15746694.

17. Cole JA, Ephross SA, Cosmatos IS, et al. Paroxetine in the first trimester and the prevalence of congenital malformations. Pharmacoepidemiol Drug Saf. 2007 Oct;16(10):1075-85. PMID: 17729379.

18. Cole JA, Modell JG, Haight BR, et al. Bupropion in pregnancy and the prevalence of congenital malformations. Pharmacoepidemiol Drug Saf. 2007 May;16(5):474-84. PMID: 16897811.

19. Colvin L, Slack-Smith L, Stanley FJ, et al. Linking a pharmaceutical claims database with a birth defects registry to investigate birth defect rates of suspected teratogens. Pharmacoepidemiol Drug Saf. 2010;19(11):1137-50. PMID: 20602344.

20. Colvin L, Slack-Smith L, Stanley FJ, et al. Dispensing patterns and pregnancy outcomes for women dispensed selective serotonin reuptake inhibitors in pregnancy.[Erratum appears in Birth Defects Res A Clin Mol Teratol. 2011 Apr;91(4):268]. Birth Defects Res Part A Clin Mol Teratol. 2011 Mar;91(3):142-52. PMID: 21381184.

21. Colvin L, Slack-Smith L, Stanley FJ, et al. Early morbidity and mortality following in utero exposure to selective serotonin reuptake inhibitors: a population-based study in Western australia. CNS Drugs. 2012;26(7):e1-e14. PMID: 2011592323. Language: English. Entry Date: 20121102. Revision Date: 20121102. Publication Type: journal article.

22. Costei AM, Kozer E, Ho T, et al. Perinatal outcome following third trimester exposure to paroxetine. Arch Pediatr Adolesc Med. 2002 Nov;156(11):1129-32. PMID: 12413342.

23. Croen LA, Grether JK, Yoshida CK, et al. Antidepressant use during pregnancy and childhood autism spectrum disorders. Arch Gen Psychiatry. 2011 Nov;68(11):1104-12. PMID: 21727247.

24. Davidson S, Prokonov D, Taler M, et al. Effect of exposure to selective serotonin reuptake inhibitors in utero on fetal growth: potential role for the IGF-I and HPA axes. Pediatr Res. 2009 Feb;65(2):236-41. PMID: 19262294.

25. Davis RL, Rubanowice D, McPhillips H, et al. Risks of congenital malformations and perinatal events among infants exposed to antidepressant medications during pregnancy. Pharmacoepidemiol Drug Saf. 2007 Oct;16(10):1086-94. PMID: 17729378.

26. De Vera MA, Bérard A. Antidepressant use during pregnancy and the risk of pregnancy-induced hypertension. Br J Clin Pharmacol. 2012;74(2):362-9. PMID: 22435711.

27. de Vries NKS, van der Veere CN, Reijneveld SA, et al. Early Neurological Outcome of Young Infants Exposed to Selective Serotonin Reuptake Inhibitors during Pregnancy: Results from the Observational SMOK Study. PLoS ONE. 2013;8(5)PMID: 23785389.

28. Diav-Citrin O, Shechtman S, Weinbaum D, et al. Paroxetine and fluoxetine in pregnancy: a prospective, multicentre, controlled, observational study. Br J Clin Pharmacol. 2008 Nov;66(5):695-705. PMID: 18754846.

29. Djulus J, Koren G, Einarson TR, et al. Exposure to mirtazapine during pregnancy: a prospective, comparative study of birth outcomes. J Clin Psychiatry. 2006 Aug;67(8):1280-4. PMID: 16965209.

30. Dubnov-Raz G, Hemila H, Vurembrand Y, et al. Maternal use of selective serotonin reuptake inhibitors during pregnancy and neonatal bone density. Early Hum Dev. 2012 Mar;88(3):191-4. PMID: 21890289.

31. Dubnov-Raz G, Juurlink DN, Fogelman R, et al. Antenatal use of selective serotonin-reuptake inhibitors and QT interval prolongation in newborns. Pediatrics. 2008 Sep;122(3):e710-5. PMID: 18762507.

32. Einarson A, Bonari L, Voyer-Lavigne S, et al. A multicentre prospective controlled study to determine the safety of trazodone and nefazodone use during pregnancy. Can J Psychiatry. 2003;48(2):106-10. PMID: 12655908.

33. Einarson A, Choi J, Einarson TR, et al. Rates of spontaneous and therapeutic abortions following use of antidepressants in pregnancy: results from a large prospective database. J Obstet Gynaecol Can. 2009;31(5):452-6. PMID: 19604427.

34. Einarson A, Choi J, Einarson TR, et al. Incidence of major malformations in infants following antidepressant exposure in pregnancy: results of a large prospective cohort study. Can J Psychiatry. 2009 Apr;54(4):242-6. PMID: 19321030.

35. Einarson A, Choi J, Einarson TR, et al. Adverse effects of antidepressant use in pregnancy: an evaluation of fetal growth and preterm birth. Depress Anxiety. 2010;27(1):35-8. PMID: 19691030.

36. Einarson A, Choi J, Koren G, et al. Outcomes of infants exposed to multiple antidepressants during pregnancy: results of a cohort study. J Popul Ther Clin Pharmacol. 2011;18(2):e390-6. PMID: 22071601.

37. El Marroun H, Jaddoe VWV, Hudziak JJ, et al. Maternal use of selective serotonin reuptake inhibitors, fetal growth, and risk of adverse birth

outcomes. Arch Gen Psychiatry. 2012 Jul;69(7):706-14. PMID: 22393202.

38. Ericson A, Kallen B, Wiholm B. Delivery outcome after the use of antidepressants in early pregnancy. Eur J Clin Pharmacol. 1999 Sep;55(7):503-8. PMID: 10501819.

39. Ferreira E, Carceller AM, Agogue C, et al. Effects of selective serotonin reuptake inhibitors and venlafaxine during pregnancy in term and preterm neonates. Pediatrics. 2007 Jan;119(1):52-9. PMID: 17200271.

40. Figueroa R. Use of antidepressants during pregnancy and risk of attention-deficit/hyperactivity disorder in the offspring. J Dev Behav Pediatr. 2010 Oct;31(8):641-8. PMID: 20613624.

41. Galbally M, Lewis AJ, Buist A. Developmental outcomes of children exposed to antidepressants in pregnancy. Aust N Z J Psychiatry. 2011 May;45(5):393-9. PMID: 21314237.

42. Galbally M, Lewis AJ, Lum J, et al. Serotonin discontinuation syndrome following in utero exposure to antidepressant medication: prospective controlled study. Aust N Z J Psychiatry. 2009 Sep;43(9):846-54. PMID: 19670058.

43. Gorman JR, Kao K, Chambers CD. Breastfeeding among Women Exposed to Antidepressants during Pregnancy. J Hum Lact. 2012;28(2):181-8. PMID: 2011521514. Language: English. Entry Date: 20120601. Revision Date: 20120817. Publication Type: journal article.

44. Grzeskowiak LE, Gilbert AL, Morrison JL. Neonatal outcomes after late-gestation exposure to selective serotonin reuptake inhibitors. J Clin Psychopharmacol. 2012;32(5):615-21. PMID: 22926594.

45. Hale TW, Kendall-Tackett K, Cong Z, et al. Discontinuation syndrome in newborns whose mothers took antidepressants while pregnant or breastfeeding. Breastfeed Med. 2010 Dec;5(4):283-8. PMID: 20807106.

46. Hanley GE, Brain U, Oberlander TF. Infant developmental outcomes following prenatal exposure to antidepressants, and maternal depressed mood and positive affect. Early Hum Dev. 2013;89(8):519-24. PMID: 23384962.

47. Heikkinen T, Ekblad U, Kero P, et al. Citalopram in pregnancy and lactation. Clin Pharmacol Ther. 2002 Aug;72(2):184-91. PMID: 12189365.

48. Jimenez-Solem E, Andersen JT, Petersen M, et al. Exposure to selective serotonin reuptake inhibitors and the risk of congenital malformations: A nationwide cohort study. BMJ Open. 2012;2(3)PMID: 22710132.

49. Jimenez-Solem E, Andersen JT, Petersen M, et al. SSRI Use During Pregnancy and Risk of Stillbirth and Neonatal Mortality. Am J Psychiatry. 2013 Mar 1;170(3):299-304 PMID: 23361562.

50. Jordan AE, Jackson GL, Deardorff D, et al. Serotonin reuptake inhibitor use in pregnancy and the neonatal behavioral syndrome. J Matern Fetal Neonatal Med. 2008 Oct;21(10):745-51. PMID: 19012191.

51. Kallen B. Neonate characteristics after maternal use of antidepressants in late pregnancy. Arch Pediatr Adolesc Med. 2004 Apr;158(4):312-6. PMID: 15066868.

52. Kallen B, Olausson PO. Maternal use of selective serotonin re-uptake inhibitors and persistent pulmonary hypertension of the newborn. Pharmacoepidemiol Drug Saf. 2008 Aug;17(8):801-6. PMID: 18314924.

53. Kallen BAJ, Otterblad Olausson P. Maternal use of selective serotonin re-uptake inhibitors in early pregnancy and infant congenital malformations. Birth Defects Res Part A Clin Mol Teratol. 2007 Apr;79(4):301-8. PMID: 17216624.

54. Kieler H, Artama M, Engeland A, et al. Selective serotonin reuptake inhibitors during pregnancy and risk of persistent pulmonary hypertension in the newborn: population based cohort study from the five Nordic countries. BMJ. 2012;344:d8012. PMID: 22240235.

55. Klieger-Grossmann C, Weitzner B, Panchaud A, et al. Pregnancy outcomes following use of escitalopram: a prospective comparative cohort study. J Clin Pharmacol. 2012 May;52(5):766-70. PMID: 22075232.

56. Klinger G, Frankenthal D, Merlob P, et al. Long-term outcome following selective serotonin reuptake inhibitor induced neonatal abstinence syndrome. J Perinatol. 2011 Sep;31(9):615-20. PMID: 21311497.

57. Kornum JB. Use of selective serotonin-reuptake inhibitors during early pregnancy and risk of

congenital malformations: updated analysis. Clin Epidemiol. 2010 Aug 9;2:29-36. PMID: 20865100.

58. Kulin NA, Pastuszak A, Sage SR, et al. Pregnancy outcome following maternal use of the new selective serotonin reuptake inhibitors: a prospective controlled multicenter study. JAMA. 1998 Feb 25;279(8):609-10. PMID: 9486756.

59. Laine K, Heikkinen T, Ekblad U, et al. Effects of exposure to selective serotonin reuptake inhibitors during pregnancy on serotonergic symptoms in newborns and cord blood monoamine and prolactin concentrations. Arch Gen Psychiatry. 2003 Jul;60(7):720-6. PMID: 12860776.

60. Latendresse G, Ruiz RJ. Maternal corticotropin-releasing hormone and the use of selective serotonin reuptake inhibitors independently predict the occurrence of preterm birth. J Midwifery Womens Health. 2011 Mar-Apr;56(2):118-26. PMID: 21429075.

61. Lennestal R, Kallen B. Delivery outcome in relation to maternal use of some recently introduced antidepressants. J Clin Psychopharmacol. 2007 Dec;27(6):607-13. PMID: 18004128.

62. Levinson-Castiel R, Merlob P, Linder N, et al. Neonatal abstinence syndrome after in utero exposure to selective serotonin reuptake inhibitors in term infants. Arch Pediatr Adolesc Med. 2006 Feb;160(2):173-6. PMID: 16461873.

63. Lewis AJ, Galbally M, Opie G, et al. Neonatal growth outcomes at birth and one month postpartum following in utero exposure to antidepressant medication. Aust N Z J Psychiatry. 2010 May;44(5):482-7. PMID: 20397792.

64. Logsdon MC, Wisner K, Sit D, et al. Depression treatment and maternal functioning. Depress Anxiety. 2011 Nov;28(11):1020-6. PMID: 21898714.

65. Louik C, Lin AE, Werler MM, et al. First-trimester use of selective serotonin-reuptake inhibitors and the risk of birth defects. N Engl J Med. 2007 Jun 28;356(26):2675-83. PMID: 17596601.

66. Lund N, Pedersen LH, Henriksen TB. Selective serotonin reuptake inhibitor exposure in utero and pregnancy outcomes.[Erratum appears in Arch Pediatr Adolesc Med. 2009 Dec;163(12):1143]. Arch Pediatr Adolesc Med. 2009 Oct;163(10):949-54. PMID: 19805715.

67. Malm H, Artama M, Gissler M, et al. Selective serotonin reuptake inhibitors and risk for major congenital anomalies. Obstet Gynecol. 2011 Jul;118(1):111-20. PMID: 21646927.

68. Manakova E, Hubickova L. Antidepressant drug exposure during pregnancy. CZTIS small prospective study. Neuroendocrinol Lett. 2011;32 Suppl 1:53-6. PMID: 22167208.

69. Maschi S, Clavenna A, Campi R, et al. Neonatal outcome following pregnancy exposure to antidepressants: a prospective controlled cohort study. BJOG. 2008 Jan;115(2):283-9. PMID: 17903222.

70. McElhatton PR, Garbis HM, Elefant E, et al. The outcome of pregnancy in 689 women exposed to therapeutic doses of antidepressants. A collaborative study of the European Network of Teratology Information Services (ENTIS). Reprod Toxicol. 1996 Jul-Aug;10(4):285-94. PMID: 8829251.

71. McFarland J, Salisbury AL, Battle CL, et al. Major depressive disorder during pregnancy and emotional attachment to the fetus. Arch Womens Ment Health. 2011;14(5):425-34. PMID: 21938509.

72. Merlob P, Birk E, Sirota L, et al. Are selective serotonin reuptake inhibitors cardiac teratogens? Echocardiographic screening of newborns with persistent heart murmur. Birth Defects Res Part A Clin Mol Teratol. 2009 Oct;85(10):837-41. PMID: 19691085.

73. Misri S, Kendrick K, Oberlander TF, et al. Antenatal depression and anxiety affect postpartum parenting stress: a longitudinal, prospective study. Can J Psychiatry. 2010 Apr;55(4):222-8. PMID: 20416145.

74. Misri S, Reebye P, Kendrick K, et al. Internalizing behaviors in 4-year-old children exposed in utero to psychotropic medications. Am J Psychiatry. 2006 Jun;163(6):1026-32. PMID: 16741203.

75. Misri S, Sivertz K. Tricyclic drugs in pregnancy and lactation: a preliminary report. Int J Psychiatry Med. 1991;21(2):157-71. PMID: 1894455.

76. Mulder EJ, Ververs FF, de Heus R, et al. Selective serotonin reuptake inhibitors affect neurobehavioral development in the human fetus. Neuropsychopharmacology. 2011 Sep;36(10):1961-71. PMID: Peer Reviewed Journal: 2011-22335-002.

77. Nakhai-Pour HR, Broy P, Berard A. Use of antidepressants during pregnancy and the risk of spontaneous abortion. CMAJ. 2010 Jul 13;182(10):1031-7. PMID: 20513781.

78. Nijenhuis CM, ter Horst PGJ, van Rein N, et al. Disturbed development of the enteric nervous system after in utero exposure of selective serotonin re-uptake inhibitors and tricyclic antidepressants. Part 2: Testing the hypotheses. Br J Clin Pharmacol. 2012 Jan;73(1):126-34. PMID: 21848990.

79. Nordeng H, van Gelder MMHJ, Spigset O, et al. Pregnancy outcome after exposure to antidepressants and the role of maternal depression: results from the Norwegian Mother and Child Cohort Study. J Clin Psychopharmacol. 2012 Apr;32(2):186-94. PMID: 22367660.

80. Nulman I, Koren G, Rovet J, et al. Neurodevelopment of children following prenatal exposure to venlafaxine, selective serotonin reuptake inhibitors, or untreated maternal depression. Am J Psychiatry. 2012 Nov 1;169(11):1165-74. . PMID: 23128923.

81. Nulman I, Rovet J, Stewart DE, et al. Neurodevelopment of children exposed in utero to antidepressant drugs. N Engl J Med. 1997 Jan 23;336(4):258-62. PMID: 8995088.

82. Nulman I, Rovet J, Stewart DE, et al. Child development following exposure to tricyclic antidepressants or fluoxetine throughout fetal life: a prospective, controlled study. Am J Psychiatry. 2002 Nov;159(11):1889-95. PMID: 12411224.

83. O. S, H. K, B. H, et al. Selective serotonin reuptake inhibitors during pregnancy and risk of stillbirth and infant mortality. JAMA. 2013;309(1):48-54. PMID: 23280224.

84. Oberlander TF, Bonaguro RJ, Misri S, et al. Infant serotonin transporter (SLC6A4) promoter genotype is associated with adverse neonatal outcomes after prenatal exposure to serotonin reuptake inhibitor medications. Mol Psychiatry. 2008 Jan;13(1):65-73. PMID: 17519929.

85. Oberlander TF, Eckstein Grunau R, Fitzgerald C, et al. Prolonged prenatal psychotropic medication exposure alters neonatal acute pain response. Pediatr Res. 2002 Apr;51(4):443-53. PMID: 11919328.

86. Oberlander TF, Misri S, Fitzgerald CE, et al. Pharmacologic factors associated with transient neonatal symptoms following prenatal psychotropic medication exposure. J Clin Psychiatry. 2004 Feb;65(2):230-7. PMID: 15003078.

87. Oberlander TF, Papsdorf M, Brain UM, et al. Prenatal effects of selective serotonin reuptake inhibitor antidepressants, serotonin transporter promoter genotype (SLC6A4), and maternal mood on child behavior at 3 years of age. Arch Pediatr Adolesc Med. 2010 May;164(5):444-51. PMID: 20439795.

88. Oberlander TF, Reebye P, Misri S, et al. Externalizing and attentional behaviors in children of depressed mothers treated with a selective serotonin reuptake inhibitor antidepressant during pregnancy. Arch Pediatr Adolesc Med. 2007 Jan;161(1):22-9. PMID: 17199063.

89. Oberlander TF, Warburton W, Misri S, et al. Neonatal outcomes after prenatal exposure to selective serotonin reuptake inhibitor antidepressants and maternal depression using population-based linked health data. Arch Gen Psychiatry. 2006 Aug;63(8):898-906. PMID: 16894066.

90. Oberlander TF, Warburton W, Misri S, et al. Effects of timing and duration of gestational exposure to serotonin reuptake inhibitor antidepressants: population-based study. Br J Psychiatry. 2008 May;192(5):338-43. PMID: 18450656.

91. Oberlander TF, Warburton W, Misri S, et al. Major congenital malformations following prenatal exposure to serotonin reuptake inhibitors and benzodiazepines using population-based health data. Birth Defects Res Part B Dev Reprod Toxicol. 2008 Feb;83(1):68-76. PMID: 18293409.

92. Okun ML, Kiewra K, Luther JF, et al. Sleep disturbances in depressed and nondepressed pregnant women. Depress Anxiety. 2011 Aug;28(8):676-85. PMID: 21608086.

93. Okun ML, Luther JF, Wisniewski SR, et al. Disturbed sleep, a novel risk factor for preterm birth? J Womens Health (Larchmt). 2012 Jan;21(1):54-60. PMID: 21967121.

94. Palmsten K, Setoguchi S, Margulis AV, et al. Elevated risk of preeclampsia in pregnant women with depression: depression or antidepressants? Am J Epidemiol. 2012 May 15;175(10):988-97. PMID: 22442287.

95. Pastuszak A, Schick-Boschetto B, Zuber C, et al. Pregnancy outcome following first-trimester exposure to fluoxetine (Prozac). JAMA. 1993;269(17):2246-8. PMID: 8474204.

96. Pawluski JL, Galea LAM, Brain U, et al. Neonatal S100B protein levels after prenatal exposure to selective serotonin reuptake inhibitors. Pediatrics. 2009 Oct;124(4):e662-70. PMID: 19786426.

97. Pearlstein TB, Zlotnick C, Battle CL, et al. Patient choice of treatment for postpartum depression: a pilot study. Arch Women Ment Health. 2006 Nov;9(6):303-8. PMID: 16932988.

98. Pearson KH, Nonacs RM, Viguera AC, et al. Birth outcomes following prenatal exposure to antidepressants. J Clin Psychiatry. 2007 Aug;68(8):1284-9. PMID: 17854255.

99. Pedersen L, Henriksen T, Bech B, et al. Prenatal antidepressant exposure and behavioral problems in early childhood - A cohort study. Acta Psychiatr Scand. 2013 Feb;127(2):126-35. PMID: Peer Reviewed Journal: 2013-00954-005.

100. Pedersen LH, Henriksen TB, Olsen J. Fetal exposure to antidepressants and normal milestone development at 6 and 19 months of age. Pediatrics. 2010 Mar;125(3):e600-8. PMID: 20176667.

101. Pedersen LH, Henriksen TB, Vestergaard M, et al. Selective serotonin reuptake inhibitors in pregnancy and congenital malformations: population based cohort study. BMJ. 2009;339:b3569. PMID: 19776103.

102. Polen KND, Rasmussen SA, Riehle-Colarusso T, et al. Association between reported venlafaxine use in early pregnancy and birth defects, national birth defects prevention study, 1997-2007. Birth Defects Res A Clin Mol Teratol. 2013;97(1):28-35. PMID: 23281074.

103. Rai D, Lee BK, Dalman C, et al. Parental depression, maternal antidepressant use during pregnancy, and risk of autism spectrum disorders: population based case-control study. BMJ. 2013 2013-04-19 12:14:20;346PMID: 23604083.

104. Ramos E, St-Andre M, Berard A. Association between antidepressant use during pregnancy and infants born small for gestational age. Can J Psychiatry. 2010 Oct;55(10):643-52. PMID: 20964943.

105. Ramos E, St-Andre M, Rey E, et al. Duration of antidepressant use during pregnancy and risk of major congenital malformations. Br J Psychiatry. 2008 May;192(5):344-50. PMID: 18450657.

106. Rampono J, Proud S, Hackett LP, et al. A pilot study of newer antidepressant concentrations in cord and maternal serum and possible effects in the neonate. Int J Neuropsychopharmcol. 2004 Sep;7(3):329-34. PMID: 15035694.

107. Rampono J, Simmer K, Ilett KF, et al. Placental transfer of SSRI and SNRI antidepressants and effects on the neonate. Pharmacopsychiatry. 2009 May;42(3):95-100. PMID: 19452377.

108. Reebye P, Morison SJ, Panikkar H, et al. Affect expression in prenatally psychotropic exposed and nonexposed mother-infant dyads. Infant Ment Health J. 2002 Jul;23(4):403-16. PMID: Peer Reviewed Journal: 2002-17492-004.

109. Reis M, Kallen B. Delivery outcome after maternal use of antidepressant drugs in pregnancy: an update using Swedish data. Psychol Med. 2010 Oct;40(10):1723-33. PMID: 20047705.

110. Salisbury AL, Wisner KL, Pearlstein T, et al. Newborn neurobehavioral patterns are differentially related to prenatal maternal major depressive disorder and serotonin reuptake inhibitor treatment. Depress Anxiety. 2011 Nov;28(11):1008-19. PMID: 21898709.

111. Salkeld E, Ferris LE, Juurlink DN. The risk of postpartum hemorrhage with selective serotonin reuptake inhibitors and other antidepressants. J Clin Psychopharmacol. 2008 Apr;28(2):230-4. PMID: Peer Reviewed Journal: 2008-03759-017.

112. Simon GE, Cunningham ML, Davis RL. Outcomes of prenatal antidepressant exposure. Am J Psychiatry. 2002 Dec;159(12):2055-61. PMID: 12450956.

113. Sit D, Perel JM, Wisniewski SR, et al. Mother-infant antidepressant concentrations, maternal depression, and perinatal events. J Clin Psychiatry. 2011 Jul;72(7):994-1001. PMID: 21824458.

114. Sivojelezova A, Shuhaiber S, Sarkissian L, et al. Citalopram use in pregnancy: prospective comparative evaluation of pregnancy and fetal outcome. Am J Obstet Gynecol. 2005 Dec;193(6):2004-9. PMID: 16325604.

115. Smith MV, Sung A, Shah B, et al. Neurobehavioral assessment of infants born at term and in utero exposure to serotonin reuptake inhibitors. Early Hum Dev. 2013;89(2):81-6. PMID: 22999988.

116. Suri R, Altshuler L, Hellemann G, et al. Effects of antenatal depression and antidepressant treatment on gestational age at birth and risk of preterm birth. Am J Psychiatry. 2007 Aug;164(8):1206-13. PMID: 17671283.

117. Suri R, Altshuler L, Hendrick V, et al. The impact of depression and fluoxetine treatment on obstetrical outcome. Arch Women Ment Health. 2004 Jul;7(3):193-200. PMID: 15241665.

118. Suri R, Hellemann G, Stowe ZN, et al. A prospective, naturalistic, blinded study of early neurobehavioral outcomes for infants following prenatal antidepressant exposure. J Clin Psychiatry. 2011 Jul;72(7):1002-7. PMID: 21672498.

119. Ter Horst PGJ, Bos HJ, De Jong-Van De Berg LTW, et al. In utero exposure to antidepressants and the use of drugs for pulmonary diseases in children. Eur J Clin Pharmacol. 2013;69(3):541-7. PMID: 22815049.

120. Toh S, Mitchell AA, Louik C, et al. Antidepressant use during pregnancy and the risk of preterm delivery and fetal growth restriction. J Clin Psychopharmacol. 2009 Dec;29(6):555-60. PMID: 19910720.

121. Toh S, Mitchell AA, Louik C, et al. Selective serotonin reuptake inhibitor use and risk of gestational hypertension. Am J Psychiatry. 2009 Mar;166(3):320-8. PMID: 19122006.

122. Ververs TF, van Wensen K, Freund MW, et al. Association between antidepressant drug use during pregnancy and child healthcare utilisation. BJOG. 2009 Nov;116(12):1568-77. PMID: 19681852.

123. Wen SW, Yang Q, Garner P, et al. Selective serotonin reuptake inhibitors and adverse pregnancy outcomes. Am J Obstet Gynecol. 2006 Apr;194(4):961-6. PMID: 16580283.

124. Wichman CL, Moore KM, Lang TR, et al. Congenital heart disease associated with selective serotonin reuptake inhibitor use during pregnancy. Mayo Clin Proc. 2009;84(1):23-7. PMID: 19121250.

125. Wilson KL, Zelig CM, Harvey JP, et al. Persistent pulmonary hypertension of the newborn is associated with mode of delivery and not with maternal use of selective serotonin reuptake inhibitors. Am J Perinatol. 2011 Jan;28(1):19-24. PMID: 20607643.

126. Wisner KL, Bogen DL, Sit D, et al. Does Fetal Exposure to SSRIs or Maternal Depression Impact Infant Growth? Am J Psychiatry. 2013 May 1;170(5):485-93. PMID: 23511234.

127. Wisner KL, Sit DKY, Hanusa BH, et al. Major depression and antidepressant treatment: impact on pregnancy and neonatal outcomes. Am J Psychiatry. 2009 May;166(5):557-66. PMID: 19289451.

128. Wogelius P, Norgaard M, Gislum M, et al. Maternal use of selective serotonin reuptake inhibitors and risk of congenital malformations. Epidemiology. 2006 Nov;17(6):701-4. PMID: 17028507.

129. Yonkers KA, Norwitz ER, Smith MV, et al. Depression and serotonin reuptake inhibitor treatment as risk factors for preterm birth. Epidemiology. 2012;23(5):677-85. PMID: 22627901.

130. Zeskind PS, Stephens LE. Maternal selective serotonin reuptake inhibitor use during pregnancy and newborn neurobehavior. Pediatrics. 2004 Feb;113(2):368-75. PMID: 14754951

Randomized Controlled Trials

1. Appleby L, Warner R, Whitton A, et al. A controlled study of fluoxetine and cognitive-behavioural counselling in the treatment of postnatal depression. BMJ. 1997 Mar 29;314(7085):932-6. PMID: 9099116.

2. Bloch M, Meiboom H, Lorberblatt M, et al. The effect of sertraline add-on to brief dynamic psychotherapy for the treatment of postpartum depression: a randomized, double-blind, placebo-controlled study. J Clin Psychiatry. 2012 Feb;73(2):235-41. PMID: 22401479.

3. Lanza di Scalea T, Hanusa BH, Wisner KL. Sexual function in postpartum women treated for depression: results from a randomized trial of nortriptyline versus sertraline. J Clin Psychiatry. 2009 Mar;70(3):423-8. PMID: 19284932.

4. Logsdon MC, Wisner K, Hanusa BH. Does maternal role functioning improve with antidepressant treatment in women with postpartum depression? J Womens Health (Larchmt). 2009 Jan-Feb;18(1):85-90. PMID: 19132881.

5. Misri S, Reebye P, Corral M, et al. The use of paroxetine and cognitive-behavioral therapy in postpartum depression and anxiety: a randomized controlled trial. J Clin Psychiatry. 2004 Sep;65(9):1236-41. PMID: 15367052.

6. Morrell CJ, Warner R, Slade P, et al. Psychological interventions for postnatal depression: cluster randomised trial and economic evaluation. The PoNDER trial. Health Technol Assess. 2009 1-153, 2009 Jun;13(30):iii-iv. PMID: 19555590.

7. Sharp DJ, Chew-Graham C, Tylee A, et al. A pragmatic randomised controlled trial to compare antidepressants with a community-based psychosocial intervention for the treatment of women with postnatal depression: the RESPOND trial. Health Technol Assess. 2010 1-153, 2010 Sep;14(43):iii-iv. PMID: 20860888.

8. Wan MW, Sharp DJ, Howard LM, et al. Attitudes and adjustment to the parental role in mothers following treatment for postnatal depression. J Affect Disord. 2011 Jun;131(1-3):284-92. PMID: 21349585.

9. Wisner KL, Hanusa BH, Perel JM, et al. Postpartum depression: a randomized trial of sertraline versus nortriptyline. J Clin Psychopharmacol. 2006 Aug;26(4):353-60. PMID: 16855451.

10. Yonkers KA, Lin H, Howell HB, et al. Pharmacologic treatment of postpartum women with new-onset major depressive disorder: a randomized controlled trial with paroxetine. J Clin Psychiatry. 2008 Apr;69(4):659-65. PMID: 18363420.

Appendix C. Excluded Studies

The following full text articles were reviewed for inclusion but failed to meet inclusion criteria for reasons specified below.

1: Foreign language, 2: ineligible outcome, 3: ineligible intervention, 4: ineligible population, 5: ineligible publication type, 6: ineligible study design, 8: outdated or ineligible systematic review.

Study	Exclusion Code
1. St John's wort and depression: slight efficacy at best, many drug interactions. Prescrire Int. 2004 Oct;13(73):187-92. PMID: 15499702.	5
2. Neonatal complications after intrauterine exposure to SSRI antidepressants. Prescrire Int. 2004 Jun;13(71):103-4. PMID: 15233148.	5
3. Bupropion (amfebutamone): caution during pregnancy. Prescrire Int. 2005 Dec;14(80):225. PMID: 16400747.	5
4. Prenatal exposure to mirtazapine and birth outcomes. 2006;8(10):5-. PMID: 2009312560. Language: English. Entry Date: 20080125. Publication Type: journal article. Journal Subset: Biomedical.	5
5. Teratogenicity of SSRI antidepressants: study 2. 2007;31(8):45-6. PMID: 2009641186. Language: English. Entry Date: 20071207. Revision Date: 20101022. Publication Type: journal article.	5
6. Selective serotonin reuptake inhibitors and birth defects. 2008;13(2):12-3. PMID: 2009951120. Language: English. Entry Date: 20080718. Publication Type: journal article.	5
7. Safety of SSRIs in pregnancy. Obstet Gynecol. 2009;113(5):1162-7.	5
8. Study: Both SSRI use and depression in pregnancy linked to risky birth outcomes. 2012;23(6):1-6. PMID: 2011552058. Language: English. Entry Date: 20120608. Revision Date: 20120608. Publication Type: journal article. Journal Subset: Biomedical.	5
9. Altamura AC, De Gaspari IF, Rovera C, et al. Safety of SSRIs during pregnancy: A controlled study. Hum Psychopharmacol. 2013;28(1):25-8. PMID: 23166037.	2
10. Ananth J. Congenital malformations with psychopharmacologic agents. Compr Psychiatry. 1975 Sep-Oct;16(5):437-45. PMID: 240643.	5
11. Andrade C. Selective serotonin reuptake inhibitors and persistent pulmonary hypertension of the newborn. J Clin Psychiatry. 2012 May;73(5):e601-5. PMID: 22697207.	5
12. Andrade SE, Raebel MA, Brown J, et al. Use of antidepressant medications during pregnancy: a multisite study. Am J Obstet Gynecol. 2008 Feb;198(2):194.e1-5. PMID: 17905176.	2
13. Appleby L, Koren G, Sharp D. Depression in pregnant and postnatal women: an evidence-based approach to treatment in primary care. Br J Gen Pract. 1999 Oct;49(447):780-2. PMID: 10885079.	5
14. Babu GN, Thippeswamy H, Chandra PS. Use of electroconvulsive therapy (ECT) in postpartum psychosis-a naturalistic prospective study. Arch Womens Ment Health. 2013 Apr 9;9:9. PMID: 23568390.	3
15. Bar-Oz B, Einarson T, Einarson A, et al. Paroxetine and congenital malformations: meta-Analysis and consideration of potential confounding factors. Clin Ther. 2007 May;29(5):918-26. PMID: 17697910.	8
16. Bellantuono C, Migliarese G, Gentile S. Serotonin reuptake inhibitors in pregnancy and the risk of major malformations: a systematic review. Hum Psychopharmacol. 2007 Apr;22(3):121-8. PMID: 17397101.	6

Study	Exclusion Code
17. Berard A. Paroxetine exposure during pregnancy and the risk of cardiac malformations: what is the evidence? Birth Defects Res Part A Clin Mol Teratol. 2010 Mar;88(3):171-4. PMID: 19950383.	5
18. Birnbaum CS, Cohen LS, Bailey JW, et al. Serum concentrations of antidepressants and benzodiazepines in nursing infants: A case series. Pediatrics. 1999 Jul;104(1):e11. PMID: 10390297.	5
19. Blier P. Pregnancy, depression, antidepressants and breast-feeding. J Psychiatry Neurosci. 2006 Jul;31(4):226-8. PMID: 16862240.	5
20. Bodnar LM, Sunder KR, Wisner KL. Treatment with selective serotonin reuptake inhibitors during pregnancy: deceleration of weight gain because of depression or drug?.[Erratum appears in Am J Psychiatry. 2006 Oct;163(10):1843]. Am J Psychiatry. 2006 Jun;163(6):986-91. PMID: 16741197.	5
21. Boucher N, Koren G, Beaulac-Baillargeon L. Maternal use of venlafaxine near term: correlation between neonatal effects and plasma concentrations. Ther Drug Monit. 2009 Jun;31(3):404-9. PMID: 19455083.	6
22. Bowen A, Bowen R, Butt P, et al. Patterns of depression and treatment in pregnant and postpartum women. Can J Psychiatry. 2012;57(3):161-7. PMID: 22398002.	6
23. Brandon AR. Ethical Barriers to Perinatal Mental Health Research and Evidence-Based Treatment: An Empirical Study. AJOB Prim Res. 2011 2011/01/01;2(1):2-12.	6
24. Bromley RL, Wieck A, Makarova D, et al. Fetal effects of selective serotonin reuptake inhibitor treatment during pregnancy: Immediate and longer term child outcomes. Fetal Matern Med Rev. 2012;23(3-4):230-75.	8
25. Brosh K, Matok I, Sheine E, et al. Teratogenic determinants of first- trimester exposure to antiepileptic medications. J Popul Ther Clin Pharmacol. 2011;18(1):e89-e98. PMID: 21467600.	3
26. Burns A, O'Mahen H, Baxter H, et al. A pilot randomised controlled trial of cognitive behavioural therapy for antenatal depression. BMC Psychiatry. 2013 Jan 22;13(1):33. PMID: 23339584.	3
27. Byatt N, Deligiannidis K, Freeman M. Antidepressant use in pregnancy: A critical review focused on risks and controversies. Acta Psychiatr Scand. 2013 Feb;127(2):94-114. PMID: Peer Reviewed Journal: 2013-00954-002.	6
28. Casper RC, Gilles AA, Fleisher BE, et al. Length of prenatal exposure to selective serotonin reuptake inhibitor (SSRI) antidepressants: effects on neonatal adaptation and psychomotor development. Psychopharmacology (Berl). 2011 Sep;217(2):211-9. PMID: 21499702.	6
29. Chaudron LH. Complex challenges in treating depression during pregnancy. Am J Psychiatry. 2013 Jan 1;170(1):12-20. doi: 10.1176/appi.ajp.2012.12040440. PMID: 23288385.	5
30. Cipriani A, Koesters M, Furukawa TA, et al. Duloxetine versus other anti-depressive agents for depression. Cochrane Database Syst Rev. 2012(10)PMID: 00075320-100000000-05164.	8
31. Cipriani A, Purgato M, Furukawa TA, et al. Citalopram versus other anti-depressive agents for depression. Cochrane Database Syst Rev. 2012(7)PMID: 00075320-100000000-05154.	8
32. Clementi M, Di Gianantonio E, Ornoy A. Teratology Information Services in Europe and Their Contribution to the Prevention of Congenital Anomalies. Public Health Genomics. 2002;5(1):8-12. PMID: 14960896.	5
33. Cohen LS, Altshuler LL, Harlow BL, et al. Relapse of major depression during pregnancy in women who maintain or discontinue antidepressant treatment.[Erratum appears in JAMA. 2006 Jul 12;296(2):170]. JAMA. 2006 Feb 1;295(5):499-507. PMID: 16449615.	4
34. Cohen LS, Altshuler LL, Stowe ZN, et al. Reintroduction of antidepressant therapy across pregnancy in women who previously discontinued treatment. A preliminary retrospective study. Psychother Psychosom. 2004 Jul-Aug;73(4):255-8. PMID: 15184721.	4

Study	Exclusion Code
35. Cohen LS, Heller VL, Bailey JW, et al. Birth outcomes following prenatal exposure to fluoxetine. Biol Psychiatry. 2000 Nov 15;48(10):996-1000. PMID: 11082474.	6
36. Cohen LS, Nonacs RM, Bailey JW, et al. Relapse of depression during pregnancy following antidepressant discontinuation: a preliminary prospective study. Arch Women Ment Health. 2004 Oct;7(4):217-21. PMID: 15338315.	4
37. Cohen LS, Rosenbaum JF. Birth outcomes in pregnant women taking fluoxetine. N Engl J Med. 1997 Mar 20;336(12):872; author reply 3. PMID: 9072682.	5
38. Cohen LS, Viguera AC, Bouffard SM, et al. Venlafaxine in the treatment of postpartum depression. J Clin Psychiatry. 2001 Aug;62(8):592-6. PMID: 11561929.	6
39. Condon J. Serotonergic symptoms in neonates exposed to SSRIs during pregnancy. Aust N Z J Psychiatry. 2003 Dec;37(6):777-8. PMID: 14636401.	5
40. Conlon O, Price J. A comparative study of pregnant women attending a tertiary obstetric unit and a district general hospital with a previous history of postnatal depression. J Obstet Gynaecol. 2006 Aug;26(6):514-7. PMID: 17000495.	2
41. Courtney K. Use of SSRIs in pregnancy: neonatal implications. Nurs Womens Health. 2009 Jun;13(3):234-8. PMID: 19523137.	5
42. Coverdale JH, McCullough LB, Chervenak FA. The ethics of randomized placebo-controlled trials of antidepressants with pregnant women: a systematic review. Obstet Gynecol. 2008 Dec;112(6):1361-8. PMID: 19037048.	6
43. D C. OPEN-LABEL TRIAL OF ESCITALOPRAM IN WOMEN WITH POSTPARTUM MOOD AND ANXIETY DISORDERS. Prim psychiatry. 2010;17(7):22-. PMID: 2011389039. Language: English. Entry Date: 20120106. Revision Date: 20120713. Publication Type: journal article.	5
44. Davis RL, Andrade S, Platt R. Risk of congenital malformations among infants exposed to antidepressants during pregnancy. Pharmacoepidemiol Drug Saf. 2008;17(4):423. PMID: 18383065.	5
45. Dennis C-LE, Stewart DE. Treatment of postpartum depression, part 1: a critical review of biological interventions. J Clin Psychiatry. 2004 Sep;65(9):1242-51. PMID: 15367053.	8
46. Desai G, Babu GN, Chandra PS. Unplanned pregnancies leading to psychotropic exposure in women with mental illness - Findings from a perinatal psychiatry clinic. Indian J Psychiatry. 2012;54(1):59-63. PMID: 22556440.	6
47. di Scalea TL, Wisner KL. Pharmacotherapy of postpartum depression. Expert Opin Pharmacother. 2009 Nov;10(16):2593-607. PMID: 19874247.	6
48. Dolk H, Jentink J, Loane M, et al. Does lamotrigine use in pregnancy increase orofacial cleft risk relative to other malformations? Neurology. 2008;71(10):714-22. PMID: 18650491.	3
49. Einarson A, Fatoye B, Sarkar M, et al. Pregnancy outcome following gestational exposure to venlafaxine: a multicenter prospective controlled study. Am J Psychiatry. 2001 Oct;158(10):1728-30. PMID: 11579012.	6
50. Einarson A, Koren G. New antidepressants in pregnancy. Can Fam Physician. 2004;50(FEB.):227-9. PMID: 15000332.	5
51. Einarson A, Pistelli A, DeSantis M, et al. Evaluation of the risk of congenital cardiovascular defects associated with use of paroxetine during pregnancy.[Erratum appears in Am J Psychiatry. 2008 Sep;165(9):1208], [Erratum appears in Am J Psychiatry. 2008 Jun;165(6):777]. Am J Psychiatry. 2008 Jun;165(6):749-52. PMID: 18381907.	6
52. Einarson TR, Einarson A. Newer antidepressants in pregnancy and rates of major malformations: a meta-analysis of prospective comparative studies. Pharmacoepidemiol Drug Saf. 2005 Dec;14(12):823-7. PMID: 15742359.	8

Study	Exclusion Code
53. Farr SL, Dietz PM, Rizzo JH, et al. Health care utilisation in the first year of life among infants of mothers with perinatal depression or anxiety. Paediatr Perinat Epidemiol. 2013;27(1):81-8.	3
54. Flynn HA, Blow FC, Marcus SM. Rates and predictors of depression treatment among pregnant women in hospital-affiliated obstetrics practices. Gen Hosp Psychiatry. 2006;28(4):289-95. PMID: 16814627.	2
55. Freeman MP. New data inform the risk/benefit analysis in antenatal depression. J Clin Psychiatry. 2007 Aug;68(8):1277-8. PMID: 17854253.	5
56. Freeman MP. Complementary and alternative medicine for perinatal depression. J Affect Disord. 2009;112(1-3):1-10. PMID: 18692251.	5
57. Galanti M, Jeffrey Newport D, Pennell PB, et al. Postpartum depression in women with epilepsy: Influence of antiepileptic drugs in a prospective study. Epilepsy Behav. 2009;16(3):426-30. PMID: 19854113.	3
58. Galbally M, Gentile S, Lewis AJ. Further findings linking SSRIs during pregnancy and persistent pulmonary hypertension of the newborn: Clinical implications. CNS Drugs. 2012;26(10):813-22. PMID: 22950489.	5
59. Gentile S. SSRIs in pregnancy and lactation: emphasis on neurodevelopmental outcome. CNS Drugs. 2005;19(7):623-33. PMID: 15984897.	5
60. Gentile S. The safety of newer antidepressants in pregnancy and breastfeeding. Drug Saf. 2005;28(2):137-52. PMID: 15691224.	5
61. Gentile S. Serotonin reuptake inhibitor-induced perinatal complications. Paediatr Drugs. 2007;9(2):97-106. PMID: 17407365.	5
62. Gentile S. On categorizing gestational, birth, and neonatal complications following late pregnancy exposure to antidepressants: the prenatal antidepressant exposure syndrome. CNS Spectr. 2010 Mar;15(3):167-85. PMID: 20414166.	6
63. Gentile S. Neonatal Withdrawal Reactions Following Late in Utero Exposure to Antidepressant Medications. Curr Womens Health Rev. 2011;7(1):18-27. PMID: 2011195182. Language: English. Entry Date: 20110729. Revision Date: 20120706. Publication Type: journal article.	6
64. Gentile S. Selective serotonin reuptake inhibitor exposure during early pregnancy and the risk of birth defects. Acta Psychiatr Scand. 2011 Apr;123(4):266-75. PMID: 21261600.	5
65. Gentile S, Bellantuono C. Selective serotonin reuptake inhibitor exposure during early pregnancy and the risk of fetal major malformations: focus on paroxetine. J Clin Psychiatry. 2009 Mar;70(3):414-22. PMID: 19254517.	5
66. Gentile S, Galbally M. Prenatal exposure to antidepressant medications and neurodevelopmental outcomes: a systematic review. J Affect Disord. 2011 Jan;128(1-2):1-9. PMID: 20303599.	5
67. Gjerdingen D. The effectiveness of various postpartum depression treatments and the impact of antidepressant drugs on nursing infants. J Am Board Fam Pract. 2003 Sep-Oct;16(5):372-82. PMID: 14645327.	5
68. Gold KJ, Marcus SM. Effect of maternal mental illness on pregnancy outcomes. Expert Rev Obstet Gynecol. 2008;3(3):391-401.	5
69. Goldfarb C, Keating G. Use of antidepressants from conception to delivery. J Med Soc N J. 1981 May;78(5):357-60. PMID: 6945438.	5
70. Goldstein DJ, Corbin LA, Sundell KL. Effects of first-trimester fluoxetine exposure on the newborn. Obstet Gynecol. 1997 May;89(5 Pt 1):713-8. PMID: 9166307.	6

Study	Exclusion Code
71. Grigoriadis S, VonderPorten EH, Mamisashvili L. Antidepressant Exposure During Pregnancy and Congenital Malformations: Is There an Association? A Systematic Review and Meta-Analysis of the Best Evidence. J Clin Psychiatry. 2013 April;74(4):e293-e308. PMID: 23656855.	8
72. Grigoriadis S, VonderPorten EH, Mamisashvili L. The Effect of Prenatal Antidepressant Exposure on Neonatal Adaptation: A Systematic Review and Meta-Analysis. J Clin Psychiatry. 2013 April;74(4):e309-e20. PMID: 23656856.	8
73. Grigoriadis S, VonderPorten EH, Mamisashvili L. The Impact of Maternal Depression During Pregnancy on Perinatal Outcomes: A Systematic Review and Meta-Analysis. J Clin Psychiatry. 2013 April;74(4):e321-e41. PMID: 23656857.	5
74. Grush LR, Cohen LS. Treatment of depression during pregnancy: balancing the risks. Harv Rev Psychiatry. 1998 Jul-Aug;6(2):105-9. PMID: 10370454.	5
75. Gunlicks ML, Weissman MM. Change in child psychopathology with improvement in parental depression: a systematic review. J Am Acad Child Adolesc Psychiatry. 2008 Apr;47(4):379-89. PMID: 18388766.	2
76. Haller E. Depression during and after pregnancy: what does the primary care physician need to know? 2005;5(1):21-6. PMID: 2005107077. Language: English. Entry Date: 20050715. Revision Date: 20090313. Publication Type: journal article.	5
77. Harrington RA, Lee LC, Crum RM, et al. Serotonin Hypothesis of Autism: Implications for Selective Serotonin Reuptake Inhibitor Use during Pregnancy. Autism Res. 2013;6(3):149-68. PMID: 23495208.	5
78. Hayes LJ, Goodman SH, Carlson E. Maternal antenatal depression and infant disorganized attachment at 12 months. Attach Hum Dev. 2013;15(2):133-53. PMID: 23216358.	3
79. Hemels MEH, Einarson A, Koren G, et al. Antidepressant use during pregnancy and the rates of spontaneous abortions: a meta-analysis. Ann Pharmacother. 2005 May;39(5):803-9. PMID: 15784808.	8
80. Hendrick V, Altshuler L. Management of major depression during pregnancy. Am J Psychiatry. 2002 Oct;159(10):1667-73. PMID: 12359670.	5
81. Hendrick V, Altshuler L, Strouse T, et al. Postpartum and nonpostpartum depression: differences in presentation and response to pharmacologic treatment. Depress Anxiety. 2000;11(2):66-72. PMID: 10812531.	4
82. Hendrick V, Smith LM, Hwang S, et al. Weight gain in breastfed infants of mothers taking antidepressant medications. J Clin Psychiatry. 2003 Apr;64(4):410-2. PMID: 12716242.	6
83. Hendrick V, Smith LM, Suri R, et al. Birth outcomes after prenatal exposure to antidepressant medication. Am J Obstet Gynecol. 2003 Mar;188(3):812-5. PMID: 12634662.	6
84. Highet N, Drummond P. A comparative evaluation of community treatments for post-partum depression: Implications for treatment and management practices. Aust N Z J Psychiatry. 2004;38(4):212-8. PMID: 15038799.	2
85. Hilli J, Heikkinen T, Rontu R, et al. MAO-A and COMT genotypes as possible regulators of perinatal serotonergic symptoms after in utero exposure to SSRIs. Eur Neuropsychopharmacol. 2009 May;19(5):363-70. PMID: 19223155.	6
86. Hoffbrand S, Howard L, Crawley H. Antidepressant treatment for post-natal depression. Nurs Times. 2001 Nov 8-14;97(45):35. PMID: 11966146.	5
87. Hoffbrand S, Howard L, Crawley H. Antidepressant drug treatment for postnatal depression. Cochrane Database Syst Rev. 2001(2):CD002018. PMID: 11406023.	8
88. Howard L. Postnatal depression. Clin Evid. 2004 Dec(12):2000-15. PMID: 15865767.	4
89. Howard L. Postnatal depression. Clin Evid. 2005 Dec(14):1764-75. PMID: 16620472.	8

Study	Exclusion Code
90. Howard L. Postnatal depression. Clin Evid. 2006 Jun(15):1919-31. PMID: 16973070.	6
91. Howard LM, Hoffbrand S, Henshaw C, et al. Antidepressant prevention of postnatal depression. Cochrane Database Syst Rev. 2005(2):CD004363. PMID: 15846711.	8
92. Huang H, Chan Y, Katon W, et al. Variations in depression care and outcomes among high-risk mothers from different racial/ethnic groups. Fam Pract. 2012;29(4):394-400. PMID: 22090192.	6
93. Hunter SK, Mendoza JH, D'Anna K, et al. Antidepressants may mitigate the effects of prenatal maternal anxiety on infant auditory sensory gating. Am J Psychiatry. 2012 Jun;169(6):616-24. PMID: 22581104.	2
94. Jermain DM. Treatment of postpartum depression. Am Pharm. 1995 Jan;NS35(1):33-8. PMID: 7887372.	5
95. Kellner CH, Pasculli RM, Briggs MC. Treatment of depression during pregnancy. J ECT. 2012;28(3):195-6. PMID: 22914631.	5
96. Kendall-Tackett K, Hale TW. The use of antidepressants in pregnant and breastfeeding women: a review of recent studies. J Hum Lact. 2010 May;26(2):187-95. PMID: 19652194.	8
97. Koke SC, Brown EB, Miner CM. Safety and efficacy of fluoxetine in patients who receive oral contraceptive therapy. Am J Obstet Gynecol. 2002;187(3):551-5. PMID: 12237626.	4
98. Koren G. ACP Journal Club. SSRIs in early pregnancy were associated with increased risk for septal heart defects but not major congenital malformations overall. Ann Intern Med. 2009;151(6):13-. PMID: 2010610620. Language: English. Entry Date: 20100430. Revision Date: 20100430. Publication Type: journal article.	5
99. Koren G. The effect of ascertainment bias in evaluating gestational antidepressant exposure. J Popul Ther Clin Pharmacol. 2011;18(1):e174-e5. PMID: 21471609.	5
100. Koren G. SSRIs and persistent pulmonary hypertension in newborns. 2012;23(5):7-8. PMID: 2011520008. Language: English. Entry Date: 20120504. Revision Date: 20120615. Publication Type: journal article. Journal Subset: Biomedical.	5
101. Koren G, Boucher N. Adverse effects in neonates exposed to SSRIs and SNRI in late gestation--Motherisk Update 2008. Can J Clin Pharmacol. 2009;16(1):e66-7. PMID: 19164848.	5
102. Koren G, Nordeng H. Antidepressant use during pregnancy: The benefit-risk ratio. Am J Obstet Gynecol. 2012;207(3):157-63. PMID: 22425404.	5
103. Koren G, Nordeng H. SSRIs and persistent pulmonary hypertension of the newborn: Observational evidence suggests a link, but causation is yet to be established. BMJ (Online). 2012;344(7842)PMID: 22240234.	6
104. Koren G, Nulman I, Addis A. Outcome of children exposed in utero to fluoxetine: a critical review. Depress Anxiety. 1998;8 Suppl 1:27-31. PMID: 9809211.	5
105. Krebs C. Depression in pregnancy. 2010;13(10):9. PMID: 2010920999. Language: English. Entry Date: 20110218. Publication Type: journal article.	5
106. Kwon P, Lefkowitz W. Neonatal extrapyramidal movements. Neonatal withdrawal due to maternal citalopram and ondansetron use. Pediatr Ann. 2008 Mar;37(3):128-30. PMID: 18411854.	5
107. Lewis JD, Schinnar R, Bilker WB, et al. Validation studies of the health improvement network (THIN) database for pharmacoepidemiology research. Pharmacoepidemiol Drug Saf. 2007;16(4):393-401. PMID: 17066486.	5
108. Logsdon MC, Wisner K, Hanusa BH, et al. Role functioning and symptom remission in women with postpartum depression after antidepressant treatment. Arch Psychiatr Nurs. 2003 Dec;17(6):276-83. PMID: 14685952.	3

Study	Exclusion Code
109. Lopez-Yarto M, Ruiz-Mirazo E, Holloway AC, et al. Do psychiatric medications, especially antidepressants, adversely impact maternal metabolic outcomes? J Affect Disord. 2012 Dec;141(2-3):120-9. PMID: Peer Reviewed Journal: 2012-05505-001.	8
110. Lorenzo L, Byers B, Einarson A. Antidepressant use in pregnancy. Expert Opin Drug Saf. 2011 Nov;10(6):883-9. PMID: 21545242.	5
111. Loughhead AM, Stowe ZN, Newport DJ, et al. Placental passage of tricyclic antidepressants. Biol Psychiatry. 2006 Feb 1;59(3):287-90. PMID: 16271264.	6
112. MacQueen GM, Ramakrishnan K, Ratnasingan R, et al. Desipramine treatment reduces the long-term behavioural and neurochemical sequelae of early-life maternal separation. Int J Neuropsychopharmacol. 2003;6(4):391-6. PMID: 14641986.	6
113. Malm H. Prenatal exposure to selective serotonin reuptake inhibitors and infant outcome. Ther Drug Monit. 2012;34(6):607-14. PMID: 23042258.	5
114. Malm H, Klaukka T, Neuvonen PJ. Risks associated with selective serotonin reuptake inhibitors in pregnancy. Obstet Gynecol. 2005 Dec;106(6):1289-96. PMID: 16319254.	4
115. Marcus SM, Flynn HA. Depression, antidepressant medication, and functioning outcomes among pregnant women. Int J Gynaecol Obstet. 2008 Mar;100(3):248-51. PMID: 18005968.	6
116. Misri S, Kendrick K. Treatment of perinatal mood and anxiety disorders: a review. Can J Psychiatry. 2007 Aug;52(8):489-98. PMID: 17955910.	6
117. Morrison JL, Riggs KW, Rurak DW. Fluoxetine during pregnancy: Impact on fetal development. Reprod Fertil Dev. 2005;17(6):641-50. PMID: 16263070.	5
118. Morrow AW. Imipramine and congenital abnormalities. N Z Med J. 1972 Apr;75(479):228-9. PMID: 4503545.	5
119. Moses-Kolko EL, Bogen D, Perel J, et al. Neonatal signs after late in utero exposure to serotonin reuptake inhibitors: literature review and implications for clinical applications. JAMA. 2005 May 18;293(19):2372-83. PMID: 15900008.	6
120. Murthy L, Shepperd S, Clarke MJ, et al. Interventions to improve the use of systematic reviews in decision-making by health system managers, policy makers and clinicians. Cochrane Database Syst Rev. 2012(9)PMID: 00075320-100000000-07759.	3
121. Myles N, Newall H, Ward H, et al. Systematic meta-analysis of individual selective serotonin reuptake inhibitor medications and congenital malformations. Aust N Z J Psychiatry. 2013 Nov;47(11):1002-12. doi: Epub 2013 Jun 12. PMID: 23761574.	8
122. Ng RC, Hirata CK, Yeung W, et al. Pharmacologic treatment for postpartum depression: a systematic review. Pharmacotherapy. 2010 Sep;30(9):928-41. PMID: 20795848.	6
123. No authorship i. Maternal SSRI Use Associated with Neurobehavioral Disruptions in Neonates. Prim psychiatry. 2004 Apr;11(4):14-5. PMID: Peer Reviewed Journal: 2004-95123-004.	4
124. No authorship i. Depression, SSRIs, and premature birth. Am J Psychiatry. 2009 May;166(5):A22. PMID: Peer Reviewed Journal: 2009-09562-001.	5
125. Oberlander TF, Grunau RE, Fitzgerald C, et al. Pain reactivity in 2-month-old infants after prenatal and postnatal serotonin reuptake inhibitor medication exposure. Pediatrics. 2005 Feb;115(2):411-25. PMID: 15687451.	2
126. O'Brien LA-M. Critical determinants of the risk-benefit assessment of antidepressants in pregnancy: Pharmacokinetic, safety and economic considerations. 2010;70(10-B):6133. PMID: Dissertation Abstract: 2010-99080-145.	2

Study	Exclusion Code
127. O'Mahen H, Himle JA, Fedock G, et al. A Pilot Randomized Controlled Trial of Cognitive Behavioral Therapy for Perinatal Depression Adapted for Women with Low Incomes. Depress Anxiety. 2013 Jan 14;14(10):22050. PMID: 23319454.	3
128. Oyebode F, Rastogi A, Berrisford G, et al. Psychotropics in pregnancy: safety and other considerations. Pharmacol Ther. 2012 Jul;135(1):71-7. PMID: 22483705.	6
129. Painuly N, Heun R, Painuly R, et al. Risk of cardiovascular malformations after exposure to paroxetine in pregnancy: meta-analysis. Psychiatrist. 2013 June 1, 2013;37(6):198-203.	8
130. Payne JL. Use of antidepressants in the second trimester is associated with reduced pregnancy duration, and third trimester antidepressant use with infant convulsions. Evid Based Nurs. 2013;16(3):74-5. PMID: 2012154183. Language: English. Entry Date: 20130705. Revision Date: 20130712. Publication Type: journal article.	6
131. Pupco A, Bozzo P, Koren G. Selective serotonin reuptake inhibitors and risk for major congenital anomalies. Obstet Gynecol. 2011;118(4):959-60. PMID: 21934468.	5
132. Rahimi R, Nikfar S, Abdollahi M. Pregnancy outcomes following exposure to serotonin reuptake inhibitors: a meta-analysis of clinical trials. Reprod Toxicol. 2006;22(4):571-5. PMID: 16720091.	6
133. Raudzus J, Misri S. Managing unipolar depression in pregnancy. Curr Opin Psychiatry. 2009 Jan;22(1):13-8. PMID: 19122529.	6
134. Reefhuis J, Rasmussen SA, Friedman JM. Selective serotonin-reuptake inhibitors and persistent pulmonary hypertension of the newborn. N Engl J Med. 2006 May 18;354(20):2188-90; author reply -90. PMID: 16707761.	5
135. Richards EM, Payne JL. The management of mood disorders in pregnancy: alternatives to antidepressants. CNS Spectr. 2013;FirstView:1-11. PMID: 23570692.	5
136. Ricke AK, Farrell CE, Chambers JE. The pharmacotherapy of perinatal mood disorders. Psychopharm Review. 2009;44(10):73-80.	5
137. Roca A, Garcia-Esteve L, Imaz ML, et al. Obstetrical and neonatal outcomes after prenatal exposure to selective serotonin reuptake inhibitors: the relevance of dose. J Affect Disord. 2011 Dec;135(1-3):208-15. PMID: 21890210.	6
138. Ross EL, Grigoriadis S, Mamisashvili L. Selected pregnancy and delivery outcomes after exposure to antidepressant medication: A systematic review and meta-analysis. JAMA Psychiatry. 2013:1-8. PMID: 23446732.	8
139. Ross LE, Grigoriadis S, Mamisashvili L, et al. Selected pregnancy and delivery outcomes after exposure to antidepressant medication: A systematic review and meta-analysis. JAMA Psychiatry. 2013;70(4):436-43. PMID: 23446732.	8
140. Ruchkin V, Martin A. SSRIs and the developing brain. Lancet. 2005 Feb 5-11;365(9458):451-3. PMID: 15705440.	5
141. Russell EJ, Fawcett JM, Mazmanian D. Risk of Obsessive-Compulsive Disorder in Pregnant and Postpartum Women: A Meta-Analysis. J Clin Psychiatry. 2013;74(4):377-85. PMID: 23656845.	3
142. Santone G, Ricchi G, Rocchetti D, et al. Is the exposure to antidepressant drugs in early pregnancy a risk factor for spontaneous abortion? A review of available evidences. Epidemiol Psichiatr Soc. 2009;18(3):240-7. PMID: 20034202.	6
143. Santos F, Sola I, Rigau D, et al. Quality assessment of clinical practice guidelines for the prescription of antidepressant drugs during pregnancy. Curr Clin Pharmacol. 2012 Feb 1;7(1):7-14. PMID: 22299765.	5

Study	Exclusion Code
144. Sanz EJ, De-las-Cuevas C, Kiuru A, et al. Selective serotonin reuptake inhibitors in pregnant women and neonatal withdrawal syndrome: a database analysis. Lancet. 2005 Feb 5-11;365(9458):482-7. PMID: 15705457.	6
145. Schroeder JW, Smith AK, Brennan PA, et al. DNA methylation in neonates born to women receiving psychiatric care. Epigenetics. 2012 Apr;7(4):409-14. PMID: 22419064.	2
146. Seifritz E, Holsboer-Trachsler E, Haberthur F, et al. Unrecognized pregnancy during citalopram treatment. Am J Psychiatry. 1993 Sep;150(9):1428-9. PMID: 8352360.	5
147. Shea AK, Kamath MV, Fleming A, et al. The effect of depression on heart rate variability during pregnancy. A naturalistic study. Clin Auton Res. 2008 Aug;18(4):203-12. PMID: 18592128.	3
148. Silvani P, Camporesi A. Drug-induced pulmonary hypertension in newborns: A review. Curr Vasc Pharmacol. 2007;5(2):129-33. PMID: 17430217.	5
149. Simoncelli M, Martin B-Z, Berard A. Antidepressant use during pregnancy: a critical systematic review of the literature. Curr Drug Saf. 2010 Apr;5(2):153-70. PMID: 19534639.	6
150. Sockol LE, Epperson CN, Barber JP. A meta-analysis of treatments for perinatal depression. Clin Psychol Rev. 2011 Jul;31(5):839-49. PMID: 21545782.	6
151. Sontheimer DL, Ables AZ. Safety of antidepressant medications during pregnancy. JAMA. 2000 Mar 1;283(9):1139. PMID: 10703770.	5
152. Speisman BB, Storch EA, Abramowitz JS. Postpartum obsessive-compulsive disorder. J Obstet Gynecol Neonatal Nurs. 2011 Nov-Dec;40(6):680-90. PMID: 22092284.	4
153. Steinberg SI, Bellavance F. Characteristics and treatment of women with antenatal and postpartum depression. Int J Psychiatry Med. 1999;29(2):209-33. PMID: 10587816.	2
154. Stewart DE. Are there special considerations in the prescription of serotonin reuptake inhibitors for women? Can J Psychiatry. 1998 Nov;43(9):900-4. PMID: 9825160.	5
155. Stowe ZN. The use of mood stabilizers during breastfeeding. J Clin Psychiatry. 2007;68(SUPPL. 9):22-8. PMID: 17764381.	5
156. Strom M, Mortensen EL, Halldorson TI, et al. Leisure-time physical activity in pregnancy and risk of postpartum depression: a prospective study in a large national birth cohort. J Clin Psychiatry. 2009 Dec;70(12):1707-14. PMID: 20141710.	2
157. Sunder KR, Wisner KL, Hanusa BH, et al. Postpartum depression recurrence versus discontinuation syndrome: observations from a randomized controlled trial. J Clin Psychiatry. 2004 Sep;65(9):1266-8. PMID: 15367055.	4
158. t Jong GW, Einarson T, Koren G, et al. Antidepressant use in pregnancy and persistent pulmonary hypertension of the newborn (PPHN): A systematic review. Reprod Toxicol. 2012;34(3):293-7. PMID: 22564982.	8
159. Ter Horst P, Smit J. Antidepressants during pregnancy and lactation. Tijdschr Psychiatr. 2009;51(5):307-14. PMID: Peer Reviewed Journal: 2011-28846-003.	1
160. Thompson BL, Levitt P, Stanwood GD. Prenatal exposure to drugs: effects on brain development and implications for policy and education. Nat Rev Neurosci. 2009 Apr;10(4):303-12. PMID: 19277053.	5
161. Thormahlen GM. Paroxetine use during pregnancy: is it safe? Ann Pharmacother. 2006 Oct;40(10):1834-7. PMID: 16926304.	5
162. Tuccori M, Montagnani S, Testi A, et al. Use of selective serotonin reuptake inhibitors during pregnancy and risk of major and cardiovascular malformations: an update. Postgrad Med. 2010 Jul;122(4):49-65. PMID: 20675971.	5

Study	Exclusion Code
163. Tuccori M, Testi A, Antonioli L, et al. Safety concerns associated with the use of serotonin reuptake inhibitors and other serotonergic/noradrenergic antidepressants during pregnancy: a review. Clin Ther. 2009 Jun;31 Pt 1:1426-53. PMID: 19698902.	5
164. Udechuku A, Nguyen T, Hill R, et al. Antidepressants in pregnancy: a systematic review. Aust N Z J Psychiatry. 2010 Nov;44(11):978-96. PMID: 21034181.	5
165. Ververs T, Kaasenbrood H, Visser G, et al. Prevalence and patterns of antidepressant drug use during pregnancy. Eur J Clin Pharmacol. 2006 Oct;62(10):863-70. PMID: 16896784.	2
166. Warburton W, Hertzman C, Oberlander TF. A register study of the impact of stopping third trimester selective serotonin reuptake inhibitor exposure on neonatal health. Acta Psychiatr Scand. 2010 Jun;121(6):471-9. PMID: 19878137.	6
167. Watanabe N, Omori IM, Nakagawa A, et al. Mirtazapine versus other antidepressive agents for depression. Cochrane Database Syst Rev. 2011(12)PMID: 00075320-100000000-05204.	8
168. Weikum WM, Oberlander TF, Hensch TK, et al. Prenatal exposure to antidepressants and depressed maternal mood alter trajectory of infant speech perception. Proc Natl Acad Sci U S A. 2012 Oct;109(Suppl 2):17221-7. PMID: Peer Reviewed Journal: 2012-28317-012.	5
169. Wenstrom KD. [Commentary on] Selective serotonin-reuptake inhibitors and risk of persistent pulmonary hypertension of the newborn. Obstet Gynecol Surv. 2006;61(6):370-1. PMID: 2009217667. Language: English. Entry Date: 20060929. Revision Date: 20070105. Publication Type: journal article.	5
170. Werler MM, Bower C, Payne J, et al. Findings on potential teratogens from a case-control study in Western Australia. Aust N Z J Obstet Gynaecol. 2003;43(6):443-7. PMID: 14712948.	3
171. Wisner KL, Gelenberg AJ, Leonard H, et al. Pharmacologic treatment of depression during pregnancy. JAMA. 1999 Oct 6;282(13):1264-9. PMID: 10517430.	6
172. Wisner KL, Perel JM, Peindl KS, et al. Prevention of postpartum depression: a pilot randomized clinical trial. Am J Psychiatry. 2004 Jul;161(7):1290-2. PMID: 15229064.	4
173. Wu J, Viguera A, Riley L, et al. Mood disturbance in pregnancy and the mode of delivery. Am J Obstet Gynecol. 2002;187(4):864-7. PMID: 12388965.	6
174. Wurst KE, Poole C, Ephross SA, et al. First trimester paroxetine use and the prevalence of congenital, specifically cardiac, defects: a meta-analysis of epidemiological studies. Birth Defects Res Part A Clin Mol Teratol. 2010 Mar;88(3):159-70. PMID: 19739149.	8
175. Yaris F, Ulku C, Kesim M, et al. Psychotropic drugs in pregnancy: A case-control study. Prog Neuropsychopharmacol Biol Psychiatry. 2005;29(2):333-8. PMID: 15694243.	1
176. Yonkers KA, Gotman N, Smith MV, et al. Does antidepressant use attenuate the risk of a major depressive episode in pregnancy? Epidemiology. 2011 Nov;22(6):848-54. PMID: 21900825.	4
177. Zeskind PS. [Commentary on] Maternal selective serotonin reuptake inhibitor use during pregnancy and newborn neurobehavior. Obstet Gynecol Surv. 2004;59(8):564-6. PMID: 2004161864. Language: English. Entry Date: 20041001. Publication Type: journal article.	5
178. Zhou S, Chan E, Pan SQ, et al. Pharmacokinetic interactions of drugs with St John's wort. J Psychopharmacol. 2004;18(2):262-76. PMID: 15260917.	5
179. Zuccotti GV, Fabiano V, Manfredini V. Neonates born to mothers using antidepressant drugs. Early Hum Dev. 2012;88(SUPPL.2):S84-S5. PMID: 22633523.	5

Appendix D. Strength of Evidence

Key Question 1a. Maternal and Child Benefits: Pharmacotherapy Compared With Placebo or No Treatment

Table 1. Fluoxetine compared with no treatment during pregnancy

Domains pertaining to strength of evidence					Magnitude of effect	Strength of evidence
Number of studies; Number of subjects	Methodological limitations	Consistency	Directness	Precision	Summary effect size (95% CI)	High, moderate, low, insufficient
Depression Symptomotology: Mean CES-D Score[1]						
1; N=46	High (1Observational/High)	Unknown	Direct	Unknown	Third trimester: 14.33 vs 25.93; P=0.0010	Insufficient

Table 2. SSRIs compared with no treatment during pregnancy

Domains pertaining to strength of evidence					Magnitude of effect	Strength of evidence
Number of studies; Number of subjects	Methodological limitations	Consistency	Directness	Precision	Summary effect size (95% CI)	High, moderate, low, insufficient
Functional capacity: SF-12 mental component score[2]						
1; N=62	Medium (1Observational/Medium)	Unknown	Direct	Unknown	45.2 vs 35.3, post-hoc Scheffé tests described as showing a significant difference, but results not reported	Insufficient
Preterm birth[3]						
2; N=266	Medium (1Observational/Medium)	Consistent	Direct	Imprecise	Unadjusted OR 1.87 (95% CI; 0.89-3.89)	Low
Infant/Child Development: Brazelton Neonatal Behavioral Assessment Scale[4]						
1; N=49	Medium (1Observational/Medium)	Unknown	Direct	Unknown	No significant differences on any summary scores for 7 major clusters	Insufficient

Table 3. Paroxetine compared with placebo during the postpartum period[5]

Number of studies; Number of subjects	Methodological Limitations	Consistency	Directness	Precision	Summary effect size (95% CI)	Strength of evidence (High, moderate, low, insufficient)
Danger to self						
1; N=70	High (RCT/High)	Unknown	Direct	Imprecise	No episodes	Insufficient
Danger to infant						
1; N=70	High (RCT/High)	Unknown	Direct	Imprecise	No episodes	Insufficient
Depression response[1]						
1; N=70	High (RCT/High)	Unknown	Direct	Imprecise	OR 1.31 (0.50-3.41)	Insufficient
Depression remission[2]						
1; N=70	High (RCT/High)	Unknown	Direct	Precise	OR 3.54 (1.10-11.41)	Insufficient
Breastfeeding						
NA	NA	NA	NA	NA	No evidence	Insufficient
Weight gain						
NA	NA	NA	NA	NA	No evidence	Insufficient

[1] Response at week 8 as measured by Clinical Global Impression-Improvement (CGI-I) of 1 or 2.
[2] Remission by week 8 as measured by the 17 Item Hamilton rating Scale for Depression (HAM-D-17) ≤ 8.

Key Question 1b. Maternal and Child Benefits: Pharmacological Treatments Compared With Each Other

Table 4. Sertraline compared with nortriptyline during the postpartum period

Number of studies; Number of subjects	Methodological Limitations	Consistency	Directness	Precision	Summary effect size (95% CI)	Strength of evidence (High, moderate, low, insufficient)
Depression response[1,6]						
1; N=109	High (RCT/High)	Unknown	Direct	Imprecise	Week 4: OR 0.79 (0.28-2.19)	Insufficient
				Imprecise	Week 8: OR 0.99 (0.29-3.42)	Insufficient
Depression remission[2,6]						
1; N=109	High (RCT/High)	Unknown	Direct	Imprecise	Week 4: OR 1.04 (0.41-2.65)	Insufficient
				Imprecise	Week 8: OR 1.75 (0.69-4.38)	Insufficient
Intention to Breastfeed						
	NA	NA	NA	NA	No evidence	Insufficient
Duration of Breastfeeding[3,7]						
1; N=70	High (RCT/High)	Unknown	Direct	Imprecise	Week 8: OR 2.78 (0.86-8.94)	Insufficient
Weight gain						
NA	NA	NA	NA	NA	No evidence	Insufficient

[1] Response is considered >= 50% reduction in Hamilton Rating Scale for Depression (HSRD).
[2] Remission is considered a Hamilton Rating Scale for Depression (HRDS) <7.
[3] Reported as breast feeding yes or no at 8th week of study.

Key Question 1d2. Maternal and Child Benefits: Pharmacological Treatments Plus Nonpharmacological Treatment Compared With Nonpharmacological Treatments Alone

Table 5. SSRIs plus psychotherapy compared with psychotherapy alone during pregnancy[8]

Domains pertaining to strength of evidence					Magnitude of effect	Strength of evidence
Number of studies; Number of subjects	Methodological limitations	Consistency	Directness	Precision	Summary effect size (95% CI)	High, moderate, low, insufficient
Depression Symptomotology: BDI maximum score[8]						
1; N=44	Medium (1Observational/Medium)	Unknown	Direct	Imprecise	21.3 vs 24.0; P=0.58	insufficient
Breastfeeding: Mean duration in months						
1; N=44	Medium (Observational/Medium)	Unknown	Direct	Imprecise	8.5 vs 6.4; P = 0.4	Insufficient

Table 6. Sertraline and brief dynamic psychotherapy compared with brief psychodynamic psychotherapy during the postpartum period[9]

Domains pertaining to strength of evidence					Magnitude of effect	Strength of evidence
Number of studies; Number of subjects	Methodological Limitations	Consistency	Directness	Precision	Summary effect size (95% CI)	High, moderate, low, insufficient
Depression response[1]						
1; N=40	Medium (RCT/Medium)	Unknown	Direct	Imprecise	Week 8: OR 1.91 (0.52-7.00)	Low
Depression remission[2]						
1; N=40	Medium (RCT/Medium)	Unknown	Direct	Imprecise	Week 8: OR 3.09 (0.78-12.14)	Low
				Imprecise	Week 12: OR 3.64 (0.34-39.02)	Low

[1] Response was defined as >50% reduction in MADRS or EPDS scores.
[2] Remission was considered as final score on the MADRS of <10 or the EPDS <7.

Table 7. Paroxetine plus cognitive behavioral therapy compared with cognitive behavioral therapy alone during the postpartum period[10]

Domains pertaining to strength of evidence					Magnitude of effect	Strength of evidence
Number of studies; Number of subjects	Methodological Limitations	Consistency	Directness	Precision	Summary effect size (95% CI)	High, moderate, low, insufficient
Depression response[1,2]:						
1; N=87	Medium (RCT/Medium)	NA	NA	NA	No evidence	Insufficient

Key Question 1d3. Maternal and Child Benefits: Comparing Pharmacological Treatments Alone With Pharmacological Treatments Used in Combination With Nonpharmacological Treatments

Table 8. Paroxetine compared with paroxetine plus cognitive behavioral therapy during the postpartum period[11]

Number of studies; Number of subjects	Domains pertaining to strength of evidence				Magnitude of effect	Strength of evidence
	Methodological Limitations	Consistency	Directness	Precision	Summary effect size (95% CI)	High, moderate, low, insufficient
Depression response[1,2]:						
1; N=35	Medium (RCT/Medium)	Unknown	Direct	Imprecise	HAM-D[1]: OR 1.87 (0.29-11.84)	Low
				Imprecise	EPDS[2]: OR 2.71 (0.73-10.04)	Low

[1] Response on Hamilton Rating Scale for Depression (HAM-D) (>= 50% score reduction).
[2] Response on Edinburgh Post Natal Depression Scale is (EDPS) (>= 50% score reduction).

Table 9. Sertraline compared with sertraline plus interpersonal psychotherapy during the postpartum period[12]

Number of studies; Number of subjects	Domains pertaining to strength of evidence				Magnitude of effect	Strength of evidence
	Methodological Limitations	Consistency	Directness	Precision	Summary effect size (95% CI)	High, moderate, low, insufficient
Depression response						
1; N=23	High (RCT/High)	Unknown	Direct	Imprecise	No significant differences *	Insufficient
Depression remission						
1; N=23	High (RCT/High)	Unknown	Direct	Imprecise	No significant differences *	Insufficient

* ANCOVA adjusted for pretreatment depression

Key Question 2a. Maternal and Child Harms: Pharmacotherapy Compared With Placebo or No Treatment

Table 10. SSRIs compared with no treatment during pregnancy

Number of studies; Number of subjects	Methodological limitations	Consistency	Directness	Precision	Magnitude of effect — Summary effect size (95% CI)	Strength of evidence — High, moderate, low, insufficient
Major malformations[2]						
1; N=72	Medium (1 Observational/Medium)	Unknown	Direct	Imprecise	No events	Insufficient
Convulsions[13]						
1; N=15,685	Medium (1 observational/Medium)	Unknown	Direct	Precise	0.14% vs 0.11%; RD 0.0005; 95% CI, -0.0015 to 0.0025)	Low
Respiratory Distress[2, 8, 13]						
3; N=15,793	Medium (3 observational/Medium)	Consistent	Direct	Precise	Pooled unadjusted OR 1.91 (95% CI, 1.63 to 2.24)	Low

Table 11. Bupropion compared with no treatment during pregnancy

Number of studies; Number of subjects	Methodological limitations	Consistency	Directness	Precision	Magnitude of effect — Summary effect size (95% CI)	Strength of evidence — High, moderate, low, insufficient
Major malformations[14]						
1; N=126	High (1 Observational/ High)	Unknown	Direct	Imprecise	No events	Insufficient

Key Question 2b. Maternal and Child Harms: Pharmacological Treatments Compared With Each Other

Table 12. SSRIs compared with TCAs (nortriptyline) during pregnancy

Number of studies; Number of subjects	Methodological limitations	Consistency	Directness	Precision	Magnitude of effect — Summary effect size (95% CI)	Strength of evidence — High, moderate, low, insufficient
Respiratory Distress[15]						
1; N=21	Medium (1 Observational/Medium)	Unknown	Direct	Imprecise	10% vs 0%; P not reported	Insufficient

Table 13. SSRIs compared with SSRIs during pregnancy

Number of studies; Number of subjects	Domains pertaining to strength of evidence				Magnitude of effect	Strength of evidence
	Methodological limitations	Consistency	Directness	Precision	Summary effect size (95% CI)	High, moderate, low, insufficient
Respiratory Distress[15]						
1; N=20	Medium (1Observational/Medium)	Unknown	Direct	Imprecise	22% vs 0%, P=NR	Insufficient

Table 14. Sertraline compared with nortriptyline during the postpartum period[6]

Number of studies; Number of subjects	Domains pertaining to strength of evidence				Magnitude of effect	Strength of evidence
	Methodological limitations	Consistency	Directness	Precision	Summary effect size (95% CI)	High, moderate, low, insufficient
Overall adverse events and withdrawals due to adverse events						
1; N=109	High (1Observational/High)	Unknown	Direct	Imprecise	No events	Insufficient

Key Question 2d2. Maternal and Child Harms: Pharmacological Treatments Plus Nonpharmacological Treatment Compared With Nonpharmacological Treatments Alone

Table 15. SSRIs plus psychotherapy compared with psychotherapy alone during pregnancy[8]

Number of studies; Number of subjects	Domains pertaining to strength of evidence				Magnitude of effect	Strength of evidence
	Methodological limitations	Consistency	Directness	Precision	Summary effect size (95% CI)	High, moderate, low, insufficient
Major malformations						
1; N=44	Medium (Observational/Medium)	Unknown	Direct	Imprecise	Unadjusted OR 0.40; 95% CI, 0.02 to 6.93	Insufficient

Table 16. Sertraline and brief dynamic psychotherapy compared with brief psychodynamic psychotherapy during the postpartum period[9]

Number of studies; Number of subjects	Domains pertaining to strength of evidence				Magnitude of effect	Strength of evidence
	Methodological Limitations	Consistency	Directness	Precision	Summary effect size (95% CI)	High, moderate, low, insufficient
% Discontinuing due to adverse events						
1; N=40	Medium (RCT/Medium)	Unknown	Direct	Precise	OR 5.54 (0.25-123.09)	Insufficient

Table 17. Fluoxetine plus cognitive behavioral therapy compared with cognitive behavioral therapy alone during the postpartum period[10]

	Domains pertaining to strength of evidence				Magnitude of effect	Strength of evidence
Number of studies; Number of subjects	Methodological Limitations	Consistency	Directness	Precision	Summary effect size (95% CI)	High, moderate, low, insufficient
% Discontinuing due to adverse events						
1; N=87	Medium (RCT/Medium)	Unknown	Direct	Imprecise	1 session: 0% vs 9%; *P* not reported 6 sessions: 5% vs 5%; *P* not reported	Insufficient

Table 18. Sertraline plus interpersonal therapy compared with interpersonal therapy alone during the postpartum period[12]

	Domains pertaining to strength of evidence				Magnitude of effect	Strength of evidence
Number of studies; Number of subjects	Methodological Limitations	Consistency	Directness	Precision	Summary effect size (95% CI)	High, moderate, low, insufficient
% Discontinuing due to adverse events						
1; N=23	High (RCT/High)	Unknown	Direct	Imprecise	No events	Insufficient

Key Question 2d3. Maternal and Child Harms: Pharmacological Treatments Alone Compared With Pharmacological Treatments Plus Nonpharmacological Treatments

Table 19. Sertraline alone compared with sertraline plus interpersonal therapy during the postpartum period[12]

	Domains pertaining to strength of evidence				Magnitude of effect	Strength of evidence
Number of studies; Number of subjects	Methodological Limitations	Consistency	Directness	Precision	Summary effect size (95% CI)	High, moderate, low, insufficient
Overall adverse events						
1; N=23	High (RCT/High)	Unknown	Direct	Imprecise	No events	Insufficient

Appendix D References

1. Suri R, Altshuler L, Hendrick V, et al. The impact of depression and fluoxetine treatment on obstetrical outcome. Archives of Women's Mental Health. 2004 Jul;7(3):193-200. PMID: 15241665.

2. Wisner KL, Sit DKY, Hanusa BH, et al. Major depression and antidepressant treatment: impact on pregnancy and neonatal outcomes. American Journal of Psychiatry. 2009 May;166(5):557-66. PMID: 19289451.

3. Yonkers KA, Norwitz ER, Smith MV, et al. Depression and serotonin reuptake inhibitor treatment as risk factors for preterm birth. Epidemiology. 2012;23(5):677-85.

4. Suri R, Hellemann G, Stowe ZN, et al. A prospective, naturalistic, blinded study of early neurobehavioral outcomes for infants following prenatal antidepressant exposure. Journal of Clinical Psychiatry. 2011 Jul;72(7):1002-7. PMID: 21672498.

5. Yonkers KA, Lin H, Howell HB, et al. Pharmacologic treatment of postpartum women with new-onset major depressive disorder: a randomized controlled trial with paroxetine. Journal of Clinical Psychiatry. 2008 Apr;69(4):659-65. PMID: 18363420.

6. Wisner KL, Hanusa BH, Perel JM, et al. Postpartum depression: a randomized trial of sertraline versus nortriptyline. Journal of Clinical Psychopharmacology. 2006 Aug;26(4):353-60. PMID: 16855451.

7. Lanza di Scalea T, Hanusa BH, Wisner KL. Sexual function in postpartum women treated for depression: results from a randomized trial of nortriptyline versus sertraline. Journal of Clinical Psychiatry. 2009 Mar;70(3):423-8. PMID: 19284932.

8. Casper RC, Fleisher BE, Lee-Ancajas JC, et al. Follow-up of children of depressed mothers exposed or not exposed to antidepressant drugs during pregnancy. Journal of Pediatrics. 2003 Apr;142(4):402-8. PMID: 12712058.

9. Bloch M, Meiboom H, Lorberblatt M, et al. The effect of sertraline add-on to brief dynamic psychotherapy for the treatment of postpartum depression: a randomized, double-blind, placebo-controlled study. Journal of Clinical Psychiatry. 2012 Feb;73(2):235-41. PMID: 22401479.

10. Appleby L, Warner R, Whitton A, et al. A controlled study of fluoxetine and cognitive-behavioural counselling in the treatment of postnatal depression. BMJ. 1997 Mar 29;314(7085):932-6. PMID: 9099116.

11. Misri S, Reebye P, Corral M, et al. The use of paroxetine and cognitive-behavioral therapy in postpartum depression and anxiety: a randomized controlled trial. Journal of Clinical Psychiatry. 2004 Sep;65(9):1236-41. PMID: 15367052.

12. Pearlstein TB, Zlotnick C, Battle CL, et al. Patient choice of treatment for postpartum depression: a pilot study. Archives of Women's Mental Health. 2006 Nov;9(6):303-8. PMID: 16932988.

13. Oberlander TF, Warburton W, Misri S, et al. Neonatal outcomes after prenatal exposure to selective serotonin reuptake inhibitor antidepressants and maternal depression using population-based linked health data. Archives of General Psychiatry. 2006 Aug;63(8):898-906. PMID: 16894066.

14. Bakker MK, Jentink J, Vroom F, et al. Drug prescription patterns before, during and after pregnancy for chronic, occasional and pregnancy-related drugs in the Netherlands. BJOG: An International Journal of Obstetrics and Gynaecology. 2006;113(5):559-68.

15. Sit D, Perel JM, Wisniewski SR, et al. Mother-infant antidepressant concentrations, maternal depression, and perinatal events. Journal of Clinical Psychiatry. 2011 Jul;72(7):994-1001. PMID: 21824458.

Appendix E. Evidence Tables

Evidence Table 1. Data abstraction of observational studies

Author Year Country Study Design/Data Source Risk of Bias	Population Characteristics 1. Race % Mean Age Socioeconomic Status Home Situation Unplanned Pregnancy % Marital/Partner Status Smoking % ETOH Substance Abuse %	2. Mental Health Comorbidities % Use of Other Psychoactive Drugs % Provider Characteristics Medical Care Environment	3. Depression Characteristics: - Percent with Diagnosis - Family History of Depressive/Mood Disorders (%) - Prior Use of Antidepressive Drugs (%, for Treatment or Prevention) - Symptom Severity - Time of Diagnosis - Diagnosis Method - When Treatment Commenced Relative to the Onset of Symptoms
Alwan 2007[1] US Arm of Case Control Studied, Population based Medium	Race: W: 60.5%; AA: 11%, Hisp 23%, other 5.5%. Age: <35y: 84%/>35y: 15%. Income: 20K: 32%/20-4999: 32.5%/ >50K: 35% Home: NR; Planned Pregnancy: NR; Partner NR	Mental health comorbidities: NR Other meds: 1% Provider characteristics: NR; Medical care environment: NR	% Dx: NR; Fam Hx NR; Prior use: NR; Sx Severity NR; Time of Dx NR; Dx method: NR. Tx began: before pregnancy/during pregnancy.
Alwan 2010[2] Canada Case-control/Data Source [CC] Medium	(cases vs. controls) Race 60% vs. 60% White, 39.4% vs. 39.7% Other Age: <35 years 84.7% vs. 86.1% >35 year 15.3% vs. 13.9% Socio economic status: Education <12 years 44.8% vs. 41.9% 1>2 years 55.2% vs. 58.1% Income: <$20,000 33.9% vs. 32.0% > $20,000 66.1% vs. 68.0% Home situation: NR Unplanned pregnancy % Marital/partner status: NR Smoking% ETOH: 37% vs. 37% Substance abuse: NR	Mental health Comorbidities NR Use of other psychoactive drugs NR Provider characteristics (primary care physician, obstetrician, psychiatrist, nurse, midwife, community worker, or pediatrician visits) Medical care environment (community/private/public clinic or hospital)	100% with diagnosis (exposed) Family history of depressive/mood disorders: NR Prior use of antidepressive drugs: NR Symptom severity: NR Time of diagnosis: NR Diagnosis method: NR
Andrade 2009[3] US Retrospective Cohort/Data Source [AD] Medium	Major: 1.51 (1.21-1.87)/0.69 (0.34-1.4)/1.18 (0.86-1.61)/1.25 (0.84-1.85)/1.41 (1.03-1.92)	Mental health Comorbidities: NR Use of other psychoactive drugs: NR Provider characteristics: NR Medical care environment: Hospital	% with diagnosis NR Family history of depressive/mood disorders: NR Prior use of antidepressive drugs (%, for treatment or prevention) NR Symptom severity: NR Time of diagnosis: NR Diagnosis method: NR

E-1

Author Year Country Study Design/Data Source Risk of Bias	Population Characteristics		
	1. Race % Mean Age Socioeconomic Status Home Situation Unplanned Pregnancy % Marital/Partner Status Smoking % ETOH Substance Abuse %	2. Mental Health Comorbidities % Use of Other Psychoactive Drugs % Provider Characteristics Medical Care Environment	3. Depression Characteristics: - Percent with Diagnosis - Family History of Depressive/Mood Disorders (%) - Prior Use of Antidepressive Drugs (%, for Treatment or Prevention) - Symptom Severity - Time of Diagnosis - Diagnosis Method - When Treatment Commenced Relative to the Onset of Symptoms
Bakker 2010[4] CC/PBD The Netherlands Medium	Race %: NR Mean Age: 30.3 Socio economic status: NR Home situation: NR Unplanned pregnancy %: NR Marital/partner status (S/M/D): NR Smoking %: 25.2% ETOH: NR Illicit Drug Use: NR	NR	NR
Bakker 2010[5] The Netherlands Case-Control Medium	Race: NR Mean Age: 31 years SES: NR Home situation: NR Unplanned pregnancy: NR Marital/partner status: NR	NR	NR
Ban 2012[6] U.K. PBD Medium	Race: NR Age: 15-17: 2.0%, 18-24: 21.4%, 25-34: 55%, 35-45: 21.6% SES: Townsend deprivation index score-1(least deprived): 22.8%, 2: 18.9%, 3:19.6%, 4: 19.0%, 5: 14.5% Home situation: NR Unplanned pregnancy: NR Marital/partner status: NR Maternal history of smoking: 40.6%	Provider characteristics: Primary care Other: NR	NR
Batton 2013[7] USA PD Medium	Race: 95% white Mean Age: 28 yrs Low socio economic status: NR Home situation: NR Unplanned pregnancy: NR Marital/partner status: NR Smoking%: NR ETOH%: NR Substance abuse%: NR	Mental health Comorbidities: NR Use of other psychoactive drugs: NR Provider characteristics: NR Medical care environment: NR	% with diagnosis: NR Family history of depressive/mood disorders (%) : NR Prior use of antidepressive drugs (%, for treatment or prevention): NR Symptom severity: NR Time of diagnosis: NR Diagnosis method: NR When treatment commenced relative to the onset of symptoms: NR

Author Year Country Study Design/Data Source Risk of Bias	Population Characteristics		
	1. Race % Mean Age Socioeconomic Status Home Situation Unplanned Pregnancy % Marital/Partner Status Smoking % ETOH Substance Abuse %	2. Mental Health Comorbidities % Use of Other Psychoactive Drugs % Provider Characteristics Medical Care Environment	3. Depression Characteristics: - Percent with Diagnosis - Family History of Depressive/Mood Disorders (%) - Prior Use of Antidepressive Drugs (%, for Treatment or Prevention) - Symptom Severity - Time of Diagnosis - Diagnosis Method - When Treatment Commenced Relative to the Onset of Symptoms
Berard 2007[8] Canada, Quebec LD Medium	Race % (white, AA, Hispanic, Asian, Other): NR Mean Age: 29.29 Socio economic status: Welfare Beneficiaries in year before pregnancy: 49.1% Home situation: Living alone in year before pregnancy: 69.3% Unplanned pregnancy %: NR Marital/partner status (S/M/D): NR Smoking%: NR ETOH: NR Substance abuse%: NR	Mental health Comorbidities % (e.g. anxiety) : NR Use of other psychoactive drugs % (antipsychotics, antianxiety agents (e.g., benzodiazepines), and drugs for insomnia): NR Provider characteristics (primary care physician, obstetrician, psychiatrist, nurse, midwife, community worker, or pediatrician visits): NR Medical care environment (community/private/public clinic or hospital): NR	Depression Characteristics: -% with diagnosis: 52.1% -Family history of depressive/mood disorders (%) : NR -Prior use of antidepressive drugs (%, for treatment or prevention) :NR -Symptom severity : NR -Time of diagnosis: NR -Diagnosis method : NR -When treatment commenced relative to the onset of symptoms: NR
Bogen 2010/companion Wen 2009[9] US PC Medium	Race % : White/Other: 79.2%, African American: 20.8% Age:<31: 50.6%, ≥31: 49.4% SES: NR Home situation: NR Unplanned pregnancy %: NR Marital/partner status (S/M/D):Married (or living as married): Yes:72.6%, No 27.4% Smoking%: 13.1%, ETOH: NR Substance abuse%: NR	Mental health comorbidities: NR Use of other psychoactive drugs: NR Provider characteristics: Obstetrician, community worker	% with diagnosis: of MDD: 23%, % of patients with 1 episode of MDD: 30% Mean HDRS score: 13.28 (SD 4.4) Others: NR
Boucher 2008[10] Canada LD Medium	Race: NR Mean Age: 29.5 Socio economic status: NR Home situation: NR Unplanned pregnancy: NR Marital/partner status: NR Smoking: 22.5% ETOH: 3% (occasional) Substance abuse: NR	Mental health comorbidities: NR Use of other psychoactive drugs: olanzapine (n=2), risperidone (n=2), alprazolam (n=3), bromazepam (n=1), clonazepam (n=7), lorazepam (n=4), Provider characteristics: NR Medical care environment: Secondary and tertiary care facilities hospital	NR

	Population Characteristics		3. Depression Characteristics:
Author Year Country Study Design/Data Source Risk of Bias	1. Race % Mean Age Socioeconomic Status Home Situation Unplanned Pregnancy % Marital/Partner Status Smoking % ETOH Substance Abuse %	2. Mental Health Comorbidities % Use of Other Psychoactive Drugs % Provider Characteristics Medical Care Environment	- Percent with Diagnosis - Family History of Depressive/Mood Disorders (%) - Prior Use of Antidepressive Drugs (%, for Treatment or Prevention) - Symptom Severity - Time of Diagnosis - Diagnosis Method - When Treatment Commenced Relative to the Onset of Symptoms
Casper 2003[11] US Cohort study Data/Source: [CC] Medium	Individual SSRIs: citalopram/escitalopram/fluoxetine/paroxetine/sertraline	Use of other psychoactive drugs: NR Provider characteristics: primary care and/or psychiatrist Medical care environment: public clinic	100% with diagnosis Family history of depressive/mood disorders: NR Prior use of antidepressive drugs: NR Symptom severity: (Likert scale, mean) exp vs. unexp: 1–3 months 4.2 (2.5) vs. 5.0 (2.5) 4–6 months 5.4 (3.2) vs. 5.0 (2.8) 7–9 months 6.1 (2.3) vs. 4.8 (3.0) Time of diagnosis: During pregnancy Diagnosis method: NR
Chambers 1996[12] US CC Medium	Race % (white, AA, Hispanic, Asian, Other): NR Mean Age: 30.87 Socio economic status: NR Home situation: NR Unplanned pregnancy %: NR Marital/partner status (S/M/D): NR Smoking%: Exposed early group: 10%, Exposed late group: 17.8%, Controls, 3.8% ETOH: Exposed early group: 5.0%, Exposed late group: 1.5%, controls: 0.0% Substance abuse%: <1%	Mental Health Comorbidities % (e.g. anxiety) : Anxiety 8.1%, panic disorder 6.4%, bipolar disorder 5.8%, obsessive-compulsive disorder 4.0% Use of other psychoactive drugs % (antipsychotics, antianxiety agents (e.g., benzodiazepines), and drugs for insomnia): benzodiazepine: 17.5%, trazodone: 5.2%, tricyclic 5.2% Provider characteristics (primary care physician, obstetrician, psychiatrist, nurse, midwife, community worker, or pediatrician visits): NR Medical care environment (community/private/public clinic or hospital): hospital	Depression Characteristics: -% with diagnosis: NR -Family history of depressive/mood disorders (%) : NR -Prior use of antidepressive drugs (%, for treatment or prevention): NR -Symptom severity: NR -Time of diagnosis: NR -Diagnosis method: NR -When treatment commenced relative to the onset of symptoms: NR

Author Year Country Study Design/Data Source Risk of Bias	Population Characteristics 1. Race % Mean Age Socioeconomic Status Home Situation Unplanned Pregnancy % Marital/Partner Status Smoking % ETOH Substance Abuse %	2. Mental Health Comorbidities % Use of Other Psychoactive Drugs % Provider Characteristics Medical Care Environment	3. Depression Characteristics: - Percent with Diagnosis - Family History of Depressive/Mood Disorders (%) - Prior Use of Antidepressive Drugs (%, for Treatment or Prevention) - Symptom Severity - Time of Diagnosis - Diagnosis Method - When Treatment Commenced Relative to the Onset of Symptoms
Chambers 2006[13] US CC Medium	Race: 68.2% white, 11.8% black, 6% Asian, 11.2% Hispanic, 2.8% other Mean Age: <25: 25.3%, 25-30: 28.4%, 30-35: 30.8%, >35: 15.5% Socio economic status (education): <13 years: 29.5%, 13-15 years: 28.1%, >15 years: 42.1% Home situation: NR Unplanned pregnancy: NR Marital/partner status: NR Smoking: Never: 59.3%, before pregnancy: 45.9%, during pregnancy: 16.7% ETOH: Never: 51.7%, before pregnancy: 23.9%, during pregnancy: 2.4% Substance abuse: NR	Mental health comorbidities: NR Use of other psychoactive drugs: NR Provider characteristics: Neonatologists Medical care environment: NICU	NR
Cole 2007[14] US Case-control/Data Source[AD] Medium	Race NR Mean Age: 31 years Socio economic status: NR Home situation: NR Unplanned pregnancy: NR Marital/partner status: NR Smoking: NR ETOH: NR Substance abuse: NR	Mental health Comorbidities: (Monotherapy exposed vs. other Mono- or Polytherapy exposed vs. other) Bipolar disorder 1.0 vs. 0.7 vs. 1.0 vs. 0.8 Use of other psychoactive drugs: Carbamazepine: 0% vs. 0.2% vs. 0.1 vs. 0.2% Provider characteristics: physician Medical care environment: NR	% with diagnosis Family history of depressive/mood disorders: NR Prior use of antidepressant drug: Women received sertraline before pregnancy, but prescription did not overlap with the first trimester Symptom severity: NR Time of diagnosis: NR Diagnosis method: NR
Cole 2007[15] US LD Low	Age: 12-19: 1.5%, 20-24: 9.0%, 25-29: 28.1%, 30-34: 35.7%, 35-39: 20.4%, 40-49: 5.1% Other characteristics NR	Mental health comorbidities: NR Use of other psychoactive drugs: NR Provider characteristics: NR Medical care environment: NR	NR
Colvin 2012[16] PBD/CC Australia Medium	(Exposed vs. Unexposed) Race 92% vs. 84% white Mean Age: 30 vs. 29 years Socio economic status: NR Home situation: NR Unplanned pregnancy: NR Marital/partner status: NR Smoking: 27% vs. 16% ETOH: NR Substance abuse: NR	Mental health Comorbidities NR Use of other psychoactive drugs % Provider characteristics: midwife, primary care Medical care environment: NR	% with diagnosis Family history of depressive/mood disorders: NR Prior use of antidepressive drugs (%, for treatment or prevention): NR Symptom severity: NR Time of diagnosis: NR Diagnosis method: NR

Author Year Country Study Design/Data Source Risk of Bias	Population Characteristics		
	1. Race % Mean Age Socioeconomic Status Home Situation Unplanned Pregnancy % Marital/Partner Status Smoking % ETOH Substance Abuse %	2. Mental Health Comorbidities % Use of Other Psychoactive Drugs % Provider Characteristics Medical Care Environment	3. Depression Characteristics: - Percent with Diagnosis - Family History of Depressive/Mood Disorders (%) - Prior Use of Antidepressive Drugs (%, for Treatment or Prevention) - Symptom Severity - Time of Diagnosis - Diagnosis Method - When Treatment Commenced Relative to the Onset of Symptoms
Colvin 2012[16] PBD/CC Australia Medium	Race % : NR Mean Age: 30.05 Socio economic status: SEIFA = 997.1 Home situation: NR Unplanned pregnancy %: NR Marital/partner status (S/M/D): NR	NR	NR
Croen 2011[17] US CC Medium	Race % (white, AA, Hispanic, Asian, Other): White, non-Hispanic: 47.8%; White, Hispanic: 19.2%; Black: 9.9%; Asian: 9.8%; Other: 13.3% Mean Age: 30.42 Socio economic status: Education: <high school: 6.9%; high school: 25.4%; college: 51.0%; postgraduate: 15.5%; Unknown: 1.2% Home situation: NR Unplanned pregnancy %: NR Marital/partner status (S/M/D): NR Smoking%: NR ETOH: NR Substance abuse%: NR	NR	Depression Characteristics: 3.4% with diagnosis Others:NR
Davidson 2009[18] Israel CC Medium	Race % (white, AA, Hispanic, Asian, Other): NR Mean Age: 29.71 Socio economic status: NR Home situation: NR Unplanned pregnancy %: NR Marital/partner status (S/M/D): NR Smoking%: NSD between groups ETOH: 0% Substance abuse%: NR	Mental health Comorbidities % (e.g. anxiety) : NR Use of other psychoactive drugs % (antipsychotics, antianxiety agents (e.g., benzodiazepines), and drugs for insomnia): NR Provider characteristics (primary care physician, obstetrician, psychiatrist, nurse, midwife, community worker, or pediatrician visits): NR Medical care environment (community/private/public clinic or hospital): hospital	Depression Characteristics: -% with diagnosis: NR -Family history of depressive/mood disorders (%) : NR -Prior use of antidepressive drugs (%, for treatment or prevention): NR -Symptom severity: NR -Time of diagnosis: NR -Diagnosis method: NR -When treatment commenced relative to the onset of symptoms: NR

Author Year Country Study Design/Data Source Risk of Bias	Population Characteristics 1. Race % Mean Age Socioeconomic Status Home Situation Unplanned Pregnancy % Marital/Partner Status Smoking % ETOH Substance Abuse %	2. Mental Health Comorbidities % Use of Other Psychoactive Drugs % Provider Characteristics Medical Care Environment	3. Depression Characteristics: - Percent with Diagnosis - Family History of Depressive/Mood Disorders (%) - Prior Use of Antidepressive Drugs (%, for Treatment or Prevention) - Symptom Severity - Time of Diagnosis - Diagnosis Method - When Treatment Commenced Relative to the Onset of Symptoms
Davis 2007[19] US LD Medium	Race % (white, AA, Hispanic, Asian, Other): NR Mean Age: NR Socio economic status: NR Home situation: NR Unplanned pregnancy %: NR Marital/partner status (S/M/D): NR Smoking%: NR ETOH: NR Substance abuse%: NR	Mental health Comorbidities % (e.g. anxiety) : NR Use of other psychoactive drugs % (antipsychotics, antianxiety agents (e.g., benzodiazepines), and drugs for insomnia): NR Provider characteristics (PCP, obstetrician, psychiatrist, nurse, midwife, community worker, or pediatrician visits): NR Medical care environment (community/private/public clinic or hospital): hospital	Depression Characteristics: -% with diagnosis: NR -Family history of depressive/mood disorders (%) : NR -Prior use of antidepressive drugs (%, for treatment or prevention): NR -Symptom severity : NR -Time of diagnosis: NR -Diagnosis method : NR –When treatment commenced relative to the onset of symptoms: NR
De Vries 2013[20] Australia PC Medium	Race: NR Mean Age: 31 Low socio economic status: NR Home situation: NR Unplanned pregnancy: NR Marital/partner status: NR Smoking%: 19% ETOH%: 5% Substance abuse%: NR	Mental health Comorbidities: Depression 23%; Anxiety 38% Use of other psychoactive drugs: NR Provider characteristics: NR Medical care environment: NR	% with diagnosis: 23% Family history of depressive/mood disorders (%): NR Prior use of antidepressive drugs (%, for treatment or prevention): NR Symptom severity: BDI score (mean (range)): 7 (0-34); State Trait Anxiety Inventory (STAI) (mean (range): 26 (20-58) Time of diagnosis: During pregnancy Diagnosis method: BDI score, State Trait Anxiety Inventory (STAI) When treatment commenced relative to the onset of symptoms: NR

Author Year Country Study Design/Data Source Risk of Bias	Population Characteristics		
	1. Race % Mean Age Socioeconomic Status Home Situation Unplanned Pregnancy % Marital/Partner Status Smoking % ETOH Substance Abuse %	2. Mental Health Comorbidities % Use of Other Psychoactive Drugs % Provider Characteristics Medical Care Environment	3. Depression Characteristics: - Percent with Diagnosis - Family History of Depressive/Mood Disorders (%) - Prior Use of Antidepressive Drugs (%, for Treatment or Prevention) - Symptom Severity - Time of Diagnosis - Diagnosis Method - When Treatment Commenced Relative to the Onset of Symptoms
Dubnov-Raz 2008[21] Israel CC Medium	Race % (white, AA, Hispanic, Asian, Other): NR Mean Age: NR Socio economic status: NR Home situation: NR Unplanned pregnancy %: NR Marital/partner status (S/M/D): NR Smoking%: NR ETOH: NR Substance abuse%: NR	Mental health Comorbidities % (e.g. anxiety): NR Use of other psychoactive drugs % (antipsychotics, antianxiety agents (e.g., benzodiazepines), and drugs for insomnia): Excluded women treated with any other chronic medication Provider characteristics (primary care physician, obstetrician, psychiatrist, nurse, midwife, community worker, or pediatrician visits): NR Medical care environment (community/private/public clinic or hospital): hospital	Depression Characteristics: -% with diagnosis: NR -Family history of depressive/mood disorders (%) : NR -Prior use of antidepressive drugs (%, for treatment or prevention): NR -Symptom severity: NR -Time of diagnosis: NR -Diagnosis method : NR -When treatment commenced relative to the onset of symptoms: NR
Dubnov-Raz 2012[22] Israel CC Medium	Race % (white, AA, Hispanic, Asian, Other): NR Mean Age: 33.2 year Socio economic status: NR Home situation: NR Unplanned pregnancy %: NR Marital/partner status (S/M/D): NR Smoking%: 10% ETOH: 0% Substance abuse%: NR	Mental health Comorbidities % (e.g. anxiety) : NR Use of other psychoactive drugs % (antipsychotics, antianxiety agents (e.g., benzodiazepines), and drugs for insomnia): NR Provider characteristics (primary care physician, obstetrician, psychiatrist, nurse, midwife, community worker, or pediatrician visits): NR Medical care environment (community/private/public clinic or hospital): Hospital	Depression Characteristics: -% with diagnosis: NR -Family history of depressive/mood disorders (%) : NR -Prior use of antidepressive drugs (%, for treatment or prevention): NR -Symptom severity : NR -Time of diagnosis: NR -Diagnosis method : NR -When treatment commenced relative to the onset of symptoms: NR
El Marroun 2012[23] The Netherlands Prospective Cohort Data Source [PC and PD] Low	Of the nervous system: 0.84 (0.21-3.37)/2.25 (0.32-16.05)/1.44 (0.36-5.79)/1.19 (0.17-8.45)/0.85 (0.12-6.07)	Mental health Comorbidities %: Anxiety Use of other psychoactive drugs: benzodiazepine %	7.4% with diagnosis Family history of depressive/mood disorders: NR Prior use of antidepressive drugs: N= 188 (excluded) Symptom severity: NR Time of diagnosis: NR Diagnosis method: NR

Author Year Country Study Design/Data Source Risk of Bias	Population Characteristics 1. Race % Mean Age Socioeconomic Status Home Situation Unplanned Pregnancy % Marital/Partner Status Smoking % ETOH Substance Abuse %	2. Mental Health Comorbidities % Use of Other Psychoactive Drugs % Provider Characteristics Medical Care Environment	3. Depression Characteristics: - Percent with Diagnosis - Family History of Depressive/Mood Disorders (%) - Prior Use of Antidepressive Drugs (%, for Treatment or Prevention) - Symptom Severity - Time of Diagnosis - Diagnosis Method - When Treatment Commenced Relative to the Onset of Symptoms
Ferreira 2007[24] US Retrospective Cohort/Data Source[AD] Medium	Neural tube defects: Only fluoxetine=3.22 (0.45-23.03)	Mental health Comorbidities: mixed disorders 26%, other anxiety disorders 16%, generalized anxiety disorders 3% Use of other psychoactive drugs: N=2 lithium .02% N=1 olanzapine .01% Provider characteristics NR Medical care environment: hospital	41 % with diagnosis Family history of depressive/mood disorders: NR Prior use of antidepressive drugs (%, for treatment or prevention) NR Symptom severity: NR Time of diagnosis: NR Diagnosis method: NR
Figueroa 2010[25] US Retrospective cohort Design/Data Source[AD] Medium	Of the eye: 2.62 (1.09-6.34)/None/0.93 (0.13-6.63)/None/1.05 (0.15-7.45)	Mental health Comorbidities: Anxiety disorder N=1978 5.20% Adjustment disorder N=1486 3.90% Other mental illness N=533 1.40% Bipolar disorder N=334 0.88% ADHD N=196 0.51% MR, PDD, or organic disorder N=168 0.44% Psychotic disorder N= 68 0.18% Use of other psychoactive drugs: Benzodiazepines during pregnancy N=311 0.82% Anticonvulsants during pregnancy N=147 0.39% Other psychotropics during pregnancy N=67 0.18% Provider characteristics: NR Medical care environment: mental health outpatient clinic	Depressive disorders N =3923 10.3% with diagnosis Anxiety disorder N=1978 5.20% Adjustment disorder N=1486 3.90% Other mental illness N= 533 1.40% Bipolar disorder N=334 .88% Family history of depressive/mood disorders: NR Prior use of antidepressive drugs (%, for treatment or prevention) NR Symptom severity: NR Time of diagnosis: NR Diagnosis method: NR

	Population Characteristics		3. Depression Characteristics:
Author Year Country Study Design/Data Source Risk of Bias	1. Race % Mean Age Socioeconomic Status Home Situation Unplanned Pregnancy % Marital/Partner Status Smoking % ETOH Substance Abuse %	2. Mental Health Comorbidities % Use of Other Psychoactive Drugs % Provider Characteristics Medical Care Environment	- Percent with Diagnosis - Family History of Depressive/Mood Disorders (%) - Prior Use of Antidepressive Drugs (%, for Treatment or Prevention) - Symptom Severity - Time of Diagnosis - Diagnosis Method - When Treatment Commenced Relative to the Onset of Symptoms
Gorman 2012[26] US Prospective cohort/TIS Medium	Race: % 66% white, %AA NR, 20% Hispanic, 9% Asian, 5% Other Mean Age: 32.2 Socio economic status: Report any available values: 14% Low, 17% Medium, 69% High Home situation: NR Unplanned pregnancy %: NR Marital/partner status (S/M/D):NR	NR	NR
Grzeskowiak 2012[27] Australia Retrospective cohort/LD Medium	Race: 79% white, 9.6% Asian, 11% Other Mean Age: 29.2 Socioeconomic status (Socio-Economic Indexes for Areas, calculated from the Australian Bureau of Statistics'): 5 (highest)=20%, 4=20%, 3=18%, 2=20%, 1 (lowest)=22% Home situation: NR Unplanned pregnancy: NR Marital/partner status: NR	Use of other psychoactive drugs: 1% anxiolytic use Provider characteristics: NR Medical care environment: NR	NR
Hanley 2013[28] Canada PC Medium	Race: NR Mean Age: 33.5 Low socio economic status: NR Home situation: NR Unplanned pregnancy: NR Marital/partner status: NR Smoking%: 1 (3.2) ETOH%: 19 (61.3) Substance abuse%: NR	Mental health Comorbidities: NR Use of other psychoactive drugs: NR Provider characteristics: NR Medical care environment: NR	% with diagnosis: 100% Family history of depressive/mood disorders (%): NR Prior use of antidepressive drugs (%, for treatment or prevention): NR Symptom severity: NR Time of diagnosis: Before conception Diagnosis method: Edinburgh Postnatal Depression Scale (EPDS); Hamilton Rating Scale for Depression (HAMD); Depression during pregnancy defined as having an EPDS≥13 or HAM-D≥14 at study recruitment When treatment commenced relative to the onset of symptoms: NR

Author Year Country Study Design/Data Source Risk of Bias	Population Characteristics 1. Race % Mean Age Socioeconomic Status Home Situation Unplanned Pregnancy % Marital/Partner Status Smoking % ETOH Substance Abuse %	2. Mental Health Comorbidities % Use of Other Psychoactive Drugs % Provider Characteristics Medical Care Environment	3. Depression Characteristics: - Percent with Diagnosis - Family History of Depressive/Mood Disorders (%) - Prior Use of Antidepressive Drugs (%, for Treatment or Prevention) - Symptom Severity - Time of Diagnosis - Diagnosis Method - When Treatment Commenced Relative to the Onset of Symptoms
Heikkinen 2002[29] Finland PC	Race: NR Mean age: 32.6 SES: NR Home situation: NR Unplanned pregnancy: NR Marital status: NR % smoking: 23.8% ETOH %: light alcohol use: 9.5%	Mental health Comorbidities % (e.g. anxiety) :NR Use of other psychoactive drugs % (antipsychotics, antianxiety agents (e.g., benzodiazepines), and drugs for insomnia): 0% Provider characteristics (primary care physician, obstetrician, psychiatrist, nurse, midwife, community worker, or pediatrician visits): Psychiatrists, pediatrician Medical care environment (community/private/public clinic or hospital):NR	% with depression: 28.6% Family history of depressive/ mood disorders: NR Prior use of antidepressive drugs: NR Symptom severity: NR Time of diagnosis: NR When treatment commenced relative to onset of symptoms: NR
Jimenez-Solem 2012[30] Denmark RC-PD Low	Race NR Age: <20=3%, 21-25=15%, 26-30=38%, 31-35=32%, >35=12% SES: Annual household income <$58,338=25%, $58335-$93-656=25%, $93,656-$119,082=25%, ≥ $119,082=25%; Education, short=33%, medium=30%, long=32% Home situation: NR Unplanned pregnancy: NR Marital/partner status: NR Smoking: Daily cigarettes 0=78%, 1-10=15%, 11-20=0.6%, >20=2.4% ETOH: NR Substance abuse: NR	NR	NR
Jimenez-Solem 2013[31] Denmark PBR Low	Race: NR Mean Age: <20: 2.9%; 21-25: 16.2%, 26-30: 38.4%, 31-35: 30.9%, >35: 11.6% Socio economic status: Education level low: 35.5%, medium: 32.5%, high: 31.8% Annual household income: <62,192: 24.9%, 62,192-89,140: 25.0%, 89,141-126,344: 25.0%, >126,344: 25.0% Home situation: NR Unplanned pregnancy: NR Marital/partner status: NR Smoking (cigarettes/day): 0: 80.9%, 1-10: 12.8%, 11-20: 5.2%, >20: <1% ETOH: NR Substance abuse: NR	Mental health comorbidities: NR Use of other psychoactive drugs: NR Provider characteristics: NR (stillbirth and neonatal mortality) Medical care environment: NR	NR

Author Year Country Study Design/Data Source Risk of Bias	Population Characteristics: 1. Race % Mean Age Socioeconomic Status Home Situation Unplanned Pregnancy % Marital/Partner Status Smoking % ETOH Substance Abuse %	2. Mental Health Comorbidities % Use of Other Psychoactive Drugs % Provider Characteristics Medical Care Environment	3. Depression Characteristics: - Percent with Diagnosis - Family History of Depressive/Mood Disorders (%) - Prior Use of Antidepressive Drugs (%, for Treatment or Prevention) - Symptom Severity - Time of Diagnosis - Diagnosis Method - When Treatment Commenced Relative to the Onset of Symptoms
Jordan 2008[32] US Clinic Appt Logs, Pediatrics records review AD Medium	W= .06%; AA 14%; Hisp 78%; Other .03% Mean Age: 27. Home Situation: NR Unplanned pregnancy: NR Partner status: NR	MH Comorbidities: Anx=12% in SRI pregnancies vs.06% non subjects; Adj DO 4% SRI gp/24% non SRI gp=15% all. BAD 4% SRI/12% non SRI = 0.8% all. Other drugs: Benzo (N=3). Med Care Envir: Hospital	% with Dx: NR Fam Hx NR; Prior use NR; Sx Severity NR; Dx method: NR; Tx/onset sxs: NR
Kallen 2004[33] Sweden PBR Medium	Race % (white, AA, Hispanic, Asian, Other): NR Age: 13-19, 0.8%; 20-24, 10.8%; 25-29, 26.8%; 30-34, 34.4%; 35-39, 22.0%; 40-44, 4.9%; ≥45, 0.2% Socio economic status: NR Home situation: Cohabitating, 84.5% Unplanned pregnancy %: NR Marital/partner status (S/M/D): NR Smoking%: 30.5% in early pregnancy ETOH: NR Substance abuse%: NR	Mental health Comorbidities % (e.g. anxiety) : NR Use of other psychoactive drugs % (antipsychotics, antianxiety agents (e.g., benzodiazepines), and drugs for insomnia): Anticonvulsants, 1.6%; Neuroleptics, sedatives, hypnotics, 18.7% Provider characteristics (primary care physician, obstetrician, psychiatrist, nurse, midwife, community worker, or pediatrician visits): NR Medical care environment (community/private/public clinic or hospital): NR	Depression Characteristics: -% with diagnosis: NR -Family history of depressive/mood disorders (%) : NR -Prior use of antidepressive drugs (% for treatment or prevention): NR -Symptom severity : NR -Time of diagnosis: NR -Diagnosis method : NR -When treatment commenced relative to the onset of symptoms: NR
Kallen 2007[34] Sweden Retrospective cohort/Data Source[PBR] Medium	Of the ear, face and neck: None/None/None/8.32 (1.16-59.81)/6.13 (0.85-44.05)	Mental Health Comorbidities %:NR Use of other psychoactive drugs: Clomipramine N=57 Trimipramine N= 2 Amitriptyline N=21 Nortriptyline N=4 Moclobemide N=3 Mianserin N=32 Nefazodone N=3 Mirtazapine N=27 Venlafaxine N=30 Reboxetine N=3 Provider characteristics NR Medical care environment NR	% with diagnosis: NR Family history of depressive/mood disorders: NR Prior use of antidepressive drugs NR Symptom severity: NR Time of diagnosis: NR Diagnosis method: NR

	Population Characteristics		
Author Year Country Study Design/Data Source Risk of Bias	1. Race % Mean Age Socioeconomic Status Home Situation Unplanned Pregnancy % Marital/Partner Status Smoking % ETOH Substance Abuse %	2. Mental Health Comorbidities % Use of Other Psychoactive Drugs % Provider Characteristics Medical Care Environment	3. Depression Characteristics: - Percent with Diagnosis - Family History of Depressive/Mood Disorders (%) - Prior Use of Antidepressive Drugs (%, for Treatment or Prevention) - Symptom Severity - Time of Diagnosis - Diagnosis Method - When Treatment Commenced Relative to the Onset of Symptoms
Kallen 2008[35] Sweden Unclear/Data Source[PBR] Medium	Of the heart: 1.91 (1.31-2.77)/1.06 (0.34-3.3)/2.05 (1.27-3.31)/1.54 (0.77-3.1)/2.73 (1.75-4.26)	Mental health Comorbidities % Use of other psychoactive drugs % Provider characteristics: NR Medical care environment: NR	% with diagnosis: NR Family history of depressive/mood disorders: NR Prior use of antidepressive drugs: NR Symptom severity: NR Time of diagnosis: NR Diagnosis method: NR
Kieler 2012[36] Nordic countries Retrospective cohort, PBD Medium	Age: ≤ 24=16.3%, 25-34=66.2%, 35-44=17.3%, ≥ 45=0.1% Others NR	NR	NR
Kornum 2010[37] Denmark PBR Medium	Race %: (white, AA, Hispanic, Asian, Other): NR Mean Age: Median Age 29.8 Socio economic status: NR Home situation: NR Unplanned pregnancy %: NR Marital/partner status (S/M/D): NR Smoking%: With SSRI in first trimester or 30 days before conception: 35.8%, With SSRI in second or third month after conception: 31.8%, No SSRI: 20.6% ETOH: NR Substance abuse%: NR	Mental health Comorbidities % (e.g. anxiety): NR Use of other psychoactive drugs % (antipsychotics, antianxiety agents (e.g., benzodiazepines), and drugs for insomnia): excluded women with both SSRI and non-SSRI antidepressants Provider characteristics (primary care physician, obstetrician, psychiatrist, nurse, midwife, community worker, or pediatrician visits): NR Medical care environment (community/private/public clinic or hospital): NR	Depression Characteristics: -% with diagnosis: NR -Family history of depressive/mood disorders (%): NR -Prior use of antidepressive drugs (%, for treatment or prevention): NR -Symptom severity: NR -Time of diagnosis: NR -Diagnosis method: NR -When treatment commenced relative to the onset of symptoms: NR
Laine 2003[38] Finland Prospective cohort/Data Source[PC] Medium	Race %: (white, AA, Hispanic, Asian, Other) Mean Age:35yrs Socio economic status: Report any available values Home situation:NR Unplanned pregnancy %: NR Marital/partner status: (S/M/D) Smoking: 60% vs 10% ETOH: 10% vs. 0% Substance abuse: NR	Mental health Comorbidities: 50% panic disorder Use of other psychoactive drugs 3% benzodiazepines Provider characteristics: primary care physician Medical care environment: private/public clinic	50% with diagnosis N=10 Family history of depressive/mood disorders: NR Prior use of antidepressive drugs (%, for treatment or prevention) NR Symptom severity: NR Time of diagnosis: NR Diagnosis method: NR

Author Year Country Study Design/Data Source Risk of Bias	Population Characteristics		
	1. Race % Mean Age Socioeconomic Status Home Situation Unplanned Pregnancy % Marital/Partner Status Smoking % ETOH Substance Abuse %	2. Mental Health Comorbidities % Use of Other Psychoactive Drugs % Provider Characteristics Medical Care Environment	3. Depression Characteristics: - Percent with Diagnosis - Family History of Depressive/Mood Disorders (%) - Prior Use of Antidepressive Drugs (%, for Treatment or Prevention) - Symptom Severity - Time of Diagnosis - Diagnosis Method - When Treatment Commenced Relative to the Onset of Symptoms
Latendresse 2011[39] US PS Medium	Ethnicity: Hispanic 24%, Race: white: 69%, Hispanic/Mexican: 13%, African American, Other: 18% Mean age: NR SES: health insurance: private 56%, state Medicaid: 33%, Uninsured/self pay: 11% Home situation: NR Unplanned pregnancy: NR Marital status: married: 64%, living with partner: 13%, single: 21%, divorced/separated: 2% Smoking:<5%, ETOH:<5%, substance abuse:<5%	Anxiety: % NR Use of other psychoactive drugs: NR Provider characteristics: NR Medical care environment: community	% with diagnosis: 1% -Family history of depressive/mood disorders (%): NR -Prior use of antidepressive drugs (%, for treatment or prevention): NR -Symptom severity: NR -Time of diagnosis: NR -Diagnosis method: NR -When treatment commenced relative to the onset of symptoms: NR
Lennestal 2007[40] Sweden PBR Medium	Race % (white, AA, Hispanic, Asian, Other): NR Mean Age: NR: Age distribution: <20: 132, 20-24: 950, 25-29: 2032, 30-34: 2347, 35-39: 1426, 40-44: 306, ≥45: 19 Socio economic status: NR Home situation: NR Unplanned pregnancy %: NR Marital/partner status (S/M/D): NR Smoking%: 27.4% ETOH: NR Substance abuse%: NR	Mental health Comorbidities % (e.g. anxiety): NR Use of other psychoactive drugs % (antipsychotics, antianxiety agents (e.g., benzodiazepines), and drugs for insomnia): Neuroleptics, sedatives, hypnotics: 21.2% of SNRI users Provider characteristics (primary care physician, obstetrician, psychiatrist, nurse, midwife, community worker, or pediatrician visits): NR Medical care environment (community/private/public clinic or hospital): NR	Depression Characteristics: -% with diagnosis: NR -Family history of depressive/mood disorders (%): NR -Prior use of antidepressive drugs (%, for treatment or prevention): NR -Symptom severity: NR -Time of diagnosis: NR -Diagnosis method : NR -When treatment commenced relative to the onset of symptoms: NR
Levinson-Castiel 2006[41] Israel PC, PBD Medium	Race: NR Maternal Mean age: 31.8 yrs Socio-economic status: NR Home situation: NR Unplanned pregnancy: NR Marital/partner status: NR % Smoking: NR ETOH: NR Substance abuse %: NR	NR	NR

E-14

	Population Characteristics		3. Depression Characteristics: - Percent with Diagnosis - Family History of Depressive/Mood Disorders (%) -Prior Use of Antidepressive Drugs (%, for Treatment or Prevention) - Symptom Severity - Time of Diagnosis - Diagnosis Method -When Treatment Commenced Relative to the Onset of Symptoms
Author Year Country Study Design/Data Source Risk of Bias	1. Race % Mean Age Socioeconomic Status Home Situation Unplanned Pregnancy % Marital/Partner Status Smoking % ETOH Substance Abuse %	2. Mental Health Comorbidities % Use of Other Psychoactive Drugs % Provider Characteristics Medical Care Environment	
Lewis 2010[42] Australia PC-Clinic Medium	Race NR Mean Age=32.3 years SES: NR Home situation: NR Unplanned pregnancy: NR Marital/partner status: Married=72%; de facto=22%; Widowed=5.6% Smoking: 15% ETOH: 48% Substance abuse: 5.6%	Mental health Comorbidities: NR Use of other psychoactive drugs: 41% medication other than antidepressants Provider characteristics: NR Medical care environment: NR	100% with diagnosis Family history of depressive/mood disorders: NR Prior use of antidepressive drugs: NR Symptom severity: NR Time of diagnosis: NR Diagnosis method: Independent psychiatric evaluation When treatment commenced relative to the onset of symptoms: NR
Logsdon 2011[43] US PC Medium	Race % (white, AA, Hispanic, Asian, Other): White 79.5%, AA 18.1%, Other 2.3% Mean Age (SD): 30.4 (5.7) Socio economic status: Education level: high school or less 18.7%, Some college 16.4%, college 40.7%, graduate school 24.3%; Employment/academic status: Not at all 33.2%, Occasional 1.9%, Part time 10.3%, Full time 54.7%, Employed/attending school 66.8% Home situation: Partner, no children 30.2%, Partner and children 46.0%, Alone, no children 11.6%, Alone with children 9.3%, Parents, no children 0.5%, Parents and children 2.3% Unplanned pregnancy %: NR Marital/partner status (S/M/D): S 21.4%, M/cohabitating 75.8%, D/separated 2.3% Smoking%: NR ETOH: NR Substance abuse%: NR	Mental health Comorbidities % (e.g. anxiety): NR Use of other psychoactive drugs % (antipsychotics, antianxiety agents (e.g., benzodiazepines), and drugs for insomnia): excluded women using benzodiazepines Provider characteristics (primary care physician, obstetrician, psychiatrist, nurse, midwife, community worker, or pediatrician visits): Psychiatrist Medical care environment (community/private/public clinic or hospital): clinic	Depression Characteristics: -% with diagnosis: NR -Family history of depressive/mood disorders (%): NR -Prior use of antidepressive drugs (%, for treatment or prevention): NR -Symptom severity: NR -Time of diagnosis: NR -Diagnosis method: NR -When treatment commenced relative to the onset of symptoms: NR

Author Year Country Study Design/Data Source Risk of Bias	Population Characteristics 1. Race % Mean Age Socioeconomic Status Home Situation Unplanned Pregnancy % Marital/Partner Status Smoking % ETOH Substance Abuse %	2. Mental Health Comorbidities % Use of Other Psychoactive Drugs % Provider Characteristics Medical Care Environment	3. Depression Characteristics: - Percent with Diagnosis - Family History of Depressive/Mood Disorders (%) - Prior Use of Antidepressive Drugs (%, for Treatment or Prevention) - Symptom Severity - Time of Diagnosis - Diagnosis Method - When Treatment Commenced Relative to the Onset of Symptoms
Lund 2009[44] Denmark PC Medium	Race: NR Maternal age:<20: 1.5%,20-24:12.1%, 25-29:38.4%, 30-34:33.8%, ≥35:14.3% Nonsmoker: 78.4% Smoking cigarettes/day: 1-4:3.8%, 5-9:5.9%,10-14:5.9%, ≥15:3.2% Home situation: NR Unplanned pregnancy: NR Marital status:Married/cohabiting:89.9%, living alone: 2.9% ETOH (alcohol intake):<1:73.4%, 1-4:19.7%, 5-9:1%, ≥10:1.3% Education, yrs:<9:15.8%, 9-12:26%, >12:37.5%	Mental health comorbidities Patients with psychiatric history but no use of SSRI group: schizophrenia: 0.2%, eating-disorder: 1%, bipolar disorder: 0.2%, OCD:0.4%, stress: 0.2%, anxiety: 0.5%, unspecified: 1.8% Use of other psychoactive drugs in SSRI use patients: benzodiazepines 2.4%, antipsychotics:4%, TCA: 3%, mirtazapine: 1.5%, venlafaxine: 2.1%, sleeping pills: 0.6%, lithium: 0.3% Use of other psychoactive drugs in psychiatric history but no SSRI use patients: psychotropics: 0.5%, antipsychotics: 0.4%, anxiolytics: 0.3%, antidepressants other than SSRI: 0.7% Provider characteristics: GP, psychiatrist, psychologist Medical care environment: hospital	% with diagnosis reported in patients with psychiatric history but no SSRI: 1.8%
Malm 2011[45] Finland TIS Low	Race % (white, AA, Hispanic, Asian, Other): NR Mean Age: Median Age 29.4 Socio economic status: NR Home situation: NR Unplanned pregnancy %: NR Marital/partner status (S/M/D): M 60.20% Smoking%: 14.67% ETOH: NR Substance abuse%: NR	Mental health Comorbidities % (e.g. anxiety): NR Use of other psychoactive drugs % (antipsychotics, antianxiety agents (e.g., benzodiazepines), and drugs for insomnia): 27.98% Provider characteristics (primary care physician, obstetrician, psychiatrist, nurse, midwife, community worker, or pediatrician visits): NR Medical care environment (community/private/public clinic or hospital): NR	Depression Characteristics: -% with diagnosis: NR -Family history of depressive/mood disorders (%): NR -Prior use of antidepressive drugs (%, for treatment or prevention): NR -Symptom severity: NR -Time of diagnosis: NR -Diagnosis method: NR -When treatment commenced relative to the onset of symptoms: NR

E-16

Author Year Country Study Design/Data Source Risk of Bias	Population Characteristics		3. Depression Characteristics: - Percent with Diagnosis - Family History of Depressive/Mood Disorders (%) - Prior Use of Antidepressive Drugs (%, for Treatment or Prevention) - Symptom Severity - Time of Diagnosis - Diagnosis Method - When Treatment Commenced Relative to the Onset of Symptoms
	1. Race % Mean Age Socioeconomic Status Home Situation Unplanned Pregnancy % Marital/Partner Status Smoking % ETOH Substance Abuse %	2. Mental Health Comorbidities % Use of Other Psychoactive Drugs % Provider Characteristics Medical Care Environment	
McFarland 2011[46] US PC Medium	Race % (white, AA, Hispanic, Asian, Other): Non White 13.04%, Hispanic 17.39% Mean Age: 29.1 Socio economic status : low SES 11.80% Home situation: NR Unplanned pregnancy %: NR Marital/partner status (S/M/D): S 32.92% Smoking%: NR ETOH: NR Substance abuse%: NR	Mental health Comorbidities % (e.g. anxiety): NR Use of other psychoactive drugs % (antipsychotics, antianxiety agents (e.g., benzodiazepines), and drugs for insomnia): NR Provider characteristics (primary care physician, obstetrician, psychiatrist, nurse, midwife, community worker, or pediatrician visits): obstetrician Medical care environment (community/private/public clinic or hospital): clinic	Depression Characteristics: -% with diagnosis: 40.37% -Family history of depressive/mood disorders (%): NR -Prior use of antidepressive drugs (%, for treatment or prevention): NR -Symptom severity: NR -Time of diagnosis: NR -Diagnosis method: NR -When treatment commenced relative to the onset of symptoms: NR
Merlob 2009[47] Israel TIS Medium	Race % (white, AA, Hispanic, Asian, Other): NR Mean Age: Median Age NR Socio economic status: NR Home situation: NR Unplanned pregnancy %: NR Marital/partner status (S/M/D): NR Smoking%: NR ETOH: NR Substance abuse%: NR	Mental health Comorbidities % (e.g. anxiety): NR Use of other psychoactive drugs % (antipsychotics, antianxiety agents (e.g., benzodiazepines), and drugs for insomnia): NR Provider characteristics (primary care physician, obstetrician, psychiatrist, nurse, midwife, community worker, or pediatrician visits): NR Medical care environment (community/private/public clinic or hospital): hospital	Depression Characteristics: -% with diagnosis: NR -Family history of depressive/mood disorders (%): NR -Prior use of antidepressive drugs (%, for treatment or prevention): NR -Symptom severity: NR -Time of diagnosis: NR -Diagnosis method: NR -When treatment commenced relative to the onset of symptoms: NR
Misri 2006[48] Canada PC-Clinic Medium	Race: NR Mean Age: 32 years SES: NR Home situation: NR Unplanned pregnancy: NR Marital/partner status: 91% married, 9% common-law Smoking% ETOH: NR Substance abuse: NR	NR	NR

E-17

Author Year Country Study Design/Data Source Risk of Bias	Population Characteristics		
	1. Race % Mean Age Socioeconomic Status Home Situation Unplanned Pregnancy % Marital/Partner Status Smoking % ETOH Substance Abuse %	2. Mental Health Comorbidities % Use of Other Psychoactive Drugs % Provider Characteristics Medical Care Environment	3. Depression Characteristics: - Percent with Diagnosis - Family History of Depressive/Mood Disorders (%) - Prior Use of Antidepressive Drugs (%, for Treatment or Prevention) - Symptom Severity - Time of Diagnosis - Diagnosis Method - When Treatment Commenced Relative to the Onset of Symptoms
Misri 2010[49] Canada PC-Clinic Medium	Race: 78% white, 0% AA, 0% Hispanic, 9% East Asian, 13% Other) Mean Age: 32.5 years SES: Education=16.5 years Home situation: NR Unplanned pregnancy: NR Marital/partner status: 83% married, 15% common-law, 1% separated, 1% divorced Smoking: NR ETOH: NR Substance abuse: NR	NR	NR
Mulder 2011[50] The Netherlands Prospective cohort/Data Source [PC] Medium	Race NR Mean Age: 31.5 (control vs. previously exposed vs. exposed) Socio economic status: NR Home situation: NR Unplanned pregnancy: NR Marital/partner status: NR Smoking :17.7% vs. 21.6% vs. 17.7% ETOH: 11.5% vs. 8.1% vs. 6.3% Substance abuse: NR	Mental health Comorbidities Panic disorder: 9% Depression and panic combined: 46% Anxiety: 3% OCD: 1.5% Use of other psychoactive drugs % Provider characteristics: physician or mid wife Medical care environment: clinic	38 % with diagnosis N=133 Family history of depressive/mood disorders: NR Prior use of antidepressive drugs: NR Symptom severity: NR Time of diagnosis: NR Diagnosis method: NR
Nakhai-Pour 2010[51] Canada CC Low	Race % (white, AA, Hispanic, Asian, Other): NR Mean Age: 27.52 Socio economic status: Recipients of social assistance: 30.90% Home situation: Urban Residences: 77.13% Unplanned pregnancy %: NR Marital/partner status (S/M/D): NR Smoking%: NR ETOH: NR Substance abuse%: NR	Mental health Comorbidities % (e.g. anxiety): Anxiety 6.79%, Bipolar 0.44% Use of other psychoactive drugs % (antipsychotics, antianxiety agents (e.g., benzodiazepines), and drugs for insomnia): NR Provider characteristics (primary care physician, obstetrician, psychiatrist, nurse, midwife, community worker, or pediatrician visits): NR Medical care environment (community/private/public clinic or hospital): NR	Depression Characteristics: -% with diagnosis: 4.93% -Family history of depressive/mood disorders (%): NR -Prior use of antidepressive drugs (%, for treatment or prevention): NR -Symptom severity: NR -Time of diagnosis: NR -Diagnosis method: NR -When treatment commenced relative to the onset of symptoms: NR

Author Year Country Study Design/Data Source Risk of Bias	Population Characteristics 1. Race % Mean Age Socioeconomic Status Home Situation Unplanned Pregnancy % Marital/Partner Status Smoking % ETOH Substance Abuse %	2. Mental Health Comorbidities % Use of Other Psychoactive Drugs % Provider Characteristics Medical Care Environment	3. Depression Characteristics: - Percent with Diagnosis - Family History of Depressive/Mood Disorders (%) - Prior Use of Antidepressive Drugs (%, for Treatment or Prevention) - Symptom Severity - Time of Diagnosis - Diagnosis Method - When Treatment Commenced Relative to the Onset of Symptoms
Nordeng 2012[52] Norway PBR Medium	Race: NR Mean Age: <20: 1.0%, 20-29: 44.2%, 30-39: 52.9%, >=40: 1.8% Socio economic status (education): primary: 3.0%, secondary: 35.4%, tertiary-short: 41.2%, tertiary- long: 20.3% Home situation: NR Unplanned pregnancy: NR Marital/partner status: Married/cohabiting: 96.5%, other: 3.5% Smoking: no: 89.9%, sometimes: 5.2%, daily: 5.0% ETOH: NR Substance abuse: NR	NR	Depressive symptoms at 17 gestational weeks: Nonexposed: 6.0% Prior-only: 22.1% Use of antidepressants during pregnancy: 39.9% Depressive symptoms at 30 gestational weeks: Nonexposed: 6.3% Prior-only: 22.1% Use of antidepressants during pregnancy: 38.4% Lifetime history of depression Nonexposed: 31.9% Prior-only: 86.8% Use of antidepressants during pregnancy: 88.7% Other characteristics: NR
Nulman 2002[53] Canada PC Medium	Mean Age: 31.2 Socioeconomic status (Score on Hollingshead index of social status): 44.1 Other characteristics: NR	Mental health comorbidities: tricyclic antidepressants were taken for pain control in 11 cases and for an anxiety disorder in 3 cases. Use of other psychoactive drugs: NR Provider characteristics: NR Medical care environment: NR	% with diagnosis: 100% Family history of depressive/mood disorders: NR Prior use of antidepressive drugs: NR Symptom severity (Mean [SD] Depression Score on CES-D Scale): 39.9 (11.3) fluoxetine, 28.0 (16.7) tricyclic antidepressants Duration of depression (Mean [SD]): 2.4 (0.5) years fluoxetine, 2.1 (1.0) years tricyclics Duration of treatment: (Mean [SD]): 1.9 (0.6) years fluoxetine, 1.8 (1.0) years tricyclics Time of diagnosis: NR Diagnosis method: Independent psychiatric evaluation

Author Year Country Study Design/Data Source Risk of Bias	Population Characteristics		
	1. Race % Mean Age Socioeconomic Status Home Situation Unplanned Pregnancy % Marital/Partner Status Smoking % ETOH Substance Abuse %	2. Mental Health Comorbidities % Use of Other Psychoactive Drugs % Provider Characteristics Medical Care Environment	3. Depression Characteristics: - Percent with Diagnosis - Family History of Depressive/Mood Disorders (%) - Prior Use of Antidepressive Drugs (%, for Treatment or Prevention) - Symptom Severity - Time of Diagnosis - Diagnosis Method - When Treatment Commenced Relative to the Onset of Symptoms
Oberlander 2002[54] Canada Prospective cohort/Data Source[PC] Medium	Race NR Mean Age: NR Socio economic status: NR Home situation: NR Unplanned pregnancy: NR Marital/partner status: NR Smoking : NR ETOH: NR Substance abuse: NR	Mental health Comorbidities NR Use of other psychoactive drugs: Clonazepam= 36% (N=14) Provider characteristics: NR Medical care environment: hospital	% with diagnosis: NR Family history of depressive/mood disorders: NR Prior use of antidepressive drugs: NR Symptom severity: NR Time of diagnosis: NR Diagnosis method: NR
Oberlander 2006[55] Canada PBR Medium	Race % (white, AA, Hispanic, Asian, Other): NR Mean Age: 29.51 Socio economic status: Drugs subsidized through welfare program in year before becoming pregnant 0.06%, Income decile: 5.6 Home situation: NR Unplanned pregnancy %: NR Marital/partner status (S/M/D): NR Smoking%: NR ETOH: NR Substance abuse%: NR	Mental health Comorbidities % (e.g. anxiety): Diagnosed with mental health disorder, excluding depression, in year before becoming pregnant : 0.6% Use of other psychoactive drugs % (antipsychotics, antianxiety agents (e.g., benzodiazepines), and drugs for insomnia): NR Provider characteristics (PCP, obstetrician, psychiatrist, nurse, midwife, community worker, or pediatrician visits): NR Medical care environment (community/private/public clinic or hospital): NR	Depression Characteristics: -% with diagnosis: 14.5% -Family history of depressive/mood disorders (%) :NR -Prior use of antidepressive drugs (%, for treatment or prevention): NR -Symptom severity : NR -Time of diagnosis: NR -Diagnosis method : NR -When treatment commenced relative to the onset of symptoms: NR
Oberlander 2008[56] Canada PC Medium	Race % (white, AA, Hispanic, Asian, Other): NR Mean Age: 32.32 Socio economic status: Maternal education: 16.46 years Home situation: NR Unplanned pregnancy %: NR Marital/partner status (S/M/D): NR Smoking%: NR ETOH: NR Substance abuse%: NR	Mental health Comorbidities % (e.g. anxiety): NR Use of other psychoactive drugs % (antipsychotics, antianxiety agents (e.g., benzodiazepines), and drugs for insomnia): Excluded all other psychotropic or antidepressant medications Provider characteristics (primary care physician, obstetrician, psychiatrist, nurse, midwife, community worker, or pediatrician visits): NR Medical care environment (community/private/public clinic or hospital): NR	Depression Characteristics: -% with diagnosis: NR -Family history of depressive/mood disorders (%): NR -Prior use of antidepressive drugs (%, for treatment or prevention): NR -Symptom severity: NR -Time of diagnosis: NR -Diagnosis method: NR -When treatment commenced relative to the onset of symptoms: NR

Author Year Country Study Design/Data Source Risk of Bias	Population Characteristics 1. Race % Mean Age Socioeconomic Status Home Situation Unplanned Pregnancy % Marital/Partner Status Smoking % ETOH Substance Abuse %	2. Mental Health Comorbidities % Use of Other Psychoactive Drugs % Provider Characteristics Medical Care Environment	3. Depression Characteristics: - Percent with Diagnosis - Family History of Depressive/Mood Disorders (%) - Prior Use of Antidepressive Drugs (%, for Treatment or Prevention) - Symptom Severity - Time of Diagnosis - Diagnosis Method - When Treatment Commenced Relative to the Onset of Symptoms
Oberlander 2008[57] (Birth Defects Res Part B) Canada PBR Medium	Race % (white, AA, Hispanic, Asian, Other): NR Mean Age: Socio economic status: NR Home situation: NR Unplanned pregnancy %: NR Marital/partner status (S/M/D): NR Smoking%: NR ETOH: NR Substance abuse%: NR	Mental health Comorbidities % (e.g. anxiety) : NR Use of other psychoactive drugs % (antipsychotics, antianxiety agents (e.g., benzodiazepines), and drugs for insomnia): NR Provider characteristics (primary care physician, obstetrician, psychiatrist, nurse, midwife, community worker, or pediatrician visits): NR Medical care environment (community/private/public clinic or hospital): hospital	Depression Characteristics: -% with diagnosis -Family history of depressive/mood disorders (%): NR -Prior use of antidepressive drugs (%, for treatment or prevention): NR -Symptom severity : NR -Time of diagnosis -Diagnosis method : NR -When treatment commenced relative to the onset of symptoms: NR
Okun 2011[58] US PC Medium	Race % (white, AA, Hispanic, Asian, Other): White 78.7%, AA 17.6%, Other 3.8% Mean Age: 29.9 Socio economic status: Employed 59.4%, Education: Less than high school 7.1%, High school 11.3%, Some college 20.0%, College 37.5%, Graduate school 24.2% Home situation: NR Unplanned pregnancy %: NR Marital/partner status (S/M/D): S 24.2%, M/cohabitating 72.1%, D/separated 3.3%, Widowed 0.4% Smoking%: 14.7% ETOH: 32.6% Substance abuse%: NR	Mental health Comorbidities % (e.g. anxiety): NR Use of other psychoactive drugs % (antipsychotics, antianxiety agents (e.g., benzodiazepines), and drugs for insomnia): NR Provider characteristics (primary care physician, obstetrician, psychiatrist, nurse, midwife, community worker, or pediatrician visits): NR Medical care environment (community/private/public clinic or hospital): community	Depression Characteristics: -% with diagnosis: 24.6% -Family history of depressive/mood disorders (%): NR -Prior use of antidepressive drugs (%, for treatment or prevention): NR -Symptom severity: NR -Time of diagnosis: NR -Diagnosis method: NR -When treatment commenced relative to the onset of symptoms: NR

Author Year Country Study Design/Data Source Risk of Bias	Population Characteristics		3. Depression Characteristics: - Percent with Diagnosis - Family History of Depressive/Mood Disorders (%) - Prior Use of Antidepressive Drugs (%, for Treatment or Prevention) - Symptom Severity - Time of Diagnosis - Diagnosis Method - When Treatment Commenced Relative to the Onset of Symptoms
	1. Race % Mean Age Socioeconomic Status Home Situation Unplanned Pregnancy % Marital/Partner Status Smoking % ETOH Substance Abuse %	2. Mental Health Comorbidities % Use of Other Psychoactive Drugs % Provider Characteristics Medical Care Environment	
Okun 2012[59] US PC Medium	Race % (white, AA, Hispanic, Asian, Other): White, 77.9% Mean Age: 30.1 Socio economic status: Employed, 59.3%; Education level: < high school 7.4%, high school 10.6%, some college 18.4%, college 40.1%, graduate school 23.5% Home situation: NR Unplanned pregnancy %: NR Marital/partner status (S/M/D): M/Cohabitating 72.8% Smoking%: Ever during pregnancy 13.0%; No. cigarettes per d: 4.9±0.9 ETOH: Ever during pregnancy 30.8%; No. drinks per occasion: 2.3±2.1 Substance abuse%: NR	Mental health Comorbidities % (e.g. anxiety) : NR Use of other psychoactive drugs % (antipsychotics, antianxiety agents (e.g., benzodiazepines), and drugs for insomnia): NR Provider characteristics (PCP, obstetrician, psychiatrist, nurse, midwife, community worker, or pediatrician visits): NR Medical care environment (community/private/public clinic or hospital): NR	Depression Characteristics: -% with diagnosis: 24.44% -Family history of depressive/mood disorders (%): NR -Prior use of antidepressive drugs (%, for treatment or prevention): NR -Symptom severity: NR -Time of diagnosis: NR -Diagnosis method: NR -When treatment commenced relative to the onset of symptoms: NR
Palmsten 2012[60] Canada RC-LD Medium	Race: NR Median Age=30 years SES: NR Home situation: NR Unplanned pregnancy: NR Marital/partner status: NR Smoking: NR ETOH: NR Substance abuse: NR	Mental Health Comorbidities: % with other mental health disorder=3.9% Use of other psychoactive drugs: 0.93% anticonvulsant dispensing; 0.76% antipsychotic dispensing; 8.4% Provider characteristics: NR Medical care environment: NR	100% with diagnosis Family history of depressive/mood disorders: NR Prior use of antidepressive drugs: Total antidepressant day's supply in the year before the LMP=265; # of antidepressant classes used in the year before the LMP, 0=12%, 1=75%, 2=14%, 3-4=2% Symptom severity: NR Time of diagnosis: NR Diagnosis method: NR When treatment commenced relative to the onset of symptoms: NR
Pearson 2007[61] US Retrospective cohort Data/Source: [AD] Medium	Race NR Mean Age: 33 vs. 33 Socio economic status: NR Home situation: NR Unplanned pregnancy: NR Marital/partner status: 97% vs. 77% M Smoking: 24% vs. 54% ETOH: NR Substance abuse: NR	Mental health Comorbidities %: 36% panic disorder 5% OCD 5% other anxiety disorders Use of other psychoactive drugs: 28.6% benzodiazepine (exposed) Provider characteristics: psychiatrist Medical care environment: hospital	53.4% with diagnosis Family history of depressive/mood disorders: NR Prior use of antidepressive drugs (%, for treatment or prevention): NR Symptom severity: NR Time of diagnosis: NR Diagnosis method: NR

Author Year Country Study Design/Data Source Risk of Bias	Population Characteristics 1. Race % Mean Age Socioeconomic Status Home Situation Unplanned Pregnancy % Marital/Partner Status Smoking % ETOH Substance Abuse %	2. Mental Health Comorbidities % Use of Other Psychoactive Drugs % Provider Characteristics Medical Care Environment	3. Depression Characteristics: - Percent with Diagnosis - Family History of Depressive/Mood Disorders (%) - Prior Use of Antidepressive Drugs (%, for Treatment or Prevention) - Symptom Severity - Time of Diagnosis - Diagnosis Method - When Treatment Commenced Relative to the Onset of Symptoms
Pedersen 2009[62] Denmark PBD, LD Medium	"Women taking an SSRI were more likely to be older, living alone, unmarried and smokers.' Data not shown. Others: NR	Mental health comorbidities: NR Use of other psychotropic drugs: 1.2% for women with no recorded use of antidepressants, 16% in SSRI group use of TCA: n=42 (0.008%, Venlafaxine: n=91, 0.02%)	NR
Pedersen 2010[63] Denmark PC Medium	Race % (white, AA, Hispanic, Asian, Other): NR Mean Age: 29.81% Socio economic status: Education level: High: 55.75%, Middle: 34.07%, Low: 9.29% Home situation: Live with partner: 94.47%, Live alone: 5.53% Unplanned pregnancy %: NR Marital/partner status (S/M/D): NR Smoking%: 47.35% ETOH: 40.60% Substance abuse%: NR	Mental health Comorbidities % (e.g. anxiety): NR Use of other psychoactive drugs % (antipsychotics, antianxiety agents (e.g., benzodiazepines), and drugs for insomnia): excluded women taking psychotropic medications other than antidepressants Provider characteristics (PCP, obstetrician, psychiatrist, nurse, midwife, community worker, or pediatrician visits): NR Medical care environment (community/private/public clinic or hospital): NR	Depression Characteristics: -% with diagnosis: NR -Family history of depressive/mood disorders (%): NR -Prior use of antidepressive drugs (%, for treatment or prevention): NR -Symptom severity: NR -Time of diagnosis: NR -Diagnosis method: NR -When treatment commenced relative to the onset of symptoms: NR
Pedersen 2013[64] (Pendersen, 2010) Denmark PBR Medium	Race: NR Mean Age: 30.2 Low socio economic status: NR Home situation: NR Unplanned pregnancy: NR Marital/partner status: living with partner = 122; alone = 5 Smoking%: 46.5% ETOH%: 35.4% Substance abuse%: NR	Mental health Comorbidities: NR Use of other psychoactive drugs: NR Provider characteristics: NR Medical care environment: NR	% with diagnosis: 14% Family history of depressive/mood disorders (%): NR Prior use of antidepressive drugs (%, for treatment or prevention):NR Symptom severity: NR Time of diagnosis: NR Diagnosis method: Interview by investigators When treatment commenced relative to the onset of symptoms: NR

Author Year Country Study Design/Data Source Risk of Bias	Population Characteristics 1. Race % Mean Age Socioeconomic Status Home Situation Unplanned Pregnancy % Marital/Partner Status Smoking % ETOH Substance Abuse %	2. Mental Health Comorbidities % Use of Other Psychoactive Drugs % Provider Characteristics Medical Care Environment	3. Depression Characteristics: - Percent with Diagnosis - Family History of Depressive/Mood Disorders (%) - Prior Use of Antidepressive Drugs (%, for Treatment or Prevention) - Symptom Severity - Time of Diagnosis - Diagnosis Method - When Treatment Commenced Relative to the Onset of Symptoms
Polen 2013[65] US PBD Medium	Race: 91.2% Mean Age: 52.8<30 years Low socio economic status: NR Home situation: NR Unplanned pregnancy: NR Marital/partner status: NR Smoking%: 23.1% ETOH%: 42.9% Substance abuse%: NR	Mental health Comorbidities: NR Use of other psychoactive drugs: NR Provider characteristics: NR Medical care environment: NR	% with diagnosis: NR Family history of depressive/mood disorders (%): NR Prior use of antidepressive drugs (%, for treatment or prevention): NR Symptom severity: NR Time of diagnosis: NR Diagnosis method: NR When treatment commenced relative to the onset of symptoms: NR
Rai 2013[66] Sweden CC Low	Race NR Mean Age: 29.5 years SES: Family income highest 5th=21%, lowest 5th=16%; parental education > 12 years=49%, 10-12 years=48%, <9 years=7.3%; occupational class: higher professionals=19%, intermediate non-manual employees=20%, lower non-manual employees=15%, skilled manual workers=14%, unskilled manual workers=14%, self-employed=4.8%, unclassified=12% Home situation: NR Unplanned pregnancy: NR Marital/partner status: NR Smoking: NR ETOH: NR Substance abuse: NR	Mental health Comorbidities: Anxiety disorder=6.2%, psychotic disorder=3.5%, other psychotic disorder=1.1% Use of other psychoactive drugs: NR Provider characteristics: NR Medical care environment: NR	0.06% with diagnosis Family history of depressive/mood disorders NR Prior use of antidepressive drugs: NR Symptom severity: NR Time of diagnosis: NR Diagnosis method: NR When treatment commenced relative to the onset of symptoms: NR
Ramos 2008[67] Canada LD Medium	Race % (white, AA, Hispanic, Asian, Other): Questionnaire subgroup, N=806; White: 87.3%, Black: 1.9%, Other: 10.8% Mean Age: 28.3 Socio economic status: Welfare Recipient, 46.2% Home situation: Living alone, 29.8% Unplanned pregnancy %: NR Marital/partner status (S/M/D): NR Smoking%: Questionnaire subgroup, 34.2% ETOH: Questionnaire subgroup, 19.7% Substance abuse%: Questionnaire subgroup, illicit drug use 6.82%	Mental health Comorbidities % (e.g. anxiety) : NR Use of other psychoactive drugs % (antipsychotics, antianxiety agents (e.g., benzodiazepines), and drugs for insomnia): At least one anxiolytic/sedative prescription: 18.8% Provider characteristics (primary care physician, obstetrician, psychiatrist, nurse, midwife, community worker, or pediatrician visits): NR Medical care environment (community/private/public clinic or hospital): NR	Depression Characteristics: -% with diagnosis: 25% -Family history of depressive/mood disorders (%): NR -Prior use of antidepressive drugs (%, for treatment or prevention): NR -Symptom severity: NR -Time of diagnosis: NR -Diagnosis method: NR -When treatment commenced relative to the onset of symptoms: NR

Author Year Country Study Design/Data Source Risk of Bias	Population Characteristics		
	1. Race % Mean Age Socioeconomic Status Home Situation Unplanned Pregnancy % Marital/Partner Status Smoking % ETOH Substance Abuse %	2. Mental Health Comorbidities % Use of Other Psychoactive Drugs % Provider Characteristics Medical Care Environment	3. Depression Characteristics: - Percent with Diagnosis - Family History of Depressive/Mood Disorders (%) - Prior Use of Antidepressive Drugs (%, for Treatment or Prevention) - Symptom Severity - Time of Diagnosis - Diagnosis Method - When Treatment Commenced Relative to the Onset of Symptoms
Ramos 2010[68] Canada LD, supplemental questionnaire Medium	Race % (white, AA, Hispanic, Asian, Other): NR Mean Age: 27.84 Socio economic status: Welfare recipient: 49.1%; Education Level >12y: 33.7% Home situation: Living Alone: 27.8% Unplanned pregnancy %: NR Marital/partner status (S/M/D): NR Smoking%: NR ETOH:NR Substance abuse%: NR	Mental health Comorbidities % (e.g. anxiety) : Number of different psychiatric disorder diagnoses: ≤2: 59.9%, 3-5: 31.2%, >5: 8.9% Use of other psychoactive drugs % (antipsychotics, antianxiety agents (e.g., benzodiazepines), and drugs for insomnia): ≥1 anxiolytic or sedative prescription: 18.5%; ≥1 anticonvulsive prescription: 13.1% Provider characteristics (primary care physician, obstetrician, psychiatrist, nurse, midwife, community worker, or pediatrician visits): NR Medical care environment (community/private/public clinic or hospital): NR	Depression Characteristics: -% with diagnosis: NR -Family history of depressive/mood disorders (%): NR -Prior use of antidepressive drugs (%, for treatment or prevention): NR -Symptom severity: NR -Time of diagnosis: NR -Diagnosis method: NR -When treatment commenced relative to the onset of symptoms: NR
Rampono 2009[69] Australia PC Medium	Race: NR Median Age (range): 31 (24-37) Socio economic status: NR Home situation: NR Unplanned pregnancy: NR Marital/partner status: NR Smoking (during pregnancy): 11% ETOH (during pregnancy): 19.8% Substance abuse: Known substance abusers were excluded	Mental health comorbidities: NR Use of other psychoactive drugs: NR Provider characteristics: NR Medical care environment: Outpatient clinics	NR
Reebye 2002[70] Canada PC Medium	White: 88.5%, Asian: 9.8%, Other: 1.6% Mean age: 31.8 years M: 93.4%, S or D: 3.3% Socio economic status: NR Home situation: NR Unplanned pregnancy %: NR	Provider characteristics: Psychiatrist 14 patients taking SSRI+benzodiazapine Mental health comorbidity: NR	NR

E-25

Author Year Country Study Design/Data Source Risk of Bias	Population Characteristics 1. Race % Mean Age Socioeconomic Status Home Situation Unplanned Pregnancy % Marital/Partner Status Smoking % ETOH Substance Abuse %	2. Mental Health Comorbidities % Use of Other Psychoactive Drugs % Provider Characteristics Medical Care Environment	3. Depression Characteristics: - Percent with Diagnosis - Family History of Depressive/Mood Disorders (%) - Prior Use of Antidepressive Drugs (%, for Treatment or Prevention) - Symptom Severity - Time of Diagnosis - Diagnosis Method - When Treatment Commenced Relative to the Onset of Symptoms
Reis 2010[71] Sweden PBR Medium	Race: NR Age: <20: 2%, 20-24: 12%, 25-29: 27%, 30-34: 34%, 35-39: 20%, 40-44: 4.6%, >=45:0.2 % Socio economic status: NR Home situation: NR Unplanned pregnancy: NR Marital/partner status: 2% unknown, 85% co-habiting, 6% living alone, 6% other Smoking: 2% unknown, 74% no, 14% <10 cigarettes/d, 9% >=10 cigarettes/d ETOH: NR Substance abuse: NR	Mental health comorbidities: NR Use of other psychoactive drugs: 11% sedatives or hypnotics Provider characteristics: NR Medical care environment: NR	NR
Salisbury 2011[72] US PC Medium	Race % (white, AA, Hispanic, Asian, Other): Hispanic 12.73%, Non-white 14.55% Mean Age: 29.3 Socio economic status: low SES 9.82% Home situation: NR Unplanned pregnancy %: NR Marital/partner status (S/M/D): not married: 34.23% Smoking%: 18.35% ETOH: 46.79% Substance abuse%: NR	Mental health Comorbidities % (e.g. anxiety) : NR Use of other psychoactive drugs (antipsychotics, antianxiety agents (e.g., benzodiazepines), and drugs for insomnia): NR Provider characteristics (PCP, obstetrician, psychiatrist, nurse, midwife, community worker, or pediatrician visits): NR Medical care environment (community/private/public clinic or hospital): Hospital	Depression Characteristics: -% with diagnosis: 50% -Family history of depressive/mood disorders (%): NR -Prior use of antidepressive drugs (%, for treatment or prevention): NR -Symptom severity: 8.0 -Time of diagnosis: NR -Diagnosis method: NR -When treatment commenced relative to the onset of symptoms: NR
Salkeld 2008[73] Canada CC-LD Low	Race: NR Mean Age=26 years SES NR Home situation: NR Unplanned pregnancy: NR Marital/partner status: NR Smoking: NR ETOH: NR Substance abuse: NR	NR	NR
Simon 2002[74] US RC-HCDB Low	NR	Mental health Comorbidities: NR Use of other psychoactive drugs: NR Provider characteristics: NR Medical care environment: Primary care facilities owned by Group Health Cooperative	NR

Author Year Country Study Design/Data Source Risk of Bias	Population Characteristics 1. Race % Mean Age Socioeconomic Status Home Situation Unplanned Pregnancy % Marital/Partner Status Smoking % ETOH Substance Abuse %	2. Mental Health Comorbidities % Use of Other Psychoactive Drugs % Provider Characteristics Medical Care Environment	3. Depression Characteristics: - Percent with Diagnosis - Family History of Depressive/Mood Disorders (%) - Prior Use of Antidepressive Drugs (%, for Treatment or Prevention) - Symptom Severity - Time of Diagnosis - Diagnosis Method - When Treatment Commenced Relative to the Onset of Symptoms
Sit 2011[75] US PC Medium	Race % (white, AA, Hispanic, Asian, Other): NR Mean Age: 31 Socio economic status: NR Home situation: NR Unplanned pregnancy %: NR Marital/partner status (S/M/D): NR Smoking%: 23.8% ETOH: excluded women with alcohol abuse Substance abuse%: excluded women with substance abuse	Mental health Comorbidities % (e.g. anxiety) : NR Use of other psychoactive drugs % (antipsychotics, antianxiety agents (e.g., benzodiazepines), and drugs for insomnia): NR Provider characteristics (primary care physician, obstetrician, psychiatrist, nurse, midwife, community worker, or pediatrician visits): Psychiatrist Medical care environment (community/private/public clinic or hospital): Clinic	Depression Characteristics: -% with diagnosis: 100% -Family history of depressive/mood disorders (%): NR -Prior use of antidepressive drugs (%, for treatment or prevention): NR -Symptom severity: Structured Interview Guide for HAM-D Atypical Depression Symptoms, Mean=16.0±7.6 -Time of diagnosis: NR -Diagnosis method: NR -When treatment commenced relative to the onset of symptoms: NR
Smith 2013[76] US PC High	Race: 100% Caucasian Mean Age: 32 years Low socio economic status: NR Home situation: NR Unplanned pregnancy: NR Marital/partner status: 83% Married Smoking%: 0% ETOH%: 0% Substance abuse%: 0%	Mental health Comorbidities: GAD = 16% Panic Disorder = 16% PTSD = 16% Use of other psychoactive drugs: NR Provider characteristics: NR Medical care environment: NR	% with diagnosis: 0% - depression is excluded in this study Family history of depressive/mood disorders (%): NR Prior use of antidepressive drugs (%, for treatment or prevention): NR Symptom severity: NR Time of diagnosis: NR Diagnosis method: NR When treatment commenced relative to the onset of symptoms: NR
Stephansson 2013[77] Sweden PBR Medium	Race: NR Mean Age: <=24: 16.3%, 25-34: 66.2%, 35-44: 17.4%, >=45: 0.1% Socio economic status: NR Home situation: NR Unplanned pregnancy: NR Marital/partner status: NR Smoking in early pregnancy: 78.1% no, 15.6% yes, 6.3% missing data ETOH: NR Substance abuse: NR	Mental health comorbidities: 3.9% had a previous psychiatric hospitalization Use of other psychoactive drugs: NR Provider characteristics: NR (stillbirth and neonatal mortality) Medical care environment: NR	NR

E-27

	Population Characteristics		3. Depression Characteristics:
Author Year Country Study Design/Data Source Risk of Bias	1. Race % Mean Age Socioeconomic Status Home Situation Unplanned Pregnancy % Marital/Partner Status Smoking % ETOH Substance Abuse %	2. Mental Health Comorbidities % Use of Other Psychoactive Drugs % Provider Characteristics Medical Care Environment	- Percent with Diagnosis - Family History of Depressive/Mood Disorders (%) - Prior Use of Antidepressive Drugs (%, for Treatment or Prevention) - Symptom Severity - Time of Diagnosis - Diagnosis Method - When Treatment Commenced Relative to the Onset of Symptoms
Suri 2007[78] US PC Medium	Race % (white, AA, Hispanic, Asian, Other): NR Mean Age: 33.8y Socio economic status: College degree 87% Home situation: NR Unplanned pregnancy %: NR Marital/partner status (S/M/D): M 90% Smoking%: 2.2% ETOH: 2.2% Substance abuse%: NR	"Mental health Comorbidities % (e.g. anxiety): NR Use of other psychoactive drugs % (antipsychotics, antianxiety agents (e.g., benzodiazepines), and drugs for insomnia): NR Provider characteristics (primary care physician, obstetrician, psychiatrist, nurse, midwife, community worker, or pediatrician visits): obstetrics, psychiatric Medical care environment (community/private/public clinic or hospital): clinic" Depression Characteristics: -% with diagnosis: 78.5% -Family history of depressive/mood disorders (%): NR -Prior use of antidepressive drugs (%, for treatment or prevention): NR -Symptom severity: HAM-D: Maximum 21-item score M=17.2, Maximum 28-item score M=23.5; Maximum Beck Depression Inventory score M=9.8; Maximum Perceived Stress Scale M=9.3 -Time of diagnosis: NR -Diagnosis method: NR -When treatment commenced relative to the onset of symptoms: NR	Depression Characteristics: -% with diagnosis: 78.5% -Family history of depressive/mood disorders (%): NR -Prior use of antidepressive drugs (%, for treatment or prevention): NR -Symptom severity: HAM-D: Maximum 21-item score M=17.2, Maximum 28-item score M=23.5; Maximum Beck Depression Inventory score M=9.8; Maximum Perceived Stress Scale M=9.3 -Time of diagnosis: NR -Diagnosis method: NR -When treatment commenced relative to the onset of symptoms: NR

Author Year Country Study Design/Data Source Risk of Bias	Population Characteristics 1. Race % Mean Age Socioeconomic Status Home Situation Unplanned Pregnancy % Marital/Partner Status Smoking % ETOH Substance Abuse %	2. Mental Health Comorbidities % Use of Other Psychoactive Drugs % Provider Characteristics Medical Care Environment	3. Depression Characteristics: - Percent with Diagnosis - Family History of Depressive/Mood Disorders (%) - Prior Use of Antidepressive Drugs (%, for Treatment or Prevention) - Symptom Severity - Time of Diagnosis - Diagnosis Method - When Treatment Commenced Relative to the Onset of Symptoms
Suri 2011[79] US PC Medium	Race % (white, AA, Hispanic, Asian, Other): NR Mean Age: 334.84% Socio economic status: Education, M=17.57y Home situation: NR Unplanned pregnancy %: NR Marital/partner status (S/M/D): NR Smoking%: NR ETOH: NR Substance abuse%: NR	Mental health Comorbidities % (e.g. anxiety): NR Use of other psychoactive drugs % (antipsychotics, antianxiety agents (e.g., benzodiazepines), and drugs for insomnia): NR Provider characteristics (primary care physician, obstetrician, psychiatrist, nurse, midwife, community worker, or pediatrician visits): NR Medical care environment (community/private/public clinic or hospital): clinic	Depression Characteristics: -% with diagnosis: lifetime diagnosis 76.6% -Family history of depressive/mood disorders (%) : NR -Prior use of antidepressive drugs (%, for treatment or prevention): NR -Symptom severity: Hamilton Depression Rating Scale, M=9
Ter Horst 2013[80] The Netherlands PD Medium	Race: NR Mean Age: NR Low socio economic status: NR Home situation: NR Unplanned pregnancy: NR Marital/partner status: NR Smoking%: ETOH%: Substance abuse%:	Mental health Comorbidities: NR Use of other psychoactive drugs: NR Provider characteristics: NR Medical care environment: NR	% with diagnosis: NR Family history of depressive/mood disorders (%): NR Prior use of antidepressive drugs (%, for treatment or prevention): NR Symptom severity: NR Time of diagnosis: NR Diagnosis method: NR When treatment commenced relative to the onset of symptoms: NR
Toh 2009[81] US CC Medium	Race: 72.6% white, 6.9% black, 13.2 % Hispanic, 7.3% other Mean Age: <25: 18.9%, 25-29: 23.2%, 30-34: 35.5%, >=35: 21.9% Socioeconomic status: Education (years): <=12: 25.7%, 13-15: 24.1%, >15: 49.2% Home situation: NR Unplanned pregnancy: NR Married or living with child's partner: 89.7% Smoking during pregnancy: Never: 59.1%, past smoker: 25.5%, <10 per d: 7.9%, >=10 per d: 8.5% ETOH during pregnancy: Never: 45.7%, past drinker: 50.3%, drank: 3.3% Substance abuse: NR	Mental health comorbidities: NR Use of other psychoactive drugs: 0.8% Provider characteristics: NR Medical care environment: Various (hospitals, clinics, PICUs)	NR

Author Year Country Study Design/Data Source Risk of Bias	Population Characteristics 1. Race % Mean Age Socioeconomic Status Home Situation Unplanned Pregnancy % Marital/Partner Status Smoking % ETOH Substance Abuse %	2. Mental Health Comorbidities % Use of Other Psychoactive Drugs % Provider Characteristics Medical Care Environment	3. Depression Characteristics: - Percent with Diagnosis - Family History of Depressive/Mood Disorders (%) - Prior Use of Antidepressive Drugs (%, for Treatment or Prevention) - Symptom Severity - Time of Diagnosis - Diagnosis Method - When Treatment Commenced Relative to the Onset of Symptoms
Ververs 2009[82] The Netherlands AD Medium	Race % (white, AA, Hispanic, Asian, Other): Mean Age: 30.3y Socio economic status: NR Home situation: NR Unplanned pregnancy %: NR Marital/partner status (S/M/D): NR Smoking%: NR ETOH: NR Substance abuse%: NR	Mental health Comorbidities % (e.g. anxiety) : NR Use of other psychoactive drugs % (antipsychotics, antianxiety agents (e.g., benzodiazepines), and drugs for insomnia): NR Provider characteristics (primary care physician, obstetrician, psychiatrist, nurse, midwife, community worker, or pediatrician visits): NR Medical care environment (community/private/public clinic or hospital): NR	Depression Characteristics: -% with diagnosis: NR -Family history of depressive/mood disorders (%) : NR -Prior use of antidepressive drugs (%, for treatment or prevention): NR -Symptom severity : NR -Time of diagnosis: NR -Diagnosis method : NR -When treatment commenced relative to the onset of symptoms: NR
Wilson 2011[83] US CC Medium	Race: NR Advanced maternal age (>=35): 10% Socio economic status: NR Home situation: NR Unplanned pregnancy: NR Marital/partner status: NR Smoking (tobacco use yes): 7.1% ETOH: NR Substance abuse: NR	Mental health comorbidities: NR Use of other psychoactive drugs: NR Provider characteristics: NR Medical care environment: Army Medical Center	NR
Wisner 2009[84] US PC Medium	Race: 67% white, 12% AA, 2% Other Mean Age: 39% < 31 years, 41% > 31 years Socio economic status: NR Home situation: NR Unplanned pregnancy %: NR Marital/partner status (S/M/D): 64% M/partner	NR	% with diagnosis: 100% Family history of depressive/mood disorders (%): NR Prior use of antidepressive drugs (%, for treatment or prevention): NR Symptom severity : HAM-D 17: 4.9 (range across groups 4.2 - 14.9), Time of diagnosis: baseline Diagnosis method: HAM-D 17, Structured Interview Guide for the Hamilton Depression Rating Scale With Atypical Depression Supplement, GAS, SF-12 Mental Component When treatment commenced relative to the onset of symptoms: NR

Author Year Country Study Design/Data Source Risk of Bias	Population Characteristics 1. Race % Mean Age Socioeconomic Status Home Situation Unplanned Pregnancy % Marital/Partner Status Smoking % ETOH Substance Abuse %	2. Mental Health Comorbidities % Use of Other Psychoactive Drugs % Provider Characteristics Medical Care Environment	3. Depression Characteristics: - Percent with Diagnosis - Family History of Depressive/Mood Disorders (%) - Prior Use of Antidepressive Drugs (%, for Treatment or Prevention) - Symptom Severity - Time of Diagnosis - Diagnosis Method - When Treatment Commenced Relative to the Onset of Symptoms
Wisner 2013[85] (Wisner 2009/Okun 2012) US PC Medium	SSRI Exposed group Race: White = 91.3; Black = 6.5; Other= 2.2 Mean Age: 31.3 Low socio economic status: NR Home situation: NR Unplanned pregnancy: NR Marital/partner status: Single = 8; Married/cohabiting = 36; Divorced/separated = 2 ; Widowed = 0 Smoking%: N= 10.9 ETOH%: Once a week or less = 23.9; More than once a week = 10.9 Substance abuse%: NR	Mental health Comorbidities: Lifetime diagnosis of anxiety disorder 45.7% Use of other psychoactive drugs: NR Provider characteristics: Primary care provider Medical care environment: Primary care office	% with diagnosis: Unclear Family history of depressive/mood disorders (%) : NR Prior use of antidepressive drugs (%, for treatment or prevention): NR Symptom severity: Time of diagnosis: Diagnosis method: When treatment commenced relative to the onset of symptoms: NR
Wogelius 2006[86] Denmark PBR Medium	Age: <25: 13%, 25-30: 46%, >30: 42.1% Smoking: 24.2% smokers Other characteristics: NR	Mental health comorbidities: NR Use of other psychoactive drugs: NR Provider characteristics: NR Medical care environment: NR	NR
Yonkers 2012[87] US Prospective Cohort [PC] Low	Race 74% White 7% Black 14% Hispanic,5% Other Mean Age: 31 Socio economic status: NR Education (years) <12, 6% 12, 14% 13-15, 23% 16+, 57% Home situation: NR Unplanned pregnancy: NR Marital/partner status: NR Smoking: 15% ETOH: NR Substance abuse: 8%	Mental health Comorbidities % PDSD 5% Anxiety 10% Panic disorder 4% Use of other psychoactive drugs % Provider characteristics: obstetrician :clinic or hospital	100% with diagnosis Family history of depressive/mood disorders: NR Prior use of antidepressive drugs (%, for treatment or prevention) NR Symptom severity: NR Time of diagnosis: NR Diagnosis method: DSM-IV and screened positive for depressive episode and antidepressant treatment.
Zeskind 2004[88] US Prospective cohort study/Data Source [PC, AD] Medium	Race: 94% white Mean Age: 33 years (1.36) Low socio economic status: N=3 Home situation: NR Unplanned pregnancy: NR Marital/partner status: NR Smoking%: ETOH: 70% Substance abuse: 2%	Mental health Comorbidities: NR Use of other psychoactive drugs: NR Provider characteristics: NR Medical care environment: NR	100% with diagnosis Family history of depressive/mood disorders: NR Prior use of antidepressive drugs (%, for treatment or prevention) NR Symptom severity: NR Time of diagnosis: NR Diagnosis method: NR

Author Year Country Study Design/Data Source Risk of Bias	4. Exposures (N, duration, dose) Controls (N)	5. Exposure Period	6. Confounders
Alwan 2007[1] US Arm of Case Control Studied, Population based Medium	Fluoxetine, Sertraline, Paroxetine. Duration: 1 month before pregnancy-3 month after conception	1 month before pregnancy - 3 months after conception	Maternal race, obesity, maternal smoking, family income
Alwan 2010[2] Canada Case-control/Data Source [CC] Medium	Bupropion N = 90 Cases: N=64 Controls: N=26 Duration: NR Unexposed N = 17353 Cases: N=11,733 Controls: N=5626	Between 1 month before and 3 months after conception.	Adjusted for maternal age, maternal race, maternal education, maternal obesity before pregnancy (body mass index 30 kg/m2, 30 kg/m2), maternal smoking and alcohol use from 1 month before to 3 months after conception, use of a dietary supplement containing folic acid from 1 month before to 1 month after conception, annual family income plurality, and parity.
Andrade 2009[3] US Retrospective Cohort/Data Source [AD] Medium	Average daily doses of sertraline, fluoxetine, and paroxetine were 113.2 ± 72.3 mg, 20 ± 11.9 mg, and 17.2 ± 10.1 mg	Third trimester exposure	None adjusted for (Data NA)
Bakker 2010[4] CC/PBD The Netherlands Medium	Paroxetine (N = 6, T1) Controls (N=605)	T1	Year of birth
Bakker 2010[5] The Netherlands Case-Control Medium	Exposure=Paroxetine; dose and duration NR Cases N=678 Controls N=615	First trimester: Any use from 4 weeks before conception through the 12th week of pregnancy	Adjusted for year of birth, pregnancy outcome, maternal age, gravidity, mother's educational level, smoking, use of alcohol, BMI, folic acid use, and pre-existing maternal diabetes or epilepsy
Ban 2012[6] U.K. PBD Medium	N= all pregnancies Exposure TCA: N= 3019 SSRI:N= 10312 Control: No history N= 390665, unmedicated mental illness : N= 3647	First trimester	Maternal age at the end of pregnancy, most recent recording of smoking status before delivery, BMI before pregnancy and quintiles of Townsend's Index of Deprivation for each woman's postcode of residence, no. of previous known live births for each pregnancy
Batton 2013[7] US PD Medium	Exposure: N=19 Paroxetine= 2; Fluoxetine = 6; Sertraline = 9; Citalopram= 2; Escitalopram = 2 Control: N=19 Unexposed	First prenatal visit through delivery	Gestational age, year of birth, birth weight, gender, age at neurodevelopmental assessment.

| Author
Year
Country
Study Design/Data Source
Risk of Bias	4. Exposures (N, duration, dose) Controls (N)	5. Exposure Period	6. Confounders
Berard 2007[8]
Canada, Quebec
LD
Medium | Paroxetine (N=542)
Dose, M=22.4mg±9.0
Duration, M=64d±2.3

Other SSRI (N=443)
Dose, Duration, NR
Sertraline, n=186
Citalopram, n=113
Fluoxetine, n=101
Fluvoxamine, n=43

Non-SSRI antidepressants (Control Group) (N=293)
Dose, Duration, NR
Venlafaxine, n=153
Amitriptyline, n=140 | First trimester: 0-14 weeks of GA | Adjusted for antidepressant exposure during the second and third trimesters, GA, maternal age, mean number of prenatal visits, visits to an obstetrician during pregnancy, pregnancy in the year before this pregnancy, diagnosis of diabetes, hypertension and depression in the year before or during pregnancy, place of residence, living alone, welfare status, calendar year, mean number of physician visits in year before pregnancy, number of different medications excluding antidepressants, number of different prescribers in year before and during pregnancy. |
| Bogen 2010/companion Wen 2009[9]
US
PC
Medium | Physically healthy but taking antidepressant during pregnancy for MDD , n=38 (SSRI), n=1 (bupropion), duration: N MDD during pregnancy but no gestational antidepressant exposure, N=NR
No current psychiatric disorder and no antidepressant, N=NR | Pregnancy to 2 years postpartum | Women's prior breast feeding experience, maternal age, race, marital statu, smoking, maternal obesity, SRI use |
| Boucher 2008[10]
Canada
LD
Medium | Exposed: N=73 (22 citalopram, 19 paroxetine, 10 sertraline, 4 fluoxetine, 2 fluvoxamine, 12 venlafaxine, 3 amitriptyline, 3 trazodone, 1 mirtazapine)
Duration NR

Controls: N=73 | Late pregnancy (last 3 weeks of pregnancy) | Gestational age at birth, maternal age and other medications taken by the mother. |
| Casper 2003[11]
US
Cohort study
Data/Source: [CC]
Medium | Any SSRI,
N= 31
23% fluoxetine, 26%paroxetine, 3.2% fluvoxamine

Duration:
Throughout: N=13
First trimester: N= 22
Third trimester: N= 23

Dose:
average daily doses
sertraline 113.2 ± 72.3 mg, fluoxetine 20 ± 11.9 mg, paroxetine 17.2 ± 10.1 mg

Control: Unexposed
N= 13 | 71% before or during pregnancy
45% throughout
71% first trimester
74% third trimester
29% after delivery | Adjusted for age at delivery, marital status, years of schooling, parity, weight gain, and self-rated levels of depression |

E-33

Author Year Country Study Design/Data Source Risk of Bias	4. Exposures (N, duration, dose) Controls (N)	5. Exposure Period	6. Confounders
Chambers 1996[12] US CC Medium	Controls (N=223) Fluoxetine, N=173 Dose M=26.73 Duration: NR	At study entry, through: Exposed Early group: 93% discontinued in first trimester 7% first and second trimester Exposed Late group: 82.2% first, second third trimester 9.6% second and third trimester 5.5% third trimester only 2.7% first and third trimester only	Adjusted for multiparity, previous spontaneous abortion, preeclampsia, eclampsia, hypertension, smoking status, maternal age, SES, race, average dose of fluoxetine, gestational diabetes, use of other psychotherapeutic drugs, alcohol use, evidence of maternal age, SES, race, average dose of fluoxetine, gestational diabetes, use of other psychotherapeutic drugs, alcohol use, evidence of maternal or neonatal infection near delivery, prematurity, mode of delivery.
Chambers 2006[13] US CC Medium	Cases N=377 (16 SSRI, 4 other antidepressant) Controls: N=836 (24 SSRI, 13 other antidepressant) Duration: NR	Before week 20 (n=32) After week 20 (n=25)	Single or multiple pregnancy, maternal diabetes, maternal smoking, maternal alcohol use, maternal NSAID use after week 20.
Cole 2007[14] US Case-control/Data Source[AD] Medium	Paroxetine vs. other antidepressants* Monotherapy N=791 Mono or Polytherapy: N=989 Other antidepressants: Monotherapy N=4072 Mono or Poly therapy: N=4767 Duration: NR Control: Exposed to other antidepressants N= 4767 (mono or poly) and 4072 (monotherapy) * including selective serotonin reuptake inhibitors, selective norepinephrine reuptake inhibitors, serotonin-2 antagonist reuptake inhibitors, tricyclics, and monoamine oxidase inhibitors)	First trimester.	Adjusted for all of the covariates derived from the medical and pharmacy claims data and indicators for paroxetine exposure, maternal age category, geographic region of the health plan, and infant sex.
Cole 2007[15] US LD Low	Exposed: N=1213 bupropion, 4743 other antidepressant Controls: N=1049 (bupropion outside first trimester)	1st trimester	Diagnoses of bipolar-disorder and eclampsia within 1 year before delivery; dispensing of lithium, phenytoin, and fluconazole within 1 year before delivery through the end of the 1st trimester, and the number of physician visits within 10-12 months before delivery; maternal age, geographic region of the health plan, and infant sex.

Author Year Country Study Design/Data Source Risk of Bias	4. Exposures (N, duration, dose) Controls (N)	5. Exposure Period	6. Confounders
Colvin 2012[16] PBD/CC Australia Medium	Any SSRI, citalopram hydrobromide, escitalopram oxalate, fluoxetine hydrochloride, fluvoxamine maleate, paroxetine hydrochloride, and sertraline N=2701 Duration and dose: NR Control: Unexposed N=94,561	Medication dispensed: T0: 76 days before to 14 days after LMP (exposures in the 90 days before conception) T1: 14 days to 104 days after LMP, or end of pregnancy whichever occurred first, (first trimester exposures) T2: 105 days to 194 days after LMP, or end of the pregnancy (second trimester exposures) T3: 195 days after LMP to end of the pregnancy event to ascertain (third trimester exposures) T2 or T3: 105 days after LMP to the end of the pregnancy (second or third trimester exposures Anytime during pregnancy: 14 days after the LMP to the end of pregnancy	Adjusted for previous preterm birth, smoking, SEIFA, parity, and maternal age
Colvin 2012[16] PBD/CC Australia Medium	Any SSRI: citalopram, paroxetine, sertraline, fluoxetine, escitalopram, fluvoxamine (N=3764, varies) Controls (N=94,561)	T1: Trimester 1 T2 or T3: Trimester 2 or 3 only Any: Any time during pregnancy	Preterm birth (<37 Weeks) was adjusted for previous preterm birth, smoked during pregnancy, SEIFA, parity, maternal age; singletons only Birth weight (<2500g) was adjusted for gestational age, smoking during pregnancy, SEIFA, sex, parity, maternal height; singletons only
Croen 2011[17] US CC Medium	SSRIs (N=49) citalopram, fluoxetine, fluvoxamine, paroxetine, sertraline Dual-action antidepressants (N=10) nefazodone, trazodone, venlafaxine, serotonin-noradrenergic-reuptake inhibitors, noradrenergic and specific serotoninergic antidepressants, and noradrenaline-reuptake inhibitors Tricyclic antidepressants (N 22) amitriptyline, desipramine, doxepin, imipramine, nortriptyline, protriptyline SSRIs only, N=38 SSRIs + tricyclic antidepressants or dual-action antidepressants, N=11	Preconception: 3 months prior to LMP First trimester: first 90 days after LMP Second trimester: 91-180 days after LMP Third trimester; 181 days after LMP to date of delivery	Adjusted for age, race/ethnicity, education of mother, birth weight, sex, birth year, birth facility

Author Year Country Study Design/Data Source Risk of Bias	4. Exposures (N, duration, dose) Controls (N)	5. Exposure Period	6. Confounders
Davidson 2009[18] Israel CC Medium	Controls (N=20) Paroxetine (N=8) Fluoxetine (N=7) Citalopram (N=6)	Entire pregnancy	Groups matched for gestational age. Excluded from study: Diabetes, chronic hypertension, CV disease.
Davis 2007[19] US LD Medium	Assessing congenital anomalies: Tricyclic Antidepressants (N=221) SSRIs (N=1047) Other antidepressants (N=173) Non-exposed (N=49,663) Assessing perinatal complications: Tricyclic Antidepressants (N=339) SSRIs (N=1602) Other antidepressants (N=260) Nonexposed (N=75,833)	Assessing congenital anomalies: First trimester exposure Assessing perinatal complications: Third trimester exposure	Unadjusted
De Vries 2013[20] Australia PC Medium	Exposure: (N=63) Paroxetine = 27; Cipramil = 14; venlafaxine = 10; fluoxetine = 8; sertraline = 2; switched med = 2; stopped med = 4 Control: (N=44)	NR	NR
Dubnov-Raz 2008[21] Israel CC Medium	Controls (N=52) Paroxetine (N=25), Citalopram (N=13), Fluoxetine (N=12), Fluvoxamine (N=1), Venlafaxine (N=1), duration and doses NR	NR, women were taking SSRI at onset of labor	Excluded gestational diabetes and hypothyroidism
Dubnov-Raz 2012[22] Israel CC Medium	SSRI (N=40); High dose: fluoxetine, citalopram ≥ 40mg/d, escitalopram ≥20mg/d ; Duration: 92.5% throughout entire pregnancy Controls (N=40)	Throughout pregnancy	Adjusted for maternal age, maternal smoking status, previous births, GA, infant sex, birth weight z-score, birth length
El Marroun 2012[23] The Netherlands Prospective Cohort Data Source [PC and PD] Low	SSRIs during pregnancy N=99,1.3% Duration: NR Control: Unexposed (with low depressive symptoms) N=7027, 91.3%	First trimester only, N=47 First trimester plus 1 additional trimester, N=52	Adjusted for BMI, educational level, maternal smoking habits, maternal age, ethnicity, fetal sex, parity, and maternal use of benzodiazepines, but not maternal drinking habits and cannabis. For effects of depressive symptoms and SSRI use on head growth also adjusted for fetal body size measures.

Author Year Country Study Design/Data Source Risk of Bias	4. Exposures (N, duration, dose) Controls (N)	5. Exposure Period	6. Confounders
Ferreira 2007[24] US Retrospective Cohort/Data Source[AD] Medium	Exposed to SSRIs or venlafaxine: N=76 46 (60.5%) paroxetine (5–40 mg) 10 (13.2%) fluoxetine (10–40 mg) 9 (11.8%) venlafaxine (75–150 mg) 6 (8%) citalopram (10–30 mg), 3 (3.9%) sertraline (125–150 mg), 2 (2.6%) fluvoxamine (50–150 mg) Mean duration SSRIs: 32 months (range: 1–132 months) Controls: Unexposed N=90	Third trimester or at least two weeks prior to delivery	Adjusted for prematurity, maternal age 35 years, smoking, illicit drug use, cesarean section, maternal hypertension, prolonged preterm rupture of membranes, history of prematurity, history of 2 miscarriages, gestational diabetes, and small for gestational age.
Figueroa 2010[25] US Retrospective cohort Design/Data Source[AD] Medium	SSRI before pregnancy N=954 2.51% SSRI during pregnancy N=916 2.41% First trimester N=564 1.48% Second trimester N=450 1.18% Third trimester N=564 1.48% SSRI after pregnancy N=1,948 5.12% Bupropion before pregnancy N=165 0.43% Bupropion during pregnancy N=114 0.30% First trimester N=79 0.21 % Second trimester N=46 0.12% Third trimester N=7 0.10% Bupropion after pregnancy N=185 0.49% Other antidepressant during pregnancy N=119 0.31% Dose: NR Controls: Unexposed N=168	Before pregnancy First trimester Second trimester Third trimester Throughout	Adjusted for maternal and paternal mental health diagnoses, presence or absence of maternal mental health-related visits by period of time (year of child's life), use of other psychotropics during pregnancy, and perinatal complications.
Gorman 2012[26] US Prospective cohort/TIS Medium	Any SSRI Exposures at delivery: 197 Unexposed: 182	Means: Exposed early: 12 weeks Exposed at deliver: 33 weeks	Maternal age, SES category, and race/ethnicity, maternal characteristics, reproductive history, (any alcohol use in pregnancy, cesarean birth, and low 5-minute Apgar scores and birth characteristics

Author Year Country Study Design/Data Source Risk of Bias	4. Exposures (N, duration, dose) Controls (N)	5. Exposure Period	6. Confounders
Grzeskowiak 2012[27] Australia Retrospective cohort/LD Medium	SSRI use N=221 Psychiatric illness/no SSRI use N=1566 No psychiatric illness N=32,004	Late gestation=Definition NR	Preterm delivery adjusted for maternal age, socioeconomic status, smoking status, race, asthma, preexisting diabetes, alcohol abuse, substance abuse, hypertension, parity, epilepsy, thyroid disorder, previous history of premature delivery, and anxiolytic use Low birth weight adjusted for same as preterm delivery plus maternal H4-SGA, neonate admitted to hospital, neonate length of hospital stay > 3 days adjusted for maternal age, socioeconomic status, smoking status, race, asthma, preexisting diabetes, alcohol abuse, substance abuse, hypertension, parity, epilepsy, thyroid disorder, and anxiolytic use.
Hanley 2013[28] Canada PC Medium	Exposure: N=31 paroxetine n=4; fluoxetine n=3; sertraline n=5; venlafaxine n=12; citalopram n=7 Control: N=52	Before conception until they stopped them with a mean of 249 (SD 58.9) days	HAM-D scores
Heikkinen 2002[29] Finland PC	Exposure: Citalopram 20-40mg QD, n=11, duration: NR Controls: n=10	During pregnancy up to 1 year	Age, gravidity, parity, time and mode of delivery
Jimenez-Solem 2012[30] Denmark RC-PD Low	Any SSRI, dose and duration NR First trimester exposure N=4183 Paused during pregnancy N=806 Unexposed: N=843,797	First trimester: Between ≥1 month before conception and d 84 Paused exposure: No exposure between 3 months before conception and 1 month after giving birth	Adjusted for mother's age, parity, income, education, smoking and year of conception. SSRI, selective serotonin reuptake inhibitor
Jimenez-Solem 2013[31] Denmark PBR Low	Exposed: N=6,378 (2,434 fluoxetine, 1,800 citalopram, 212 escitalopram, 734 paroxetine, 1,654 sertraline) Unexposed: N=908,214	1st trimester (n=3982) 1st and 2nd trimesters (n=2065) All trimesters: (n=6378)	Smoking, birth year, prior stillbirths, mother's age, annual household income, education level, parity
Jordan 2008[32] US Clinic Appt Logs, Pediatrics records review AD Medium	SRI Any N=49. Duration NR; controls= unexposed and discontinued last month of pregnancy	NR	Analyzed 3 pregnancies with Benzos separately

Author Year Country Study Design/Data Source Risk of Bias	4. Exposures (N, duration, dose) Controls (N)	5. Exposure Period	6. Confounders
Kallen 2004[33] Sweden PBR Medium	SSRI (N=558): Citalopram, n=285 Paroxetine, n=106 Fluoxetine, n=91 Sertraline, n=77 Other antidepressants (N=63) Venlafaxine, n=24	throughout pregnancy; weeks of pregnancy NR, n=387 drug stopped before week 24, n=70 drug started or continued past week 23, n=561	Adjusted for year of birth, maternal age, parity, and maternal smoking in early pregnancy
Kallen 2007[34] Sweden Retrospective cohort/Data Source[PBR] Medium	Exposed SSRIs N = 6,481, 96.5% only one SSRI Fluoxetine N=860 Citalopram N=2,579 Paroxetine N=908 Sertraline N=1,807 Fluvoxamine N=36 Escitalopram N= 66 Duration: NR Dose: NR	First trimester	Adjusted for maternal age, parity, smoking, previous miscarriage, BMI, years of subfertility and maternal country of birth.
Kallen 2008[35] Sweden Unclear/Data Source[PBR] Medium	Exposed: N= 7587 SSRIs: 39% Citalopram 31% Sertraline 15% Fluoxetine 13% Paroxetine 2% Fluvoxamine or escitalopram Dose: NR Controls: All other registered births N= 831,324 Other: Mirtazapine N=1	First trimester, some late exposure	Adjusted for maternal age, parity, BMI, and smoking.
Kieler 2012[36] Nordic countries Retrospective cohort, PBD Medium	Any SSRI, fluoxetine, citalopram, paroxetine, sertraline, or escitalopram N = 2145 Duration NR Control: Unexposed N = 2300	Ever: 3 months before pregnancy until birth Early: 3 months before pregnancy until pregnancy length of 55 days Late: From 140 days after the start of pregnancy until birth	Adjusted for maternal age, dispensed non-steroidal anti-inflammatory drugs and anti diabetes drugs, pre-eclampsia, chronic diseases during pregnancy, country of birth, birth year, level of delivery hospital and birth order

Author Year Country Study Design/Data Source Risk of Bias	4. Exposures (N, duration, dose) Controls (N)	5. Exposure Period	6. Confounders
Kornum 2010[37] Denmark PBR Medium	No SSRI (N= 213,049) Any SSRI (N= 2,993, duration and dose NR)	Early: From 30 days prior to conception to the end of the first trimester Second/Third month: During the second or third month of pregnancy	Excluded from study: Antiepileptics within 90 days prior to conception or during first trimester Antidiabetic drugs at any time prior to conception or during pregnancy ORs adjusted for maternal smoking status, maternal age, birth order and birth year.
Laine 2003[38] Finland Prospective cohort/Data Source[PC] Medium	SSRIs: Citalopram, Fluoxetine N = 20 Duration: exposure during pregnancy ranged from 7- 41 weeks Dose: mean (range) Citalopram: 20mg (20-40) Fluoxetine: 20mg (20-40) Control: Unexposed N = 20	During pregnancy and lactation	Adjustment NR Controls matched age, gravidity, parity, duration of pregnancy and time and mode of delivery.
Latendresse 2011[39] US PS Medium	Total N: exposed and non exposed: 100 SSRI: n, dose and duration: NR Control: Unexposed patients, n, dose, duration NR	NR	Pregnancy related anxiety, corticotropin releasing hormone and SSRI use for depression and anxiety, age, antepartum complications (including previous history of Pre-term birth
Lennestal 2007[40] Sweden PBR Medium	SNRI Use (N=732) Mianserin, n=61 Mirtazapine, n=144 Venlafaxine, n=501 Reboxetine, n=14 Venlafaxine + mirtazapine, n=9 Venlafaxine + mianserin or reboxetine, n=3 SSRI Use comparison group (N=6481) No. women in register, controls (N=860,215) Doses, durations NR	Throughout pregnancy; "Early" exposure: maternal use of the drug prior to first antenatal care visit (usually near end of first trimester) "Late" exposure: maternal use of the drug after the "early" exposure period.	Adjusted for year of delivery, maternal age, parity, and smoking in early pregnancy, BMI class
Levinson-Castiel 2006[41] Israel PC, PBD Medium	SSRIs (n=60)N, dose range : paroxetine:37, 10-40mg; fluoxetine:12, 20-60mg; citalopram: 8,10-40mg; venlafaxine:2, 37.5-75mg Duration, mean, SD, wks: 35.5 (8.7) Control-non-SSRI exposed neonates: n=60	During entire pregnancy or at least during the third trimester	Adjusted for sex, gestational age (±1 wk), birth weight, mode of delivery

Author Year Country Study Design/Data Source Risk of Bias	4. Exposures (N, duration, dose) Controls (N)	5. Exposure Period	6. Confounders
Lewis 2010[42] Australia PC-Clinic Medium	Medication group N=27 Control group N=27 Types, doses, duration NR	NR	No adjustment for confounders
Logsdon 2011[43] US PC Medium	Control (no SSRI, no MDD): N=144 Responder (SSRI, no MDD): N=48 Untreated (MDD, no SSRI): N=12 Nonresponder (Both MDD and SSRI): N=11	NR	Excluded from study: active substance abuse, benzodiazepines, prescription drugs in FDA-defined categories of D or X.
Lund 2009[44] Denmark PC Medium	SSRI, N=329, duration and dose NR Control: Psychiatric history, no SSRI use: 4902 Control, No psychiatric history, no SSRI use: 51770	NR	Parity, maternal age, BMI, smoking habit, alcohol intake, marital status, education
Malm 2011[45] Finland TIS Low	SSRI (N=6,881, duration and dose NR) No SSRI (N=618,727, duration and dose NR)	1 month prior to pregnancy or during the first trimester	Adjusted for maternal age at end of pregnancy, parity, year of pregnancy ending, marital status, smoking during pregnancy, purchase of other reimbursed psychiatric drugs during the first trimester, maternal prepregnancy diabetes.
McFarland 2011[46] US PC Medium	Dose and duration NR MDD SRI (N=37) No SRI (N=28) Non-MDI SRI (N=15) No SRI (81)	During pregnancy	Excluded Axis I diagnosis Women with current anxiety disorder diagnosis or PTSD were included in MDD and non-MDD groups
Merlob 2009[47] Israel TIS Medium	SSRI (N=235, duration and dose NR) No-SSRI (67,636, duration and dose NR)	First-trimester exposure	Excluded chromosomal defects

Author Year Country Study Design/Data Source Risk of Bias	4. Exposures (N, duration, dose) Controls (N)	5. Exposure Period	6. Confounders
Misri 2006[48] Canada PC-Clinic Medium	SSRIs only (N=13) During Pregnancy: Fluoxetine 20.00 mg Paroxetine 23.57 mg Sertraline 91.67 mg Duration: 191 days During breastfeeding: Fluoxetine 26.67 mg Paroxetine 27.50 mg Sertraline 91.67 mg Duration: 59.46 days SSRIs plus clonazepam (N=9) During Pregnancy: Fluoxetine 15.00 mg Paroxetine 23.57 mg SSRI Duration: 167.78 days Clonazepam dose/duration: 0.67 mg/136.63 days During breastfeeding: Fluoxetine 26.56 mg Paroxetine 15.00 mg Sertraline 28.57 mg Duration: 60.13 days Clonazepam dose/duration: 0.71 mg/41.22 days	During pregnancy and breastfeeding	Depression, anxiety
Misri 2010[49] Canada PC-Clinic Medium	Depressed and treated with antidepressants N=39 Individual drugs, % patients, mean dosages: Fluoxetine: 17%, 3.14 mg Paroxetine: 44%, 25.6 mg Sertraline: 15%, 91.7 mg Citalopram: 17%, 57.3 mg Venlafaxine: 7%, 87.5 mg days on SSRIs and/or SNRIs=222 Exposed to SSRIs and/or SNRIs at 3-month visit=26% and 6-month visit=11% Depressed and not treated with antidepressants, N=13 Not depressed and not treated with antidepressants	NR	NR

Author Year Country Study Design/Data Source Risk of Bias	4. Exposures (N, duration, dose) Controls (N)	5. Exposure Period	6. Confounders
Mulder 2011[30] The Netherlands Prospective cohort/Data Source [PC] Medium	Exposed N=96, previously exposed N=37 44% paroxetine, 21% fluoxetine, 20% citalopram, 7% venlafaxine, 4% fluvoxamine, 4%sertraline median mDDD: 1 (range 0.2–3.0 mDDD) Duration: 6 months Control: Unexposed N =130	Throughout pregnancy	Adjusted for fetal behavioral states and gestation.
Nakhai-Pour 2010[31] Canada CC Low	Exposures: Selective Serotonin Reuptake Inhibitors (SSRI): citalopram, fluoxetine, fluvoxamine, paroxetine, sertraline; Tricyclic Antidepressants: amitriptyline, desipramine, imipramine, nortriptyline; Serotonin-norepinephrine reuptake inhibitors: venlafaxine; Serotonin modulators; dopamine and norepinephrine reuptake inhibitors. Doses and Duration: NR Cases N= 5124 Controls N= 51240	Cases: First day of gestation through the calendar date of spontaneous abortion Controls: First d of gestation through the same gestation age as matched case	Adjusted for maternal age, social assistance status, place of residence, gestational age at index date, comorbidities (diabetes mellitus, CV disease, asthma, untreated thyroid disease, depression, anxiety and bipolar disorder), history of spon taneous abortion and therapeutic abortion, visits to psychiatrists, number of prescribers, number of visits to physicians, duration of exposure to antidepressants and other medications in the year before pregnancy, number of prenatal visits, visits to obstetricians and other medication use during pregnancy.
Nordeng 2012[32] Norway PBR Medium	Exposed: N= 699 antidepressant use during pregnancy, 1,048 use prior to pregnancy only Unexposed: N=61,648	6 months before pregnancy; 1st trimester, 2nd and/or 3rd trimester, total pregnancy (includes use when timing during pregnancy unknown)	Level of maternal depression, maternal age at delivery, education, parity, prepregnancy BMI, maternal asthma or CV disease, NSAID use, folic acid use, and smoking during pregnancy.
Nulman 2002[33] Canada PC Medium	Exposed: N=46 tricyclic antidepressants, 40 fluoxetine Unexposed: N=36 nondepressed women	Throughout pregnancy	Mother's IQ, socioeconomic status, ethanol use and cigarette smoking, depression severity, depression duration, treatment duration, number of depressive episodes after delivery, and medications used for depression treatment.

| Author
Year
Country
Study Design/Data Source
Risk of Bias	4. Exposures (N, duration, dose) Controls (N)	5. Exposure Period	6. Confounders
Oberlander 2002[54]
Canada
Prospective cohort/Data Source[PC]
Medium | Exposed group 1, N=22, and Group 2, N=16
Group 1:
Paroxetine: 11
Fluoxetine: 7
Sertraline: 4
Group 2:
Paroxetine + Clonazepam: 2
Fluoxetine + Clonazepam: 14

Dose: (median mg/day)
Paroxetine: 20 (10-30)
Fluoxetine: 20 (10-30)
Sertraline: 62.5 (50-150)
Group 2:
Paroxetine + Clonazepam: 20 (10-30) + 05 (.25-1.175)
Fluoxetine + Clonazepam: 20 (10-30) +.43 (.1-.75)
Duration: NR
Control: Unexposed
N = 23 | Pre and post partum | Not reported |
| Oberlander 2006[55]
Canada
PBR
Medium | Any SSRI (N=1451), fluoxetine 44.7%, sertraline 25.6%, fluvoxamine 4.6%, citalopram 3.3%.

Depression, No SSRI (N=14234)

No depression, No SSRI (N=92192) | SSRI prescription filled more than 49 days after conception | Propensity score matching used to draw a comparison sub-group from the depressed, no SSRI group that was similar in all measured maternal characteristics to the SSRI exposed group. |
| Oberlander 2008[56]
Canada
PC
Medium | SRI Exposure, N=37
Paroxetine, n=18 (Median dose, 27.5mg)
Fluoxetine, n=6 (Median dose, 35mg)
Sertraline, n=5 (Median dose, 100mg)
Venlafaxine, n=3 (Median dose, 75mg)
Citalopram, n=5 (Median dose, 30mg)
Duration: 94.6% continued from prior to recruitment to delivery

No Exposure, N=47 | Throughout pregnancy | NR |

Author Year Country Study Design/Data Source Risk of Bias	4. Exposures (N, duration, dose) Controls (N)	5. Exposure Period	6. Confounders
Oberlander 2008[37] (Birth Defects Res Part B) Canada PBR Medium	Controls Depression alone: N=7,883 No exposure: N=10,702 Medication Groups SRI only Benzodiazepines only SRI + Benzodiazepines SRIs: Paroxetine, 37.0%; Sertraline, 24.3%; Fluoxetine, 24.2%; Venlafaxine, 7.1%; Fluvoxamine, 4.6%; Citalopram, 2.8%	First trimester: LMP to LMP plus 90 days	Controlled for maternal illness characteristics, diseases, and complications of pregnancy diagnosed more than 60 days before birth, depression in the first trimester, and a dummy variable indicating that the mother filled a prescription after she knew that she was pregnant, and a variable indicating whether the patient had been prescribed methadone, exposure to clonazepam or clobazam (sometimes used as anticonvulsants), exposure to antipsychotics, non-SRI antidepressants.
Okun 2011[58] US PC Medium	SSRI vs. No SSRI Total N: 240 20 weeks: 46 vs. 194 30 weeks: 46 vs. 159 36 weeks: 36 vs. 143 duration, doses NR	At 20, 30 and 36 weeks	NR
Okun 2012[59] US PC Medium	At enrollment (20 weeks) No MDD, No SSRI (N=135) No MDD, taking SSRI (N=26) MDD, No SSRI (N=35) MDD, taking SSRI (N=16) Dose, duration NR	At 20 and 30 weeks of pregnancy	Adjusted for the effect of depression and SSRI status at the time of assessment (week 20 or 30), as well as history of pre-term birth, age, marital status, and employment status.
Palmsten 2012[60] Canada RC-LD Medium	SSRI monotherapy, N=3,169 SSRI polytherapy, N=333 SNRI monotherapy, N=408 TCA monotherapy, N=146 No antidepressant therapy, N=65,392	During estimated gestational weeks 10 and 20	Adjusted for delivery year, age, diabetes, multifetal gestation, obesity, primiparity, and physician visits, number of depression claims, number of psychiatrist visits/mental health hospitalizations, and dispensing of benzodiazepines, anticonvulsants, and antipsychotics

Author Year Country Study Design/Data Source Risk of Bias	4. Exposures (N, duration, dose) Controls (N)	5. Exposure Period	6. Confounders
Pearson 2007[61] US Retrospective cohort Data/Source: [AD] Medium	Exposed: N=84 Total SSRI: N= 42 Escitalopram N= Fluoxetine N= 17 Sertraline N= 13 Paroxetine N= 12 Total Tricyclic Antidepressants: N= 37 Amitriptyline N= 2 Desipramine N= 7 Imipramine N= 11 Nortriptyline N= 13 Other: N= 5 Bupropion N= 2 Dose: NR Controls: Unexposed N=168	Conception only: 7.6% First and second trimesters: 15% Third trimester: 67% Throughout: 70%	Conception only: 7.6% First and second trimesters: 15% Third trimester: 67% Throughout: 70%
Pedersen 2009[62] Denmark PBD, LD Medium	SSRI: fluoxetine n=348, citalopram n=460, Paroxetine n=299, Sertraline: n=259, more than 1 type of SSRI n=193, dose and duration NR Control: No unexposed infants n=493113	28 days before to 112 days after beginning of gestation	Adjusted for maternal age, calendar time, marital status, income and smoking.
Pedersen 2010[63] Denmark PC Medium	Exposed N=415, SSRI only n=336, fluoxetine n=88, citalopram n=86, paroxetine n=76, sertraline n=86 Untreated N=489, depression with no psychotropic medication Unexposed N=81042, no exposure to psychotropic medication and no severe symptoms of depression	Entire pregnancy	Adjusted for maternal age, gender, age at interview, breastfeeding, problems during pregnancy, mother-child connection, postnatal symptoms of depression, and postnatal difficulties.
Pedersen 2013[64] (Pendersen, 2010) Denmark PBR Medium	Exposure: N= 127 Fluoxetine = 50; citalopram = 37; paroxetine =38; sertraline=47; 10 >1 AD; TCA = 10, other = 13 Depressed no exposure: N=98 Control (no exposure, no depression): N=723	During pregnancy (could have been before or after also)	Smoking, alcohol use, social class, child's gender
Polen 2013[65] US PBD Medium	Case (one of 30 major birth defects): N=19,043 Venlafaxine used in 77 of 19,043 Control (no major birth defect): N=8,002 Venlafaxine used in 14 of 8002	1 month before conception through the third month of pregnancy	Maternal age, Race

Author Year Country Study Design/Data Source Risk of Bias	4. Exposures (N, duration, dose) Controls (N)	5. Exposure Period	6. Confounders
Rai 2013[66] Sweden CC Low	SSRIs=fluoxetine, citalopram, paroxetine, sertraline Non-selective monoamine reuptake inhibitors (MRIs)=clomipramine, amitriptyline, nortriptyline Dose, duration NR Cases N=4,429 Controls N=43,277	During pregnancy	Adjusted for history of psychiatric disorders other than depression, parental ages, income, education, occupation, migration status, and parity.
Ramos 2008[67] Canada LD Medium	Doses, durations NR Antidepressant use: First trimester, N=1101 Second trimester, N=510 Third trimester, N=476 Drugs: SSRIs (citalopram, fluoxetine, fluvoxamine, paroxetine, sertraline); Tricyclics (amitriptyline, clomipramine, desipramine, doxepin, imipramine, nortriptyline, trimipramine); Other Antidepressants (bupropion, mirtazapine, moclobemide, nefazodone, trazodone, venlafaxine)	Throughout pregnancy	Adjusted for maternal age, being on welfare, urban dweller, living alone, measures related to psychiatric disorders and measures of comorbidities not related to psychiatric disorders before and during pregnancy, hypertension and diabetes diagnoses before and during pregnancy, gender of baby, prenatal visits and year of pregnancy.

Author Year Country Study Design/Data Source Risk of Bias	4. Exposures (N, duration, dose) Controls (N)	5. Exposure Period	6. Confounders
Ramos 2010[68] Canada LD, supplemental questionnaire Medium	Doses, durations NR SSRIs (citalopram, fluoxetine, fluvoxamine, paroxetine, sertraline): First trimester, N=851 Second trimester, N=458 Third trimester, N=434 Tricyclics (amitriptyline, clomipramine, desipramine, doxepin, imipramine, nortriptyline, trimipramine) First trimester, N=85 Second trimester, N=29 Third trimester, N=24 Other Antidepressants (bupropion, mirtazapine, moclobemide, nefazodone, trazodone, venlafaxine) First trimester, N=211 Second trimester, N=70 Third trimester, N=62 Co-exposure (2 classes or more) First trimester, N=109 Second trimester, N=33 Third trimester, N=30 No Antidepressants First trimester, N=1450 Second trimester, N=2116 Third trimester, N=2156	Throughout pregnancy	Adjusted for: in the year prior to pregnancy: the number of different medications used other than ADs, the number of visits to the emergency department or hospitalizations, and the BMI; and on the first d of gestation and during pregnancy: maternal age, race, being a welfare recipient or not, area of residence, parity, income, marital status, maternal weight gain, tobacco, alcohol, and illicit drug use, and finally caffeine intake, pre-pregnancy and gestational diabetes, pre-pregnancy and gestational hypertension, and asthma. The following proxies were used: the number of days on antidepressants and the number of visits to the psychiatrist in the year prior to pregnancy; the number of different psychiatric disorder diagnoses received prior to and during pregnancy; the use of an anxiolytic or sedative such as benzodiazepines; and the use of an anticonvulsant such as carbamazepine during pregnancy. Stratified according to antidepressant dosage used during pregnancy.
Rampono 2009[69] Australia PC Medium	Exposed: N=9 citalopram (median daily dose 20 mg), 8 escitalopram (20 mg), 6 sertraline (50 mg, fluoxetine (30 mg), 1 fluvoxamine (150 mg), 1 paroxetine (30 mg), 11 venlafaxine Controls: N=18	"During pregnancy". Not specified.	None
Reebye 2002[70] Canada PC Medium	Exposure SSRI: N=24, duration: median 192 d, dose: 20mg/d SSRI+: N=14d, duration median: 161 days, SSRI mean dose 19mg/d, Rivotril mean dose: 0.48mg/dog Nonexposed, non-depressed: N=24	During pregnancy	NR

Author Year Country Study Design/Data Source Risk of Bias	4. Exposures (N, duration, dose) Controls (N)	5. Exposure Period	6. Confounders
Reis 2010[71] Sweden PBR Medium	Exposed (early use): N=1364 tricyclics, 10,170 SSRIs, 37 MOAIs, 1,351 SNRIs, 10 unspecified antidepressants Exposed (later use): N=784 tricyclics, 4,809 SSRIs, 18 MOAIs, 538 SNRIs, 0 unspecified antidepressants	Early=before the first antenatal visit Later=during pregnancy	Year of delivery, maternal age, parity, smoking, BMI
Salisbury 2011[72] US PC Medium	Controls (N=56) MDD (N=20) MDD plus SRI (N=36): sertraline 52.8%, fluoxetine 25.0%, paroxetine 8.3%, venlafaxine 2.8%	SRI use for at least 4 consecutive weeks during the second and/or third trimesters	Adjusted for gestational age at birth, age at NNNS assessment.
Salkeld 2008[73] Canada CC-LD Low	SSRI or non-SSRI: dose and duration NR Cases N=2460 Controls N=23,943	Third trimester: Prescription within 90 days of delivery	Adjusted for previous postpartum hemorrhage, multiple pregnancy, prolonged labor, abnormalities of the forces of labor, obstructed labor, perineal laceration or other gynecologic laceration, other obstetric trauma, placenta previa, placental abruption, and hypertensive disorders of pregnancy
Simon 2002[74] US RC-HCDB Low	Tricyclic antidepressants (N=209): Amitriptyline N=66, imipramine N=49, doxepin N=36, nortriptyline N=33, desipramine N=22 SSRIs (N=185): Fluoxetine N=129, sertraline N=32, paroxetine N=28 Dose, duration NR	Any antidepressant prescription during the 270 days before delivery	Matched based on maternal age, year of delivery, lifetime use of antidepressants, and lifetime history of psychiatric treatment. Adjustment for maternal tobacco use, other substance use, race, and number of prior births.
Sit 2011[75] US PC Medium	SRI (N=21) Sertraline, n=9 Venlafaxine, n=2 Escitalopram, n=2 Citalopram, n=1 Nortriptyline, n=1 Fluvoxamine, n=1 Fluoxetine, n=5 Doses, durations NR	Throughout pregnancy	Smoking
Smith 2013[76] US PC High	Exposure: N=6 Within 6 months before pregnancy and more than one month in the third trimester Control: N=61	Within 6 months before pregnancy and more than one month in the third trimester	NR

Author Year Country Study Design/Data Source Risk of Bias	4. Exposures (N, duration, dose) Controls (N)	5. Exposure Period	6. Confounders
Stephansson 2013[77] Sweden PBR Medium	Exposed: N=29,228 Controls: N=1,604,649	T0 (from 3 months before until last menstrual period before pregnancy), 1st trimester, 2nd trimester, 3 trimester	Smoking, country and year of birth, maternal age, birth order, maternal diabetes and hypertension, previous psychiatric hospitalization
Suri 2007[78] US PC Medium	Durations, NR Dose Groups: High (≥ 300mg bupropion; ≥ 225mg venlafaxine; ≥ 150mg sertraline; ≥ 100mg nortriptyline; ≥ 40mg citalopram, fluoxetine, paroxetine; ≥ 20mg escitalopram) Low-Medium: Any doses lower than in high group. MDD, antidepressant >50% of pregnancy (N=49) Monotherapies: Sertraline, n=15; Fluoxetine, n=13; Citalopram, n=4; Paroxetine, n=4; Venlafaxine, n=2; Nortriptyline, n=1 Sequential therapy: Citalopram/fluoxetine, n=1; Paroxetine/sertraline, n=1; Escitalopram/citalopram, n=1; Nefazodone/fluoxetine, n=1; Venlafaxine/sertraline, n=1; Fluoxetine/citalopram/sertraline, n=1; Citalopram/fluoxetine/sertraline, n=1; Venlafaxine/fluoxetine/sertraline, n=1 Concurrent therapy: Sertraline/venlafaxine, bupropion, n=1 Venlafaxine/nefazodone, then sertraline, n=1 MDD, no antidepressant or discontinued during first trimester and/or <10 days exposure (N=22) First trimester only: Sertraline, n=3; Venlafaxine, n=2; Fluoxetine, n=1 6 weeks of first trimester + 9 days second trimester, Citalopram, n=1 Second trimester, seven days, sertraline, n=1 No psychiatric history, controls (N=19)	Entire pregnancy	Controlled for maternal age, number of previous pregnancies, historical and developing risk factors for preterm birth, hypertension, pregnancy-induced hypertension, pre-eclampsia and maternal weight gain.

Author Year Country Study Design/Data Source Risk of Bias	4. Exposures (N, duration, dose) Controls (N)	5. Exposure Period	6. Confounders
Suri 2011[79] US, California PC Medium	MDD, with antidepressant (N=33) Fluoxetine: 38%, Daily dose M=22.5mg/d Sertraline: 36%, Daily dose M=90.5mg/d MDD, no antidepressant (N=16) No MDD, no antidepressant (N=15)	Throughout pregnancy	Adjusted for GA at delivery
Ter Horst 2013[80] The Netherlands PD Medium	SSRI Exposure: N= 436 Paroxetine N=0266; fluoxetine N= 111; citalopram N=91; fluvoxamine N=70; sertraline N=034; and escitalopram N=011; TCA Exposure: N=67 Clomipramine N=43; amitriptyline N=031 Control: N=35,033	Anytime during pregnancy Only first trimester Only 2nd and 3rd trimester At least 2nd and 3rd trimester	In utero exposure to antibiotics, benzodiazepines, insulin, or drugs for pulmonary disease. Maternal age > 30 at delivery.
Toh 2009[81] US CC Medium	Exposed: N=92 who continued SSRI exposure, 107 who discontinued SSRI exposure Controls: N=5,532 with no SSRI exposure	Discontinued exposure=Treated 2 months before pregnancy but discontinued before the end of the 1st trimester Continued exposure=Treated 2 months before pregnancy and continued after the 1st trimester	Region, birth year, maternal age, race/ethnicity, education, family income, gravidity, number of fetuses, prepregnancy BMI, age at menarche, diabetes mellitus, infertility treatment, cigarette smoking, coffee and alcohol intake, use of illicit drugs or other psychotherapeutic medications during pregnancy.
Ververs 2009[82] The Netherlands AD Medium	Any antidepressant (N=784) SSRI total, n=557 Paroxetine, n=305 Fluoxetine, n=110 Tricyclic antidepressant, n=109 Other antidepressant, n=118 Dose, Duration, NR	Continuous Users: Used antidepressant before and throughout pregnancy Starters: No antidepressant use in the 6 months prior to pregnancy, but used them during pregnancy Stoppers: Antidepressant used before pregnancy, but did not do so during pregnancy Irregular Users: Any other pattern of antidepressant use during pregnancy Non-Users: No antidepressant use before or during pregnancy	NR
Wilson 2011[83] US CC Medium	Cases: N=20 Controls: N=120	After 20 weeks gestation	Maternal age, parity, neonatal gender, tobacco use, mode of delivery, diabetes (preexisting and gestational), chorioamnionitis, obesity

Author Year Country Study Design/Data Source Risk of Bias	4. Exposures (N, duration, dose) Controls (N)	5. Exposure Period	6. Confounders
Wisner 2009[84] US Prospective cohort Medium	Any SSRI No SSRI, no depression (N=131) 2. Continuous SSRI exposure (N=48)— 3. Continuous SSRI exposure, no SSRI (N=14) 4. Partial SSRI exposure (N=23) 5. Partial depression, no SSRI (N=22)	Groups formed by the following definitions: No SSRI, no depression: no exposure to any antidepressant or to major depressive disorder. 2. Continuous SSRI exposure: treatment with an SSRI during the entirety of pregnancy or for the majority of each of the three trimesters. 3. Continuous depression, no SSRI: the presence of major depression throughout pregnancy or for the majority of each of the three trimesters, without SSRI treatment. 4. Partial SSRI exposure : treatment with an SSRI at some point during pregnancy but at least one full trimester without exposure; this group was equally split between women treated with an SSRI in the first and/or second trimester, but not the third, and women treated in the second and/or third trimester, but not the first. 5. Partial depression, no SSRI : major depressive disorder at some point during pregnancy but no depression for at least one trimester, without SSRI treatment	Maternal age and race, Prepregnancy BMI, weight gain at week 36, and infant birth weight, preterm birth, NICU admission, 1- and 5-minute Apgar scores of 7 or less, Peripartum Events Scale subscale ratings of 2 or higher, and respiratory signs
Wisner 2013[85] (Wisner 2009/Okun 2012) US PC Medium	Exposure to SSRI: N=71 Individual medications NR Depression no exposure to SSRI: N=36 no depression, no exposure to SSRI: N=131	The majority (N=30) of women with SSRI exposure were treated continuously throughout gestation. This group also included women exposed to SSRIs in the first and/or second trimester but not the third (N=10) and women exposed in the second and/or third trimester but not the first (N=6).	NR
Wogelius 2006[86] Denmark PBR Medium	Exposed: N=1051 within 1st trimester or 30 days before, 453 within 2nd or 3rd month after conception Controls: N=150,780	Within 1st trimester or 30 days before, within 2nd or 3rd month after conception	Maternal smoking during pregnancy, birth order, maternal age, prescriptions for antiepileptics, antidiabetics and NSAIDS during pregnancy, birth year, country, length of gestation
Yonkers 2012[87] US Prospective Cohort [PC] Low	Exposed: N= 320 SSRI: Citalopram N=26 Escitalopram N=47 Fluoxetine N=68 Sertraline N=121 Paroxetine N=21 Other: Venlafaxine N=29 Duloxetine N=8 Dose: NR	First trimester only Second trimester and third trimester only Throughout	Adjusted for mother's age, education, race, smoking, illicit drug use, history of preterm birth. Second adjusted analysis additionally included psychiatric illness history, severity of disease, concurrent diagnoses.

Author Year Country Study Design/Data Source Risk of Bias	4. Exposures (N, duration, dose) Controls (N)	5. Exposure Period	6. Confounders
Zeskind 2004[88] US Prospective cohort study/Data Source [PC, AD] Medium	N=17 Celexa N= 5, Prozac N= ‹, Paxil N= 3, Zoloft N= 5; sequential combination of Paxil, Prozac, and Zoloft N= 1 or Paxil N= 1; or Paxil and Zoloft N= 1 in combination with Wellbutrin. Duration NR Control: Unexposed N = 17	Throughout pregnancy	NR

Author Year Country Study Design/Data Source Risk of Bias	7. Fetus/infant/child outcomes up to 12 months of age	8. Child outcomes after 12 months of age	9. Maternal Outcomes
Alwan 2007[1] US Arm of Case Control Studied, Population based Medium	No increase in congenital heart defects with SSRI. + association anencephaly, craniosynostosis, omphalocele	NR	NR
Alwan 2010[2] Canada Case-control/Data Source [CC] Medium	Maternal Bupropion use among infants with categories of heart defects: Adjusted OR (95% CI) Conotruncal heart defects: 0.9 (0.3–2.6) Tetralogy of Fallot: 1.5 (0.4–5.1) Left outflow tract heart defects: 2.6 (1.2–5.7) Coarctation of aorta: 2.6 (1.0–6.9) Hypoplastic left heart : 2.7 (0.8–9.1) Right outflow tract heart defects: 1.2 (0.4–3.4) Pulmonary valve stenosis: 1.1 (0.3–3.8) Septal heart defects: 1.4 (0.7–2.8) Perimembranous VSD: 1.2 (0.5–3.4) ASD secundum: 1.1 (0.4–3.0) ASD nos: 2.2 (0.6–7.5) All groups of heart defects in NBDPS: 1.4 (0.8–2.5)	NR	NR
Andrade 2009[3] US RC/Data Source [AD] Medium	Persistent pulmonary hypertension, (unadjusted) Prevalence ratio (95% CI) SSRI: PPHN among exposed was 2.14 per 1000 (95% confidence interval (CI) 0.26, 7.74) vs. not exposed was 2.72 per 1000 (95%CI 0.56, 7.93)	NR	NR
Bakker 2010[4] CC/PBD Netherlands Medium	Congenital defects, comparison to not exposed: All heart defects: OR, 1.5; P=0.476; 95% CI, 0.5 to 4.0 VSD: AOR, 0.5; P=0.528; 95% CI, 0.1-4.2 ASD: AOR, 5.7: P=0.016; 95% CI, 1.4-23.7 Septal defects (includes ASD and VSD): AOR, 1.6; P=0.493; 95% CI, 0.4-5.6 Right-sided defects: AOR, 0.9; P=0.926; 95% CI, 0.1-7.6 Left-sided defects: AOR, 2.1; P=0.292; 95% CI, 0.5-8.7 Other defects: AOR, 1.0; P=0.967; 95% CI, 0.2-5.2	NR	NR

E-54

| Author
Year
Country
Study Design/Data Source
Risk of Bias	7. Fetus/infant/child outcomes up to 12 months of age	8. Child outcomes after 12 months of age	9. Maternal Outcomes
Bakker 2010[5]
The Netherlands
Case-Control
Medium | Adjusted ORs (95% CI) for cases and controls:
All heart defects: 1.5 (0.5-4.0)
VSD: 0.5 (0.1-4.2)
ASD: 5.7 (1.4-23.7)
Septal defects: 1.6 (0.4-5.6)
Right-sided defects: 0.9 (0.1-7.6)
Left-sided defects: 2.1 (0.5-8.7)
Other defects: 1.0 (0.2-5.2) | NR | NR |
| Ban 2012[6]
U.K.
PBD
Medium | Adjusted RRR (99% CI)
Referent category: No history of or current depression or anxiety
A. Unmedicated mental illness
B. TCA
C. SSRI
Perinatal death: A: 1.4 (0.8 to 2.5), B: 1.6 (0.9 to 2.9), C:1.6 (1.1 to 2.4)
Miscarriage: A: 1.0 (0.9 to 1.2), B: 1.3 (1.1 to 1.5), C:1.5 (1.3 to 1.6)
Termination: A: 1.0 (0.9 to 1.2), B: 1.7 (1.5 to 1.9), C: 2.2 (2.1 to 2.4)

Referent category: Unmedicated depression or anxiety during 1st trimester of pregnancy
Perinatal death: B: 1.2 (0.5 to 2.7), C. 1.2 (0.6 to 2.3)
Miscarriage: B. 1.3 (1.1 to 1.5), C: 1.4 (1.2 to 1.7)
Termination:B.1.4 (1.2 to 1.7). C: 2.0 (1.8 to 2.3) | NR | NR |
| Batton 2013[7]
US
PD
Medium | 24-Months
BINS - Bayley Infant Neurodevelopmental Screener
high-risk 4 (21%) vs. 8 (42%)
moderate risk 5 (26%) vs. 7 (37%)
low risk vs. 10 (53%) vs. 4 (21%)

36 months
BINS - Bayley Infant Neurodevelopmental Screener (10 (33%) were assessed using the BSID-II and 20 (67%)were assessed with the Bayley-III.)
Mean (range) Mental Developmental Index/Cognitive Composite score on the BSID-II/Bayley-III
94 (62-118) vs 91 (75-110) (p=0.46)

Mean (range) Psychomotor Developmental Index/Motor Composite score on the BSID-II/Bayley-III
79 (50-103) vs. 75 (50-112) (p=0.72) | NR | NR |

Author Year Country Study Design/Data Source Risk of Bias	7. Fetus/infant/child outcomes up to 12 months of age	8. Child outcomes after 12 months of age	9. Maternal Outcomes
Berard 2007[8] Canada LD Medium	Adjusted ORs for Major Congenital malformations: Paroxetine vs. Other antidepressants: OR, 1.32; 95%CI, 0.79 to 2.20 Other SSRI vs. Other antidepressants: OR, 0.93; 95% CI, 0.53 to 1.62 2nd trimester exposure to any antidepressants vs. no 2nd trimester exposure: OR, 1.23; 95%CI, 0.62 to 2.43 3rd trimester exposure to any antidepressants vs. no 3rd trimester exposure: OR, 0.53; 95%CI, 0.25 to 1.11 Adjusted ORs for Major Cardiac Malformations: Paroxetine vs. Other antidepressants: OR, 1.38; 95%CI, 0.49 to 3.92 Other SSRI vs. Other antidepressants: OR, 0.89; 95%CI, 0.28 to 2.84 2nd trimester exposure to any antidepressants vs. no 2nd trimester exposure: OR, 0.72; 95%CI, 0.17 to 3.01 3rd trimester exposure to any antidepressants vs. no 3rd trimester exposure: OR, 0.46; 95%CI, 0.09 to 2.30 Adjusted ORs by Dose of Paroxetine (mg/d vs. no use) Major Congenital Malformations >0 to 20: OR, 0.71; 95%CI, 0.29 to 1.71 >20-25: OR, 1.30; 95%CI, 0.76 to 2.25 >25: OR, 2.23; 95%CI, 1.19 to 4.17 Major Cardiac Malformations >0 to 20: OR, 1.76; 95%CI, 0.45 to 6.82 >20-25: OR, 0.61; 95%CI, 0.13 to 2.88 >25: OR, 3.07; 95%CI, 1.00 to 9.42	NR	NR

Author Year Country Study Design/Data Source Risk of Bias	7. Fetus/infant/child outcomes up to 12 months of age	8. Child outcomes after 12 months of age	9. Maternal Outcomes
Bogen 2010/companion Wen 2009[9] US PC Medium	NR	NR	SRI at enrolment and infant feeding intention (N=168) RRR, 95%CI Breast and formula: 2.55 (0.85 to 7.66) Formula only: 12.31 (2.50 to 60.66), p=0.002 Unsure: 4.72 (1.01 to 21.9) Association between breastfeeding initiation and SRI use at enrolment and delivery: p>0.22 Association between breastfeeding at 2 weeks and not taking SRI at 2 weeks postpartum: p=0.04 SRI use at 2 weeks postpartum and its correlation to breastfeeding status at 12 weeks postpartum (n=99) HDRS<9: stopped breast feeding 12.0 (1.64 to 88.3) HDRS>9: Stopped breast feeding 0.28 (0.04 to 1.71)
Boucher 2008[10] Canada LD Medium	Adjusted OR (95% CI) Symptoms in neonates exposed vs not exposed to antidepressants in late pregnancy: Alertness: 37 (8-174) Muscular tone: 20 (5-71) Neurological function: OR not computed because of 0 value in unexposed group, P<0.006 (unadjusted) Feeding, GI: 3.8 (1.7-8.1) Respiratory function: 2.5 (1.1-5.3) Serotonergic/adrenergic activity: 4.1 (1.1-15.5) Global (one or more of the above symptoms): 7.0 (3.2-15.3)	NR	NR

E-57

Author Year Country Study Design/Data Source Risk of Bias	7. Fetus/infant/child outcomes up to 12 months of age	8. Child outcomes after 12 months of age	9. Maternal Outcomes
Casper 2003[1] US Cohort study Data/Source: [CC] Medium	Mean birth weight: Not exposed= 3363 (498.5) vs. exposed= 3394 (432.2) P=0.84 Birth length (cm): 49.7 (7.2) vs. 50.3 (2.5) P=0.78 Gestational age (wk): 38.7 (1.5) vs. 39.1 (1.1) P=0.38 Weight (%): 46.7 (27.4) vs. 48.4 (29.4) P=0.86 Height (%): 49.7 (30.1) vs. 41.9 (28.0) P= 0.42 Fronto-occipital circumference(%): 50.3 (28.1) vs. 54.2 (25.9) P=0.66 Bayley scales: mean (SD) MDI 94.3 (7.5) vs. 91.0 (13.3) P= 0.27 PDI 98.2 (9.1) vs. 90.0 (11.4) P= 0.76 BRS 89.5 (15.4) vs. 76.0 (24.6) P=0.72 Major structural anomalies: 1 bilateral lacrimal duct stenosis (unexposed infant) 1 small asymptomatic ventricular septal defect (exposed infant) (χ^2 = 0.13; P=0.72) Minor structural anomalies: 54% unexposed and 76% of exposed infants (χ^2 = 0.18; P =0.17). 3 or more minor structural anomalies: 15% of unexposed 29% of exposed infants (χ^2 = 0.19; P =0.37).	Gross motor movement: mean (SD) 4.77 (0.44) 4.43 (0.68) P=0.17 Fine motor movement: mean (SD) 5.00 (0) 4.71 (0.46) P=0.15 Control of movement: mean (SD) 4.77 (0.44) 4.60 (0.56) P =0.46 Tremulousness: mean (SD) 5.00 (0) 4.87 (0.34) P=0.08 Slow and delayed movement: mean (SD) 4.92 (0.28) 4.83 (0.38) P= -06 0.81 Frenetic movement: mean (SD) 5.00 (0) 4.87 (0.43) P=0.15 Hypertonicity: mean (SD) 5.00 (0) 4.97 (0.18) P=0.40 Hypotonicity: mean (SD) 4.92 (0.28) 4.90 (0.31) P=0.83	Delivery and postpartum parameters: Breastfeeding average duration 6.4 ± 5.9 months (unexp) vs. 8.5 ± 7.2 (exp) t = 0.85; P = .4

Author Year Country Study Design/Data Source Risk of Bias	7. Fetus/infant/child outcomes up to 12 months of age	8. Child outcomes after 12 months of age	9. Maternal Outcomes
Chambers 1996[12] US CC Medium	Infants Exposed in First Trimester vs. Control Infants: Major malformations (ventricular septal defect, ventricular septal defect with bilateral cryptorchidism, atrial septal defect, nasal dermoid sinus, coccygeal dermal sinus, hypospadias, bilateral inguinal hernia, cleft palate): 3.7% vs. 2.7%, p=0.57 Deformations (sagitta synostosis, bilateral hip dysplasia, unilateral hip dysplasia): 1.8% vs. 0.9%, p=0.65 All major structural anomalies combined: 5.5% vs. 4.0%, p=0.63 Infants Exposed in Exposed Early group vs. Exposed Late group vs. Control group Pre-term birth (<37 weeks): 4.1% vs. 14.3% vs. 5.9%, p=0.03 Admission to special care nursery: 11.9% vs. 31.5% vs. 8.8%, p<0.001 Birth weight, g: 3589 vs. 3392 vs. 3556, p=0.04 Birth weight <10th percentile: 3.2% vs. 11.5% vs. 3.3%, p=0.02 Birth length, cm: 51.5 vs. 50.4 vs. 51.5, p=0.01 Head circumference, cm: 34.8 vs. 34.3 vs. 34.5, p=0.19 Microcephaly, <3rd percentile: 2.2% vs. 3.3% vs. 1.0%, p=0.41 Adjusted RRs for Infants Exposed Late vs. Infants Exposed Early Prematurity: RR, 4.3; 95% CI, 1.1 to 20.8 Admission to special care nursery: RR, 2.6; 95% CI, 1.1 to 6.9 Poor neonatal adaption: RR, 8.7; 95% CI, 2.9 to 26.6	NR	NR

Author Year Country Study Design/Data Source Risk of Bias	7. Fetus/infant/child outcomes up to 12 months of age	8. Child outcomes after 12 months of age	9. Maternal Outcomes
Chambers 2006[13] US CC Medium	Definite PPHN, adjusted OR (95% CI): Maternal use of antidepressants Never used during pregnancy: 1.0 Any time during pregnancy: 1.4 (0.8, 2.5); P=0.30 SSRI: 1.6 (0.8, 3.2); P=0.16 Other antidepressants:1.8 (0.2, 2.7); P=0.76 Maternal use of antidepressants Never during pregnancy: 1.0 Before week 20: 0.6 (0.2, 1.5); P=0.28 After week 20: 3.2 (1.3, 7.4); P=0.008 Maternal use of SSRIs Never during pregnancy: 1.0 Before week 20: 0.3 (0.1, 1.2); P=0.08 After week 20: 6.1 (2.2, 16.8); P=0.001	NR	NR
Cole 2007[14] US Case-control/Data Source[AD] Medium	All congenital malformations: Monotherapy paroxetine group compared with other: Adjusted odd ratio: 1.89 (95%CI 1.20–2.98) Mono- or polytherapy paroxetine group compared with other: Adjusted odd ratio: 1.76 (95%CI 1.18–2.64) Cardiovascular malformations: Monotherapy paroxetine group compared with other Adjusted odd ratio: 1.46, 95%CI 0.74–2.88 Mono or polytherapy paroxetine group compared with other Adjusted odd ratio: 1.68, 95%CI 0.95–2.97 Prevalence of all congenital malformations: Monotherapy paroxetine group compared with other: Adjusted odd ratio:1.89, 95%CI 1.20–2.98 Mono- or polytherapy paroxetine group compared with other: Adjusted odd ratio: 1.76, 95%CI 1.18–2.64 Subset of infants without maternal drugs known or suspected to be teratogenic: Monotherapy paroxetine group compared with other Adjusted odd ratio: 2.03, 95%CI 1.26–3.25 Mono or polytherapy paroxetine group compared with other Adjusted odd ratio: 1.79, 95%CI 1.17–2.73	NR	NR

Author Year Country Study Design/Data Source Risk of Bias	7. Fetus/infant/child outcomes up to 12 months of age	8. Child outcomes after 12 months of age	9. Maternal Outcomes
Cole 2007[15] US LD Low	Congenital malformations, adjusted OR (95% CI) All congenital malformations Bupropion, 1st trimester: -- Other antidepressant, 1st trimester: 0.95 (0.62, 1.45) Bupropion, outside 1st trimester: 1.00 (0.57, 1.73) CV malformations Bupropion, 1st trimester: -- Other antidepressant, 1st trimester: 0.97 (0.52, 1.80) Bupropion, outside 1st trimester: 1.07 (0.48, 2.40)	NR	NR
Colvin 2012[16] PBD/CC Australia Medium	Preterm birth <37 weeks: Adjusted Odd Ratio (95% CI) Any SSRI:1.4; (1.2–1.7) Sertraline:1.62 (1.30–2.03) Citalopram:1.38 (1.03–1.77) Paroxetine:1.41 (1.02–1.96) Fluoxetin:1.31 (0.84–2.05)	NR	NR

E-61

| Author
Year
Country
Study Design/Data Source
Risk of Bias	7. Fetus/infant/child outcomes up to 12 months of age	8. Child outcomes after 12 months of age	9. Maternal Outcomes
Colvin 2012[16]
PBD/CC
Australia
Medium | APGAR at 5 minutes
THIS IS NOT ON OUR LIST OF OUTCOMES
Preterm birth (<37 weeks), adjusted OR (95% CI), comparison to not exposed:
T1: AOR, 1.10; 95% CI, 0.88 to1.37
T2 or T3: AOR, 1.28; 95% CI, 0.97 to 1.70
Any: AOR, 1.48 ; 95% CI, 1.28 to 1.72
I LEFT THE NON-ADJUSTED DATA OFF THE CHART
Birthweight (<2500g) adjusted OR (95% CI), comparison to not exposed:
T1: AOR, 1.10; 95% CI, 0.88 to 3.8
T2 or T3: AOR, 1.46; 95% CI, 1.06 to 2.02
Any: AOR, 1.19; 95% CI 0.99 to1.43
I LEFT THE NON-ADJUSTED DATA OFF THE CHART
Birth length (<=1798), OR (95% CI), comparison to not exposed:
T1: OR, 1.52; 95% CI, 1.40 to1.65
T2 or T3: OR, 1.53; 95% CI, 1.34 to 1.74
Any: OR, 1.52; 95% CI, 1.42 to 1.63
Mean gestation, wks, t-test, comparison to not exposed:
T1: <0.0001
T2 or T3: <0.0001
Any: <0.0001
Mean birth weight, g, t-test, comparison to not exposed:
T1: <0.0001
T2 or T3: <0.0001
Any: <0.0001
Mean birth length, cm, t-test, comparison to not exposed:
T1: <0.0001
T2 or T3: <0.0001
Any: <0.0001 | NR | NR |

Author Year Country Study Design/Data Source Risk of Bias	7. Fetus/infant/child outcomes up to 12 months of age	8. Child outcomes after 12 months of age	9. Maternal Outcomes
Colvin 2012[16] PBD/CC Australia Medium ....(Cont)	Death before one year, comparison to not exposed: overall: OR, 1.38; 95% CI, 1.06 to 1.81 citalopram: OR, 1.08 95% CI, 0.64 to 1.84 paroxetine: OR, 1.44; 95% CI, 0.79 to 2.63 sertraline: OR, 1.45; 95% CI, 0.95 to 2.22 fluoxetine: OR, 1.45; 95% CI, 0.65 to 3.26 escitalopram: OR, 1.85; 95% CI, 0.76 to 4.49 fluvoxamine: OR, 1.89; 95% CI, 0.60 to 5.95 Stillbirths, comparison to not exposed: overall: OR, 1.07; 95% CI, 0.72 to 1.58 citalopram: OR, 0.93; 95% CI, 0.44 to 1.97 paroxetine: OR, 0.90. 95% CI, 0.34 to 2.42 sertraline: OR, 1.48; 95% CI, 0.85 to 2.57 fluoxetine: OR, 0.83; 95% CI, 0.21 to 3.35 escitalopram: OR, 0.63; 95% CI, 0.09 to 4.51 fluvoxamine: 0		
Croen 2011[17] US CC Medium	Any major birth defect: OR, 0.52; 95% CI, 0.21 to 1.28 NR	Adjusted OR for Risk of Autism Spectrum Disorder vs. Unexposed in year before delivery Any antidepressant: OR, 2.0; 95%CI, 1.2 to 3.6 Any SSRI: OR, 2.2; 95%CI, 1.2 to 4.3 SSRI only: OR, 2.6; 95%CI, 1.3 to 5.4 Tricyclics and/or Dual-Action: OR, 1.6; 95%CI, 0.5 to 4.5 Adjusted OR for Risk of Autism Spectrum Disorder for SSRI use by trimester vs. Unexposed in year before delivery Preconception period: OR, 2.1; 95%CI, 1.1 to 4.2 First trimester: OR, 3.8; 95%CI, 1.8 to 7.8 Second trimester: OR, 1.9; 95%CI, 0.7 to 5.6 Third trimester: OR, 2.9; 95%CI, 1.0 to 8.0 year before delivery: OR, 2.2; 95%CI, 1.2 to 4.2	NR
Davidson 2009[18] Israel CC Medium	SSRI vs. Controls GA: 38.6 vs. 38.9, NSD Birth weight, g: 3173 vs. 3333, NSD Birth length, cm: 49.0 vs. 50.4, p=0.008 Head circumference, cm: 33.8 vs. 34.4, p=0.08 Birth weight <10th percentile: 29% vs. 5%, p=0.045 Birth length <10th percentile: 14% vs. 0%, p=0.08 Head circumference <10th percentile: 19% vs. 0%, p<0.04 Discharge d: 3.9 vs. 2.7, p=0.005	NR	SSRI vs. Controls Weight gain (kg): 62.7 vs. 64.5, NSD

E-63

Author Year Country Study Design/Data Source Risk of Bias	7. Fetus/infant/child outcomes up to 12 months of age	8. Child outcomes after 12 months of age	9. Maternal Outcomes
Davis 2007[19] US LD Medium	At 30 days: RRs, SSRI vs. No SSRI Preterm delivery: RR, 1.45; 95%CI, 1.25 to 1.68 One or more perinatal event of interest: RR, 1.16; 95%CI, 1.06 to 1.26 Fetal distress: RR, 6.00; 95%CI, 1.88 to 19.18 Excessive fetal growth: RR, 6.27; 95%CI, 0.83 to 47.43 Polyhydramnios: RR, 29.35; 95%CI, 3.30 to 261.08 Polyhydramnios and oligohydramnios: RR, 8.34; 95%CI, 1.94 to 35.80 Complications of placenta, cord, and membranes: RR, 0.69; 95%CI, 0.31 to 1.54 Complications of delivery, including malpresentation and malformation: RR, 1.42; 95%CI, 1.05 to 1.93 Disorders related to gestational age and birth weight: RR, 0.92; 95%CI, 0.68 to 1.26 Birth trauma: RR, 1.51; 95%CI, 1.04 to 2.20 Intrauterine hypoxia and asphyxia: RR, 1.38; 95%CI, 0.93 to 2.06 Respiratory distress syndrome and other respiratory conditions: RR, 1.97; 95%CI, 1.65 to 2.35 Neonatal hemorrhage and hemolytic diseases of the newborn: RR, 1.09; 95%CI, 0.69 to 1.70 Other causes of perinatal jaundice: RR, 0.91; 95%CI, 0.76 to 1.09 Endocrine and metabolic disturbances specific to newborn, including neonatal hypoglycemia: RR, 1.61; 95%CI, 1.15 to 2.27 Disorders of the digestive system: RR, 0.52; 95%CI, 0.07 to 3.68 Disorders of temperature regulation, including hypothermia: RR, 1.56; 95%CI, 1.06 to 2.31 Convulsions in the newborn: RR, 2.60; 95%CI, 1.16 to 5.84 Feeding problems in the newborn: RR, 1.26; 95%CI, 0.97 to 1.65 Other conditions: RR, 1.41; 95%CI, 1.12 to 1.78 Observation and evaluation of newborns for suspected condition not found: RR, 2.22; 95%CI, 1.70 to 2.90 One or more perinatal event of interest: RR, 1.16; 95%CI, 1.06 to 1.26	At 365 days: RRs, SSRI vs. No SSRI One or more malformation of interest: RR, 0.97; 95%CI, 0.81 to 1.16 Spina Bifida: RR, 2.21; 95%CI, 0.30 to 16.00 Other congenital anomalies of nervous system: RR, 1.98; 95% CI, 0.94 to 4.19 Congenital anomalies of the eye: RR, 1.33; 95%CI, 0.82 to 2.17 Congenital anomalies of ear, face and neck: RR, 0.37; 95%CI, 0.27 to 2.60 Bulbus Cordis anomalies and anomalies of cardiac septal closure: RR, 0.93; 95%CI, 0.50 to 1.73 Other congenital anomalies of the heart: RR, 0.88; 95%CI, 0.42 to 1.86) Other congenital anomalies of circulatory system: RR, 1.55; 95%CI, 0.83 to 2.90 Congenital anomalies of respiratory system: RR, 0.23; 95%CI, 0.03 to1.68 Cleft palate and cleft lip: RR, 2.22; 95%CI, 0.69 to 7.08 Other congenital anomalies of upper alimentary tract: RR, 1.25; 95%CI, 0.65 to 2.42 Other congenital anomalies of digestive system: RR, 1.37; 95%CI, 0.44 to 4.27 Congenital anomalies of genital organs: RR, 0.82; 95%CI, 0.50 to 1.34 Congenital anomalies of urinary system: RR, 0.93; 95%CI, 0.44 to 1.96 Certain congenital musculoskeletal deformities: RR, 0.76; 95%CI, 0.46 to 1.26 Other congenital anomalies of limbs: RR, 0.67; 95%CI, 0.35 to 1.29 Other congenital musculoskeletal anomalies: RR, 0.60; 95%CI, 0.29 to 1.27 Congenital anomalies of the integument: RR, 0.89; 95%CI, 0.46 to 1.71 Other and unspecified congenital anomalies: RR, 0.84; 95%CI, 0.32 to 2.24	NR

Author Year Country Study Design/Data Source Risk of Bias	7. Fetus/infant/child outcomes up to 12 months of age	8. Child outcomes after 12 months of age	9. Maternal Outcomes
Davis 2007[19] US LD Medium ....(Cont)	CONTINUED........ RRs, Tricyclics vs. No tricyclics Preterm delivery: RR, 1.67; 95%CI, 1.25 to 2.22 One or more perinatal event of interest: RR, 1.25; 95%CI, 1.03 to 1.51 Complications of placenta, cord, and membranes: RR, 1.44; 95%CI, 0.36 to 5.72 Complications of delivery, including malpresentation and malformation: RR, 1.46; 95%CI, 0.70 to 3.02 Disorders related to gestational age and birth weight: RR, 1.29; 95%CI, 0.67 to 2.51 Birth trauma: RR, 1.81; 95%CI, 0.76 to 4.30 Intrauterine hypoxia and asphyxia: RR, 1.03; 95%CI, 0.34 to 3.13 Respiratory distress syndrome and other respiratory conditions: RR, 2.02; 95%CI, 1.33 to 3.06 Neonatal hemorrhage and hemolytic diseases of the newborn: RR, 2.12; 35%CI, 0.97 to 4.64 Other causes of perinatal jaundice: RR, 1.02; 95%CI, 0.67 to 1.54 Endocrine and metabolic disturbances specific to newborn, including neonatal hypoglycemia: RR, 2.15; 95%CI, 1.04 to 4.44 Disorders of the digestive system: RR, 3.08; 95%CI, 0.43 to 21.89 Disorders of temperature regulation, including hypothermia: RR, 2.36; 95%CI, 1.08 to 5.16 Convulsions in the newborn: RR, 2.76; 95%CI, 0.39 to 19.54 Feeding problems in the newborn: RR, 1.69; 95%CI, 0.96 to 2.97 Other conditions: RR, 1.71; 95%CI, 1.02 to 2.86 Observation and evaluation of newborns for suspected condition not found: RR, 1.07; 95%CI, 0.41 to 2.81 One or more perinatal event of interest: RR, 1.25; 95%CI, 1.03 to 1.51	CONTINUED........ RRs, Tricyclics vs. No tricyclics One or more malformation of interest: RR, 0.86; 95%CI, 0.57 to 1.30 Spina bifida: RR, 12.43; 95%CI, 1.70 to 90.66 Other congenital anomalies of nervous system: RR, 1.27; 95%CI, 0.18 to 8.99 Bulbus Cordis anomalies and anomalies of cardiac septal closure: RR, 0.92; 95%CI, 0.23 to 3.70 Other congenital anomalies of circulatory system: RR, 0.74; 95%CI, 0.10 to 5.29 Congenital anomalies of respiratory system: RR, 1.09; 95%CI, 0.15 to 7.72 Other congenital anomalies of upper alimentary tract: RR, 1.29; 95%CI, 0.32 to 5.15 Other congenital anomalies of digestive system: RR, 2.49; 95%CI, 0.35 to 17.50 Congenital anomalies of genital organs: RR, 0.77; 95%CI, 0.25 to 2.38 Congenital anomalies of urinary system: RR, 0.64; 95%CI, 0.09 to 4.53 Certain congenital musculoskeletal deformities: RR, 1.42; 95%CI, 0.65 to 3.12 Other congenital anomalies of limbs: RR, 2.55; 95%CI, 1.23 to 5.29 Other congenital musculoskeletal anomalies: RR, 0.82; 95%CI, 0.21 to 3.24 Other and unspecified congenital anomalies: RR, 0.92; 95%CI, 0.13 to 6.49	

E-65

Author Year Country Study Design/Data Source Risk of Bias	7. Fetus/infant/child outcomes up to 12 months of age	8. Child outcomes after 12 months of age	9. Maternal Outcomes
De Vries 2013[20] Australia PC Medium	Motor Performance: SSRI vs Non-SSRI General Movements (GM) General Movements (GM) quality during first week: Abnormal, n (%): 34 (59) vs 14 (33) p=0.009 Poor repertoire, n (%): 30 (52) vs 14 (33) p=0.11 Chaotic, n (%) / ChF, n (%): 4 (7) / 11 (19) vs 0 (0) / 1 (2) p= 0.14 /p= 0.012 Cramped synchronized, n (%): 0 (0) vs 0 (0) MOS (motor optimality score), median (min-max) during first week: 13 (9-18) vs 18 (10-18) p<0.001 Monotonous sequence, n (%): 36 (62) vs 13 (30) p=0.001 Amplitude abnormalities, n (%): 13 (22) vs 3 (7) p=0.052 Speed abnormalities, n (%): 26 (45) vs 16 (36%) p=0.042 Not using up full space, n (%): 11 (19) vs 0 (0) p=0.002 No rotations, or just a few, n (%): 28 (31) vs 7 (16) p=0.001 Abrupt onset and/or offset, n (%): 16 (28) vs 5 (11) p=0.051 Tremulous movements, n (%): 35 (60) vs 13 (30) p=0.012 GMs quality at 3 to 4 months of age Abnormal quality, n (%): 3 (5) vs 0 (0) p=0.27 Abnormal fidgety, n (%): 2 (3) vs 0 (0) Absent fidgety, n (%): 1 (2) vs 0 (0) MOS, median (min-max) at 3 to 4 months of age: 26 (7–28) vs 28 (21–28) p=0.035 Monotonous movements, n (%): 30 (48) vs 9 (20) p=0.005 Abnormal GMs during the first week For depression - aORdepre+; 95% CI (p value) = 4.1; 1.6–10.5 (0.003) For anxiety - aORdepre+; 95% CI (p value) = 4.2; 1.6–10.9 (0.003)	NR	NR

Author Year Country Study Design/Data Source Risk of Bias	7. Fetus/infant/child outcomes up to 12 months of age	8. Child outcomes after 12 months of age	9. Maternal Outcomes
De Vries 2013[20] Australia PC Medium ....(Cont)	Monotonous movements at 3 to 4 months of age For depression - aORdepre+; 95% CI (p value) = 6.4; 2.1–19.2 (0.001) For anxiety - aORdeore+; 95% CI (p value) = 5.8; 1.9–17.7 (0.002)	NR	
Dubnov-Raz 2008[21] Israel CC Medium	SSRI vs. Control GA: 39 vs. 39, p=0.84 Birth weight, g: 3135 vs. 3365, p=0.04 ECG results, SSRI vs. Control Heart rate, bpm: 129 vs. 138, p=0.01 PR interval, ms: 98 vs 100, p=0.31 QRS duration, ms: 51 vs. 52, p=0.28 QT interval, ms: 280 vs. 261, p<0.001 QTc interval, ms: 409 vs. 392, p=0.02 JT interval, ms: 229 vs. 209, p<0.001 Pathologically prolonged QTc interval (462-543ms): 10% vs. 0.0%, p=0.057	NR	NR
Dubnov-Raz 2012[22] Israel CC Medium	Adjusted Difference scores for infant birth outcomes, SSRI vs. Control: Birth weight, g: -96; 95% CI, -257 to 65; p=0.20 Birth weight, z-score: -0.31; 95% CI, -0.71 to 0.10; p=0.14 Length: -0.74; 95%CI, -1.53 to 0.06; p=0.07 Head circumference: -0.72; 95%CI, -1.22 to 0.22 Adjusted Difference scores for infant tibial bone density, SSRI vs. Control: Speed of sound (m/s): 3.8; 95%CI, -52 to 60 Speed of sound (z-score): 0.01; 95%CI, -0.47 to 0.50	NR	NR

| Author
Year
Country
Study Design/Data Source
Risk of Bias	7. Fetus/infant/child outcomes up to 12 months of age	8. Child outcomes after 12 months of age	9. Maternal Outcomes
El Marroun 2012[23]
The Netherlands
Prospective Cohort Data Source [PC and PD]
Low | "Exposed higher risk for preterm birth (OR=2.14; 95% CI: 1.08 to 4.25; P=.03)

Fetal Weight Gain:
(Adjusted decrease weight, g 95% CI)
Exposed:-2.3 (−7.0 to 2.3) P=.32
Unexposed: −4.4g (−6.3 to −2.4) p<.001

Fetal Head Growth:
(Adjusted decrease circumference, mm, 95% CI)
Exposed: −0.18 (−0.32 to −0.07) P=.003
Unexposed: −0.08 (−0.14 to −0.03) P=.003

Head Circumference at Birth:
Exposed: −5.88 (−11.45 to −0.30) p=.04
Unexposed: 0.05 (−3.48 to 4.43) P=.81

Control group (reference)" | NR | NR |
| Ferreira 2007[24]
US
Retrospective Cohort/Data Source[AD]
Medium | Neonatal behavioral signs (Adjusted OR, 95% CI): 3.1 (1.3–7.1)

Prematurity (Adjusted OR, 95% CI):
3.9 (1.6–9.5) 2.4 (0.9–6.3)

Admission to specialized care (Adjusted OR, 95% CI): 2.4 (0.8–6.9)

Malformations:
phenotypic dimorphisms N=2
absence of septum pellucidum N=1
sagittal craniosynostosis N=1
pulmonary peripheral stenosis N=1
hypospadias N=1
persistent pulmonary hypertension N=0
Unexposed:
phenotypic dimorphisms N=3
angioma N=1
heart murmur N=1
crypt orchidia N=1 | NR | NR |

Author Year Country Study Design/Data Source Risk of Bias	7. Fetus/infant/child outcomes up to 12 months of age	8. Child outcomes after 12 months of age	9. Maternal Outcomes
Figueroa 2010[25] US Retrospective cohort Design/Data Source[AD] Medium	NR	ADHD by age of 5 years: (OR 95%CI) SSRI before pregnancy: 1.20 (0.70–2.04) P= .50 SSRI during pregnancy: 0.91 (0.51–1.60) P=.74 First trimester :1.62 (0.79–3.32) P=.19 Second trimester: .59 (0.58–4.35) P= .37 Third trimester: 0.38 (0.14–1.03) P=.06 SSRI after pregnancy: 2.04 (1.43–2.91) P<.001 Bupropion before pregnancy: 0.49 (0.12–2.02) P=.32 Bupropion during pregnancy : 3.63 (1.20–11.04) P=.02 First trimester: 2.06 (0.35–12.16) P=.42 Second trimester:14.66 (3.27–65.73) P<.001 Third trimester: <0.01 (<0.01–>99.9) P=.94 Bupropion after pregnancy: 0.90 (0.32–2.53) P=.84 Other antidepressant during pregnancy: 0.65 (0.09–4.79) P=.68 Anticonvulsants during pregnancy: 0.36 (0.05–2.65) P=.32 Benzodiazepines during pregnancy:1.82 (0.86–3.85) P=.12 Other psychotropics during pregnancy : <0.01 (<0.01–>99.9) P= .96	NR
Gorman 2012[26] US Prospective cohort/TIS Medium	Exposed vs Unexposed: **Initiating breastfeeding:** SSRI Before delivery: Adjusted OR, 0.43; 95% CI, 0.20-0.94 SSRI At time of delivery: Adjusted OR 0.34; 95% CI, 0.16-0.72 Analysis by race, maternal age, alcohol use, low Apgar: NSD Cesarean birth 0.36 (0.20-0.66) Compared to high SES: Medium 0.46 (0.22-0.99) Low 0.23 (0.11-0.48) **Full breast-feeding at 2 weeks:** Before delivery 0.73 (0.41-1.32) At time of delivery 0.67 (0.39-1.15) Analysis by race, maternal age, BMI, SES = NSD	NR	NR

Author Year Country Study Design/Data Source Risk of Bias	7. Fetus/infant/child outcomes up to 12 months of age	8. Child outcomes after 12 months of age	9. Maternal Outcomes
Grzeskowiak 2012[27] Australia Retrospective cohort/LD Medium	(A) SSRI use vs psychiatric illness/no SSRI use (B) SSRI use vs no psychiatric illness Preterm delivery (<37 weeks): (A)=2.68 (1.83-3.93), (B) 2.46 (1.75-3.50) Low birth weight (<2500 g): (A)=2.26 (1.31-3.91), (B) 2.57 (1.57-4.21) SGA: (A)=1.13 (0.65-1.94), (B)=1.17 (0.71-1.94) Neonate admitted to hospital: (A)=1.92 (1.39-2.65), (B)=2.37 (1.76-3.19) Neonate length of stay > 3 days: (A)=1.93 (1.11-3.36), (B)=2.20 (1.34-3.59)	NR	NR
Hanley 2013[28] Canada PC Medium	Infant development by SRI exposure status (BSID-III) Unexposed (N = 52) vs. Exposed (N = 31). p-value* Cognitive: 10.9 (2.1) vs. 11.5 (2.4), 0.38 Communication, Receptive: 10.2 (2.3) vs. 10.2 (2.2), 0.57 Communication, Expressive: 9.8 (1.6) vs. 9.9 (2.1), 0.69 Motor, Fine: 11.2 (1.7) vs. 11.3 (2.2), 0.55 Motor, Gross: 9.5 (2.8) vs. 8.3 (3.3), 0.03 Social-emotional: 9.6 (2.5) vs. 8.5 (2.2), 0.04 Adaptive behavior: 73.3 (10.3) vs. 68.4 (12.4), 0.05 *Estimates are adjusted for alcohol use, smoking, depression during pregnancy (36 weeks) and postpartum (10 months).	NR	Maternal positive affect was significantly correlated with maternal depressed mood at 36 weeks gestations (−0.42 ,P<0.01) and at 10 months postpartum (−0.44, P<0.01).
Heikkinen 2002[29] Finland PC Medium	Citalopram vs control Gestational age at birth (wk) mean, range: 39 (37 to 41) vs 40 (38 to 41) Malformations: 0% vs 0% Weight at birth (g) mean (range): 3460 (2830 to 4380) vs 3560 (3220 to 4260) Weight at 12 months (g), mean(range): 10560 (11810 to 9420) vs 9810 (10860 to 8900)	NR	Citalopram vs Control -Delivery mode Vaginal: 91% vs 90% Cesarean: 9.1% vs 10% Breast-fed%: 81.8% vs 90%

| Author
Year
Country
Study Design/Data Source
Risk of Bias	7. Fetus/infant/child outcomes up to 12 months of age	8. Child outcomes after 12 months of age	9. Maternal Outcomes
Jimenez-Solem 2012[30]
Denmark
RC-PD
Low | Comparisons to women with no exposure, adjusted ORs (95% CI)
First trimester/Paused during pregnancy
Major malformations: 1.33 (1.16 to 1.53)/1.27 (0.91-1.78)
Congenital malformations of the heart: 2.01 (1.60 to 2.53)/1.85 (1.07-3.20)
Septal defects: 2.04 (1.53-2.72)/2.56 (1.41-4.64)
Ventricular septal defects: 1.62 (1.05-2.50)/3.74 (1.93-7.23)
Atrial septal defects: 2.60 (1.84-3.68)/2.61 (1.17-5.84)
Congenital malformations of the digestive system: 1.80 (1.04-3.12)/0.75 (0.11-5.35)
Congenital malformations of the internal urinary system: 0.84 (0.45-1.57)/None
Congenital malformations of the external genital organs: 1.55 (0.99-2.44)/0.89 (0.22-3.59)
Congenital malformations of the limbs: 0.93 (0.71-1.23)/1.37 (0.80-2.32)
Low-dose/high-dose SSRI during pregnancy
Major malformations: 1.26 (1.05-1.51)/1.44 (1.15-1.79)
Congenital malformations of the heart: 1.83 (1.35-2.48)/2.25 (1.60-3.19)
Congenital malformations of the digestive system: 1.78 (0.89-3.58)/1.80 (0.75-4.35)
Congenital malformations of the internal urinary system: 0.82 (0.37-1.83)/0.88 (0.33-2.34)
Congenital malformations of the external genital organs: 1.32 (0.72-2.46)/1.91 (0.99-3.68)
Congenital malformations of the limbs: 0.94 (0.67-1.33)/0.91 (0.59-1.42)
Septal defects: 1.86 (1.15-3.00)/1.12 (0.28-4.51)/1.73 (0.89-3.33)/1.89 (0.85-4.23)/3.09 (1.82-5.25)
When analyses were further adjusted for comedications, the results showed no considerable change in the estimates or their level of significance.
Individual SSRIs:
citalopram/escitalopram/fluoxetine/paroxetine/sertraline
Major: 1.51 (1.21-1.37)/0.69 (0.34-1.4)/1.18 (0.86-1.61)/1.25 (0.84-1.85)/1.41 (1.03-1.92)
Of the nervous system: 0.84 (0.21-3.37)/2.25 (0.32-16.05)/1.44 (0.36-5.79)/1.19 (0.17-8.45)/0.85 (0.12-6.07)
Neural tube defects Only fluoxetine=3.22 (0.45-23.03)
Of the eye: 2.62 (1.09-6.34)/None/0.93 (0.13-6.63)/None/1.05 (0.15-7.45)
Of the ear, face and neck: None/None/None/8.32 (1.16-59.81)/6.13 (0.85-44.05)
Of the heart: 1.91 (1.31-2.77)/1.06 (0.34-3.3)/2.04)/1.54 (0.77-3.1)/2.73 (1.75-4.26) | NR | NR |

Author Year Country Study Design/Data Source Risk of Bias	7. Fetus/infant/child outcomes up to 12 months of age	8. Child outcomes after 12 months of age	9. Maternal Outcomes
Jimenez-Solem 2012[30] Denmark RC-PD Low ……(Cont)	……(CONT)…… Septal defects: 1.86 (1.15-3)/1.12 (0.28-4.51)/1.73 (0.89-3.33)/1.89 (0.85-4.23)/3.09 (1.82-5.25) Ventricular septal defects: 1.41 (0.67-2.96)/0/1.03 (0.33-3.2)/1.13 (0.28-4.54)/3.6 (1.86-6.96) Atrial septal defects: 2.41 (1.36-4.26)/1.01 (0.14-7.23)/2.53 (1.2-5.32)/3.51 (1.57-7.87)/2.85 (1.35-5.99) Atrioventricular septal: 0/8.71 (1.21-62.64)/0/0/3.22 (0.45-23.03) Of the respiratory system: 1.03 (0.26-4.11)/2.66 (0.37-19.02)/0.94 (0.13-6.67)/1.52 (0.21-10.8)/2.09 (0.52-8.38) Oro-facial clefts: 1.8 (0.67-4.81)/0/0.76 (0.11-5.4)/0/0.88 (0.12-6.24) Of the digestive system: 2.5 (1.19-5.27)/0/1.25 (0.31-5)/2.09 (0.52-8.39)/1.43 (0.36-5.74) Abdominal wall defects: 2.54 (0.35-18.3)/0/0/0/0 Of the internal urinary system: 2.02 (1.05-3.89)/0/0/0/0.44 (0.06-3.11) Of the external genital organs: 1.7 (0.85-3.41)/1.08 (0.15-7.67)/1.09 (0.35-3.38)/3.83 (1.71-8.57)/0.41 (0.06-7.93) Of the limbs: 1.13 (0.76-1.7)/0.25 (0.04-1.75)/0.76 (0.41-1.42)/0.91 (0.43-1.92)/1 (0.55-1.81) Of the musculoskeletal system: 1.25 (0.4-3.88)/2.18 (0.31-15.57)/1.46 (0.36-5.85)/1.2 (0.17-8.55)/0.83 (0.12-5.9) Chromosomal abnormalities: 0.59 (0.08-4.19)/0/0.97 (0.14-6.92)/4.65 (1.49-14.53)/2.35 (0.59-9.45) Other malformations: 1.32 (0.42-4.12)/0/3.08 (1.15-8.23)/0/0.88 (0.12-6.28) And teratogenic syndromes: 3.58 (0.49-26.33)/0/0/10.13 (1.36-75.44) Genetic syndromes: 0.39 (0.06-2.78)/0/1.79 (0.25-12.76)/0/0 Non-SSRI antidepressants: TCAs/other antidepressants: Any congenital malformation: 1.04 (0.53-2.03)/0.70 (0.47-1.05) Malformations of the heart: 1.33 (0.42-4.15)/0.99 (0.51-1.91)		

Author Year Country Study Design/Data Source Risk of Bias	7. Fetus/infant/child outcomes up to 12 months of age	8. Child outcomes after 12 months of age	9. Maternal Outcomes
Jimenez-Solem 2013[31] Denmark PBR Low	Stillbirth/neonatal mortality, adjusted OR (95% CI) Unexposed: 1.00 (reference) Any SSRI 1st trimester: 0.77 (0.43,1.36)/0.56 (0.25,1.24) 1st and 2nd trimester: 0.84 (0.40,1.77)/0.90 (0.37, 2.17) All trimesters: 1.06 (0.71, 1.58)/1.27 (0.82, 1.99) Fluoxetine 1st trimester: 1.37 (0.56, 3.31)/1.18(0.38, 3.67) 1st and 2nd trimester: 0.65 (0.16, 2.63)/1.98 (0.74, 5.31) All trimesters: 0.97 (0.50, 1.87)/0.63 (0.24, 1.69) Citalopram 1st trimester: 0.60 (0.25, 1.45)/0.71 (0.27, 1.91) 1st and 2nd trimester: 0.26 (0.04, 1.88)/0.83(0.21, 3.32) All trimesters: 1.44 (0.74, 2.79)/2.49 (1.33, 4.65) Escitalopram 1st trimester: --/0.86 (0.12, 6.12) 1st and 2nd trimester: 1.29 (0.18, 9.28)/-- All trimesters: --/2.07 (0.29, 14.85) Paroxetine 1st trimester: 0.94(0.23, 3.78)/-- 1st and 2nd trimester: 2.28 (0.73, 7.17)/2.08 (0.52, 8.40) All trimesters: 0.66 (0.17, 2.67)/1.95 (0.73, 5.23) Sertraline 1st trimester: 1.05 (0.34, 3.28)/0.98 (0.24, 3.92) 1st and 2nd trimester: 0.54 (0.08, 3.87)/0.82(0.12, 5.85) All trimesters: 1.02 (0.46, 2.29)/0.26 (0.04, 1.81)	NR	NR
Jordan 2008[32] US Clinic Appt Logs, Pediatrics records review AD Medium	HARMS: 28% SRI reonates: Newborn Behavioral Syndrome. No more likely to be admitted to NICU, have respiratory abnormalities, prolonged hospitalization	NR	NR

Author Year Country Study Design/Data Source Risk of Bias	7. Fetus/infant/child outcomes up to 12 months of age	8. Child outcomes after 12 months of age	9. Maternal Outcomes
Kallen 2004[33] Sweden PBR Medium	ORs for type and timing of antidepressant use, vs. total population Preterm Delivery (<37 week) All antidepressants: OR, 1.96; 95%CI, 1.60 to 2.41 ≥24 week: OR, 2.02; 95%CI, 1.54 to 2.63 Tricyclic drugs: OR, 2.50; 95%CI, 1.87 to 3.34 SSRIs: OR, 2.06; 95%CI, 1.58 to 2.69 Low Birth Weight (<2500 g) All antidepressants: OR, 1.98; 95%CI, 1.55 to 2.52 ≥24 week: OR, 1.66; 95%CI, 1.18 to 2.34 Tricyclic drugs: OR, 1.88; 95%CI, 1.28 to 2.76 SSRIs: OR, 1.98; 95%CI, 1.42 to 2.76 Small for GA (≤2 SDs) All antidepressants: OR, 0.83; 95%CI, 0.53 to 1.30 ≥24 week: OR, 0.96; 95%CI, 0.56 to 1.65 Tricyclic drugs: OR, 1.00; 95%CI, 0.52 to 1.94 SSRIs: OR, 0.80; 95%CI, 0.44 to 1.44 Large for GA (≥2 SDs) All antidepressants: OR, 1.20; 95%CI, 0.93 to 1.56 ≥24 week: OR, 1.20; 95%CI, 0.85 to 1.70 Tricyclic drugs: OR, 1.18; 95%CI, 0.79 to 1.74 SSRIs: OR, 1.19; 95%CI, 0.83 to 1.70 Respiratory Distress All antidepressants: OR, 2.21; 95%CI, 1.71 to 2.86 ≥24 week: OR, 2.12; 95%CI, 1.50 to 3.00 Tricyclic drugs: OR, 2.20; 95%CI, 1.44 to 3.35 SSRIs: OR, 1.97; 95%CI, 1.38 to 2.83 Jaundice All antidepressants: OR, 1.13; 95%CI, 0.84 to 4.27	NR	NR

Author Year Country Study Design/Data Source Risk of Bias	7. Fetus/infant/child outcomes up to 12 months of age	8. Child outcomes after 12 months of age	9. Maternal Outcomes
Kallen 2004[33] Sweden PBR Medium ....(Cont)	CONTINUED........ ≥24 week: OR, 1.05; 95%CI, 0.70 to 1.59 Tricyclic drugs: OR, 1.37; 95%CI, 0.88 to 2.12 SSRIs: OR, 0.96; 95%CI, 0.63 to 1.46 Hypoglycemia All antidepressant: CR, 1.62; 95%CI, 1.22 to 2.16 ≥24 week: OR, 1.49; 95%CI, 1.00 to 2.23 Tricyclic drugs: OR, 2.07; 95%CI, 1.36 to 3.13 SSRIs 24 539 1.35 (0.90-2.03) Low Apgar Score All antidepressants: OR, 2.33; 95%CI, 1.49 to 3.64 ≥24 week: OR, 3.36; 95%CI, 2.05 to 5.49 Tricyclic drugs: OR, 2.99; 95%CI, 1.58 to 5.65 SSRIs: OR, 2.28; 95%CI, 1.27 to 4.10 RR for Convulsions vs. No antidepressants All antidepressants: RR, 4.7; 95%CI, 2.2 to 9.0 ≥24 week: RR, 4.4; 95%CI, 1.4 to 10.3 Tricyclic drugs: RR, 6.8; 95%CI, 2.2 to 16.0 SSRIs: RR, 3.6; 95%CI, 1.0 to 9.3 Crude ORs, Paroxetine vs. Other SSRIs Preterm delivery (<37 week): OR, 1.28; 95%CI, 0.57 to 2.67 Low birth weight (<2500 g): OR, 1.44; 95%CI, 0.40 to 4.24 Small for GA: OR, 0.90; 95%CI, 0.09 to 4.34 Large for GA: OR, 1.77; 95%CI, 0.70 to 4.11 Respiratory distress: OR, 1.23; 95%CI, 0.44 to 3.05 Jaundice: OR, 0.87; 95%CI, 0.21 to 2.71 Hypoglycemia: OR, 0.83; 95%CI, 0.20 to 2.55 Convulsions: OR, 1.40; 95%CI, 0.03 to 15.70		

Author Year Country Study Design/Data Source Risk of Bias	7. Fetus/infant/child outcomes up to 12 months of age	8. Child outcomes after 12 months of age	9. Maternal Outcomes
Kallen 2007[34] Sweden Retrospective cohort/Data Source[PBR] Medium	Risk for congenital malformations*: (Adjusted OR**, 95% CI): Any SSRI: 0.89 (0.79–1.07) Fluoxetine: 0.85 (0.61–1.19) Citalopram: 0.94 (0.78–1.13) Paroxetine: 1.03 (0.76–1.38) Sertraline: 0.78 (0.61–1.00) Fluvoxamine: 1.05 (0.13–3.80)** Escitalopram: 0.91 (0.19–2.66)** *Adjustments were made for year of birth, maternal age, parity, smoking, and > 3 previous miscarriages **Risk ratios	NR	NR
Kallen 2008[35] Sweden Unclear/Data Source[PBR] Medium	PPHN: Maternal use of SSRI and PPHN in births after 34 completed weeks: (Adjusted Risk Ratio, 95% CI) 2.4, (1.2–4.3) Risk for an infant to have PPHN exposed SSRI during pregnancy: Exposed in early pregnancy (Adjusted Risk Ratio, 95% CI) All infants: 2.01 (1.00–3.60) >34 weeks: 2.38 (1.19–4.25) >37 weeks: 2.36 (1.08–4.78) Exposed in early pregnancy with known exposure also in late pregnancy: (Adjusted Risk Ratio, 95% CI) All infants: 2.91 (0.94–6.78) >34 weeks: 1.40 (3.57 1.16–8.33) >37 weeks:1.24 (3.70 1.01–9.48)	NR	NR

Author Year Country Study Design/Data Source Risk of Bias	7. Fetus/infant/child outcomes up to 12 months of age	8. Child outcomes after 12 months of age	9. Maternal Outcomes
Kieler 2012[36] Nordic countries Retrospective cohort, PBD Medium	Small for gestational age (< 2 SDs of sex-specific mean birth weight: Exposed=3% vs not exposed=2.4%, P=NR Apgar score at 5 min: 0-6: Exposed=1.1% vs not exposed=0.6% 7-10: Exposed=61.0% vs not exposed=61.3%, P=NR Persistent pulmonary hypertension, adjusted OR (95% CI), comparison to not exposed: Late exposure: Any SSRI: 2.1 (1.5 to 3.0) Fluoxetine: 2.0 (1.0 to 3.8) Citalopram: 2.3 (1.2 to 4.1) Paroxetine: 2.8 (1.2 to 6.7) Sertraline: 2.3 (1.3 to 4.4) Escitalopram: 1.3 (0.2 to 9.5) Early exposure: Any SSRI: 1.4 (1.0 to 2.0) Fluoxetine: 1.3 (0.6 to 2.8) Citalopram: 1.8 (1.1 to 3.0) Paroxetine: 1.3 (0.5 to 3.5) Sertraline: 1.9 (1.0 to 3.6) Escitalopram: 0.3 (0.0 to 2.2)	NR	NR

| Author
Year
Country
Study Design/Data Source
Risk of Bias	7. Fetus/infant/child outcomes up to 12 months of age	8. Child outcomes after 12 months of age	9. Maternal Outcomes
Kornum 2010[37]
Denmark
PBR
Medium | Escitalopram (n=5): OR, 2.0; 95% CI, 0.8 to 4.9
Non-SSRI antidepressant (n=6): OR, 0.6; 95% CI, 0.3 to 1.3

Cardiac malformations:
Any SSRI (n=26): OR, 1.7; 95% CI, 1.1 to 2.5
Fluoxetine (n=6): OR, 1.9; 95% CI, 0.8 to 4.3
Sertraline (n=7): OR, 3.0; 95% CI, 1.4 to 6.4
Paroxetine (n=1): OR, 0.5; 95% CI, 0.1 to 3.6
Citalopram (n=6): OR, 1.1; 95% CI, 0.5 to 2.7
Escitalopram (n=3): OR, 3.3; 95% CI, 0.8 to 13.4
Non-SSRI antidepressant (n=0)

Septal heart defects:
Any SSRI (n=18): OR, 1.4; 95% CI, 0.8 to 2.3
Fluoxetine (n=4): OR, 1.6; 95% CI, 0.6 to 4.4
Sertraline (n=6): OR, 3.3; 95% CI, 1.5 to 7.5
Paroxetine (n=1): OR, 0.7; 95% CI, 0.1 to 4.6
Citalopram (n=2): OR, 0.3; 95% CI, 0.0 to 2.1
Escitalopram (n=3): OR, 4.2; 95% CI, 1.0 to 17.1
Non-SSRI antidepressant (n=0) | NR | NR |
| Laine 2003[38]
Finland
Prospective cohort/Data Source[PC]
Medium | Pregnancy and delivery outcomes:
mean (SD) or median (range), exposed vs controls

Duration of pregnancy (days):
274 (251-291) vs. 279 (254-289)
Mode of delivery: (number of patients)
Vaginal 16 vs 17
Cesarean 4 vs 3

Weight at birth 3455 g (457) vs 3534 g (438)
Total infant weight at 2 months
5423g (476) vs 5458g (626)
Full breastfeeding 9 weeks (0-43) vs 9 weeks (0-26)
Total breastfeeding 17 weeks (0-52) vs 24 weeks (2-52) | NR | NR |
| Latendresse 2011[39]
US
PS
Medium | Comparison to the unexposed
OR, 95% CI:
SSRI use and prediction of preterm birth
11.7 (2.2 to 60.7), p=0.004 | NR | NR |

| Author
Year
Country
Study Design/Data Source
Risk of Bias	7. Fetus/infant/child outcomes up to 12 months of age	8. Child outcomes after 12 months of age	9. Maternal Outcomes
Lennestal 2007[40]
Sweden
PBR
Medium | ORs for Birth Outcomes for singleton births, vs. all deliveries in the register
Preterm birth (<37 wk.)
SNRI/NRI exposure: OR, 1.60; 95%CI, 1.19 to 2.15
SSRI exposure: OR, 1.24; 95%CI, 1.11 to 1.39

Low birth weight (<2500 g)
SNRI/NRI exposure: OR, 1.12; 95%CI, 0.74 to 1.68
SSRI exposure: OR, 1.06; 95%CI, 0.92 to 1.23

Small for GA (≤2 SD)
SNRI/NRI exposure: OR, 0.68; 95%CI, 0.37 to 1.24
SSRI exposure: OR, 0.99; 95%CI, 0.83 to 1.18

Large for GA (>2 SD)
SNRI/NRI exposure: OR, 1.02; 95%CI, 0.70 to 1.49
SSRI exposure: OR, 1.14; 95%CI, 1.02 to 1.28

ORs/Relative Risks for Neonatal Diagnoses by exposure, vs. all deliveries in the registry
Respiratory problems*
SNRI/NRI exposure
Early: OR, 1.39; 95%CI, 0.99 to 1.96
Late: RR, 2.01; 95%CI, 0.96 to 3.69
SSRI exposure
Early: OR, 1.17; 95%CI, 1.03 to 1.23
Late: OR, 1.72; 95%CI, 1.41 to 2.11

Low Apgar score (<7 at 5 min)
SNRI/NRI exposure
Early: RR, 1.54; 95%CI, 0.74 to 2.84
Late: RR, 1.71; 95%CI, 0.21 to 6.17
SSRI exposure
Early: OR, 1.35; 95%CI, 1.08 to 1.68
Late: OR, 2.22; 95%CI, 1.58 to 3.12

Hypoglycemia
SNRI/NRI exposure
Early: OR, 1.42; 95%CI, 1.00 to 1.99
Late: RR, 2.11; 95%CI, 1.01 to 3.89
SSRI exposure
Early: OR, 1.17; 95%CI, 1.02 to 1.33
Late: OR, 1.32; 95%CI, 1.05 to 1.68 | NR | NR |

Author Year Country Study Design/Data Source Risk of Bias	7. Fetus/infant/child outcomes up to 12 months of age	8. Child outcomes after 12 months of age	9. Maternal Outcomes
Lennestal 2007[40] Sweden PBR Medium ....(Cont)	Neonatal convulsions SNRI/NRI exposure Early: RR, 0.71; 95%CI, 0.02 to 3.95 Late: RR, 4.55; 95%CI, 0.12 to 25.3 SSRI exposure Early: OR, 1.39; 95%CI, 0.85 to 2.26 Late: OR, 2.94; 95%CI, 1.34 to 5.58 Infant Survival after Maternal Use of SNRI/NRI or SSRI, vs. all deliveries in the register Intrauterine Deaths SNRI/NRI exposure Early: RR, 1.7; 95%CI, 0.6 to 3.6 Late: RR, 0.0; 95%CI, 0.0 to 6.4 SSRI exposure Early: RR, 0.8; 95%CI, 0.5 to 1.2 Late: RR, 1.2; 95%CI, 0.5 to 2.3 All Deaths <1y of Age SNRI/NRI exposure Early: RR, 1.3; 95%CI, 0.5 to 2.8 Late: RR, 0.0; 95%CI, 0.0 to 4.4 SSRI exposure Early: RR, 0.8; 95%CI, 0.6 to 1.2 Late: RR, 1.2; 95%CI, 0.7 to 2.0 Congenital Malformations, vs. all women in the register SNRI/NRI: OR, 0.85; 95%CI, 0.58 to 1.24 SSRI: OR, 0.89; 95%CI, 0.79 to 1.07	NR	

Author Year Country Study Design/Data Source Risk of Bias	7. Fetus/infant/child outcomes up to 12 months of age	8. Child outcomes after 12 months of age	9. Maternal Outcomes
Levinson-Castiel 2006[41] Israel PC, PBD Medium	Infants exposed to SSRI vs no SSRI Congenital anomalies: 5% vs 1.7%, p=0.60 Head circumference, cm, mean (SD): 34.0 (1.2) vs 34.1 (1.2), p=0.65 % of patients with NAS: 30% vs 0%, p<0.001 Symptoms of NAS High-pitched cry: 30% vs 0% Sleep disturbances: 35% vs 3% Exaggerated moro reflex: 0.5% vs 0% Tremor: 61.7% vs 8.3% Hypertonicity or myoclonus: 23% vs 1.7% Convulsions: 3% vs 0% Sweating: 1.7% vs 0% Fever: 1.7% vs 0% Autonomic nervous system: 6.7% vs 3.3% Tachypnea: 20% vs 0% GI disturbance: 56.7% vs 3.3% Mean duration of hospital stay for neonates with severe NAS (n=8) exposed to SSRI: 5.3 days	NR	NR
Lewis 2010[42] Australia PC-Clinic Medium	Unadjusted ORs (95% CI) for medication vs control Clinical range for low birth weight: 8.33 (1.11-62.67) Clinical range for prematurity: 4.51 (0.47-43.41) Birth means: Gestational age, weeks: 38.86 vs 39.86; P=0.005 Weight, g: 3273.65 vs 3671.19; P=0.010 Length, cm: 49.30 vs 51.44; P=0.001 Head circumference, cm: 34.10 vs 34.87, P=0.084 One month: Age (days): 31.05 vs 28.55, P=0.038 Weight, g: 4032.05 vs 4582.95, P=0.006 Length, cm: 53.34 vs 54.70, P=0.042 Head circumference, cm: 36.96 vs 37.64, P=0.089 Mean rates of change over 1 month: Change in weight (g d -1): 22.71 vs 31.81, P=0.02 Change in length (mm d -1): 1.26 vs 1.15, P=0.590 Change in head circumference (mm d-1): 0.84 vs 0.86, P=0.800	NR	NR

Author Year Country Study Design/Data Source Risk of Bias	7. Fetus/infant/child outcomes up to 12 months of age	8. Child outcomes after 12 months of age	9. Maternal Outcomes
Logsdon 2011[43] US PC Medium	NR	NR	Inventory of Functional Status after Childbirth Scale: NSD between groups: p=0.0549 Significant interaction with time: All groups, M(SD): p<0.0001 2-week, 2.9 (0.4); 12-week, 3.2(0.3); 26-week, 3.2(0.2); 52-week, 3.5(0.4)
Lund 2009[44] Denmark PC Medium	Comparisons to women with no exposure, adjusted ORs (95% CI) Preterm delivery: 2.02 (1.29 to 3.16) Birth weight<2500g: 0.63 (0.15-2.67) NICU admission:2.39 (1.69 to 3.39) Adjusted difference (95% CI) Gestational age, d: -4.5 (-6.2 to -2.8) Birth weight, g: 21 (-51 to 94) Head circumference: -0.0 (-0.2 to 0.2)	NR	NR
Malm 2011[45] Finland TIS Low	Adjusted OR for risk of major congenital anomalies, any SSRI (n, offspring=6,976): Overall Congenital Anomalies: OR, 1.08; 95%CI, 0.96 to 1.22 CV Anomalies: All major CV anomalies: OR, 1.09; 95%CI, 0.90 to 1.32 Organ system-specific anomalies: CNS: OR, 1.03; 95%CI, 0.68 to 1.57 Neural tube defects: OR, 1.85; 95%CI, 1.07 to 3.20 Respiratory tract: OR, 0.61; 95%CI, 0.28 to 1.30 Cleft lip with or without cleft palate: OR, 0.62; 95%CI, 0.25 to 1.51 Cleft palate: OR, 1.18; 95%CI, 0.67 to 2.08 Digestive system: OR, 0.87; 95%CI, 0.54 to 1.38 Urogenital: OR, 1.09; 95%CI, 0.80 to 1.50 Musculoskeletal: OR, 0.96; 95%CI, 0.75 to 1.23 Omphalocele: OR, 0.47; 95%CI, 0.11 to 1.94 Craniosynostosis: OR, 1.53; 95%CI, 0.61 to 3.87	NR	NR
McFarland 2011[46] US PC Medium	NR	NR	NSD for SRI use on Maternal Fetal Attachment Scale total score, p<0.66

Author Year Country Study Design/Data Source Risk of Bias	7. Fetus/infant/child outcomes up to 12 months of age	8. Child outcomes after 12 months of age	9. Maternal Outcomes
Merlob 2009[47] Israel TIS Medium	SSRI vs. Controls Nonsyndromic congenital heart malformations: N= 8/235 (3.4%) vs. 1,083/67,636 (1.60%); p=0.023 Risk of mild congenital heart defects: RR, 2.17; 95% CI, 1.07 to 4.39)	NR	NR

| Author
Year
Country
Study Design/Data Source
Risk of Bias	7. Fetus/infant/child outcomes up to 12 months of age	8. Child outcomes after 12 months of age	9. Maternal Outcomes
Misri 2006[48]
Canada
PC-Clinic
Medium | NR | Internalizing behaviors at age 4 years, ORs (95% CI):
All exposed (including clonazepam) vs unexposed
Maternal depression-controlled (parent/caregiver):
Emotionally reactive: 1.73 (0.25-11.80)/0.56 (0.08-4.01)
Anxious/depressed: Parent NR/2.70 (0.25-29.30)
Somatic complaints: 0.18 (0.02-1.48)/Caregiver NR
WDn: 1.23 (0.09-17.40)/Caregiver NR
Total internalizing problems: 0.99 (0.13-7.88/2.85 (0.26-31.20)
Clinician's ratings: Irritability=0.65 (0.07-5.69), WDal=2.45 (0.60-10.00), positivity=0.46 (0.10-1.98)

Maternal anxiety-controlled (parent/caregiver):
Emotionally reactive: 2.10 (0.33-13.40)/0.44 (0.06-3.19)
Anxious/depressed: Parent NR/3.21 (0.31-33.70)
Somatic complaints: 0.32 (0.06-1.84)/Caregiver NR
WD: 1.74 (0.15-20.10)/Caregiver NR
Total internalizing problems: 1.08 (0.15-7.89)/3.45 (0.32-36.80)
Clinician's ratings: Irritability=0.64 (0.08-5.51), wd=2.43 (0.59-9.84), positivity=0.46 (0.11-1.93)

SSRIs only vs SSRIs plus clonazepam:
Maternal depression-controlled (parent/caregiver):
Emotionally reactive: 1.63 (0.23-11.80)/8.00 (0.25-255.00)
Anxious/depressed: 1.67 (0.17-16.70)/1.29 (0.13-12.90)
Somatic complaints: 4.79 (0.36-64.50)/Caregiver NR
WDn: 2.26 (0.15-34.20)/Caregiver NR
Total internalizing problems: 4.60 (0.36-57.90)/1.53 (0.15-15.60)
Clinician's ratings: WDal=0.89 (0.15-5.06), positivity=4.57 (0.65-31.90)
>Maternal anxiety-controlled (parent/caregiver):
Emotionally reactive: 1.46 (0.20-10.50)/6.00 (0.18-196.00)
Anxious/depressed: 1.32 (0.14-12.60/1.57 (0.15-16.20)
Somatic complaints: 4.09 (0.29-56.30)/Caregiver NR
WDn: 2.00 (0.13-29.80)/Caregiver NR
Total internalizing problems: 3.28 (0.25-42.60)/1.99 (0.19-21.10)
Clinician's ratings: WDal=0.99 (0.17-5.69), positivity=5.59 (0.59-52.50) | NR |

| Author
Year
Country
Study Design/Data Source
Risk of Bias	7. Fetus/infant/child outcomes up to 12 months of age	8. Child outcomes after 12 months of age	9. Maternal Outcomes
Misri 2010[49]
Canada
PC-Clinic
Medium | NR | NR | Exposure to prenatal SSRIs and SNRIs was not a significant predictor of parenting stress at 3-months or 6-months:
β (P)
Model 1: -0.145 (0.209)/-0.024 (0.843)
Model 2: -0.086 (0.438)/0.038 (0.743) |
| Mulder 2011[50]
The Netherlands
Prospective cohort/Data Source [PC]
Medium | (control vs. previously exposed vs. exposed)

Birth weight in grams: mean (SD)
3463 (444) vs. 3392 (561) vs. 3395 (584)

% with delivery at < 37 weeks:
0% vs. 5.4% vs. 8.3%

Weeks gestation at delivery: mean (SD)
40.0 (1.1) vs. 39.4 (1.9) vs. 39.1 (2.1) | NR | NR |

Author Year Country Study Design/Data Source Risk of Bias	7. Fetus/infant/child outcomes up to 12 months of age	8. Child outcomes after 12 months of age	9. Maternal Outcomes
Nakhai-Pour 2010[51] Canada CC Low	Risk of spontaneous abortion (Adjusted OR) Duration of exposure during year before pregnancy vs. no exposure: 1 month, OR, 1.18; 95% CI, 0.95 to 1.45; 2-6 month, OR, 0.98; 95% CI, 0.80 to 1.21; >6 month, OR, 0.72; 95% CI, 0.54 to 0.95. Use from first day of gestation to index date vs. no use: OR, 1.68; 95% CI, 1.38 to 2.06 Class of antidepressant vs. no use: SSRI alone, OR, 1.61; 95% CI, 1.28 to 2.04; Tricyclic antidepressant alone, OR, 1.27; 95% CI, 0.85 to 1.91; Serotonin-norepinephrine reuptake inhibitor alone, OR, 2.11; 95% CI, 1.34 to 3.30; Other (serotonin modulators, monoamine oxidase inhibitors, tetracyclic perazino-azepines, dopamine and norepinephrine reuptake inhibitors), OR, 1.53; 95% CI, 0.86 to 2.72; Combined use of ≥ 2 classes of antidepressants, OR, 3.51; 95% CI, 2.20 to 5.61. Type of SSRI vs. no use: Paroxetine, OR, 1.75; 95% CI, 1.31 to 2.34; Sertraline, OR, 1.33; 95% CI, 0.85 to 2.08; Fluoxetine, OR, 1.44; 95% CI, 0.86 to 2.43; Citalopram, OR, 1.55; 95% CI, 0.89 to 2.68; Fluvoxamine, OR, 2.19, 95 CI, 0.79 to 6.08; Venlafaxine, OR, 2.11; 95% CI, 1.34 to 3.30; Combined use of ≥ 2 SSRIs, OR, 2.47; 95% CI, 0.62 to 9.83.	NR	NR

Author Year Country Study Design/Data Source Risk of Bias	7. Fetus/infant/child outcomes up to 12 months of age	8. Child outcomes after 12 months of age	9. Maternal Outcomes
Nordeng 2012[52] Norway PBR Medium	Any malformation/Major malformation/CV malformation, Adjusted OR (95% CI) Nonexposed: Reference Prior-only group: 1.14 (0.86, 1.51)/1.12 (0.78, 1.62)/0.69 (0.31, 1.55) Any antidepressant: 1.09(0.74, 1.62)/0.96 (0.55, 1.69)/1.24 (0.55, 2.32) SSRIs: 1.22 (0.81, 1.34)/1.07 (0.60, 1.91)/1.51 (0.67, 3.43) Citalopram/escitalopram: 1.47 (0.88, 2.46)/0.99 (0.44, 2.25)/1.51 (0.48, 4.77) Sertraline: 0.93 (0.34, 2.53)/--/-- Paroxetine: 0.95 (0.30, 3.02)/1.70 (0.55, 5.63)/-- Fluoxetine: 2.17 (0.47, 5.06)/--/-- Preterm birth, Adjusted OR (95% CI) Prior-only group: 1.12 (0.84, 1.49) Any antidepressant during pregnancy: 1.21(0.87, 1.69) SSRI during pregnancy: 1.28 (0.90, 1.84) Depressive symptoms week 17: 1.13 (1.03, 1.25) Low birthweight, Adjusted OR (95% CI) Prior-only group: 0.93 (0.55, 1.58) Any antidepressant during pregnancy: 0.62 (0.33, 1.16) SSRI during pregnancy: 0.64 (0.32, 1.26) Depressive symptoms week 17: 1.12 (0.95, 1.32)	NR	NR

Author Year Country Study Design/Data Source Risk of Bias	7. Fetus/infant/child outcomes up to 12 months of age	8. Child outcomes after 12 months of age	9. Maternal Outcomes
Nulman 2002[53] Canada PC Medium	NR	Cognitive outcomes (at 15-71 months) of children of women who took tricyclic antidepressants or fluoxetine throughout pregnancy: No difference in global IQ between antidepressant groups or nondepressed comparison women (as measured by either Bayley or McCarthy test). Children in the tricyclic antidepressant group scored slightly higher on the Reynell Developmental Language Scales, but all 3 groups scored within the normal range. Multiple regression analysis showed the duration of maternal depression was a significant negative predictor for McCarthy global cognitive index. Antidepressant drugs themselves did not predict cognitive achievement. Number of depressive episodes after delivery had a negative relationship with language scores. Treatment for maternal depression was a positive predictor for language development. No differences among the 3 groups across 9 temperament scales (P=0.83) or 3 behavioral scales (P=0.83) of the Child Behavior Checklist.	NR
Oberlander 2002[54] Canada Prospective cohort/Data Source[PC] Medium	(exposed vs. exposed vs. control) Birth age: mean (SE) 39.5 (37.3-42.0) vs. 39.6 (37.6-41.6) vs. 39.2 (37.0-41.6) Birth weight in grams: mean (SE) 3401 (2703-4270) vs. 3490 (2865-4240) vs.3485 (2690-4150) Head circumference: 34.3 (32-37) vs. 34.53 (uninterruptable in table 1) vs. 35.0 (38.5-32) Length: 51.84 (47-64) vs. 51.5(49-54.5) vs. 51.6(47-57)	NR	Breastfeeding: N= 17 vs. 13 vs. 20

E-88

Author Year Country Study Design/Data Source Risk of Bias	7. Fetus/infant/child outcomes up to 12 months of age	8. Child outcomes after 12 months of age	9. Maternal Outcomes
Oberlander 2006[55] Canada PBR Medium	Outcome Mean, Depressed, with SSRI vs. Depressed, No SSRI vs. Not depressed, No SSRI; Difference score (95% CI), Depressed, with SSRI vs. Depressed, No SSRI Birth Weight, g: 3397 vs. 3429 vs. 3453; Difference, -32; 95%CI, -1 to -64; p=0.05 GA: 38.8 vs. 39.1 vs. 39.2; Difference, -0.35; 95%CI, -0.2 to -0.45; p<0.001 Preterm birth (<37weeks): 0.090 vs. 0.065 vs. 0.059; Difference, 0.02; 95%CI, 0.009 to 0.04; p<0.001 Birth Weight <10th %: 0.085 vs. 0.081 vs. 0.074; Difference, 0.005; 95%CI, -0.01 to 0.02; p=0.51 Length of hospital stay, d: 3.31 vs. 2.88 vs. 2.76; Difference, 0.43; 95%CI, 0.12 to 0.74; p=0.007 Respiratory Distress: 0.139 vs. 0.078 vs. 0.074; Difference, 0.063; 95%CI, 0.042 to 0.079; p<0.001 Feeding Problems: 0.039 vs. 0.024 vs. 0.021; Difference, 0.015; 95%CI, 0.005 to 0.025; p=0.002 Jaundice: 0.094 vs. 0.075 vs. 0.079; Difference, 0.019; 95% CI, 0.003 to 0.034; p=0.01 Convulsions: 0.0014 vs. 0.0009 vs. 0.0011: Difference, 0.0005; 95% CI, -0.0015 to 0.0025; p=0.64 Propensity Score Matching: only birth weight <10th % (Difference, 0.033; 95%CI, 0.007 to 0.059; p=0.02) and respiratory distress (Difference, 0.044; 95%CI, 0.013 to 0.077; p=0.006) remained significantly different.	NR	NR
Oberlander 2008[56] Canada PC Medium	SRI Exposed vs. Not Exposed GA, weeks: 39.34 vs. 40.14, p<0.05 Birth weight, g: 3404.95 vs. 3605.94, NSD Small for GA: 3 vs. 1, NSD Apgar, 1 minute (M): 7.54 vs. 8.13, NSD, not moderated by SLC6A4 genotype. Apgar, 5 minutes (M): 8.70 vs. 9.06, p<0.05, significant interaction between SRI exposure and SLC6A4 genotype (F=3.28, P=0.043);	NR	NR

Author Year Country Study Design/Data Source Risk of Bias	7. Fetus/infant/child outcomes up to 12 months of age	8. Child outcomes after 12 months of age	9. Maternal Outcomes
Oberlander 2008[57] (Birth Defects Res Part B) Canada PBR Medium	Adjusted risk differences, exposure group compared to no exposure group Major Congenital Anomalies, adjusted risk difference (95% CI) SRIs only: -0.61 (-1.44 to 0.21) SRIs + benzodiazepines: 1.65 (-0.49 to 3.79) CV Congenital Defects, adjusted risk difference (95% CI) SRIs only: 0.21 (-0.14 to 0.56) SRIs + benzodiazepines: 1.18 (0.18 to 2.18) Ventricular Septal Defects, adjusted risk difference (95% CI) SRIs only: 0.10 (-0.12 to 0.33) SRIs + benzodiazepines: 0.35 (-0.26 to 0.9) Atrial Septal Defects, adjusted risk difference (95% CI) SRIs only: 0.21 (0.05 to 0.36) SRIs + benzodiazepines: -0.01 (-0.31 to 0.30) SRI monotherapy Major Congenital Anomalies, adjusted risk difference (95% CI) Citalopram: 0.40 (-3.13 to 3.93) Fluoxetine: -0.26 (-1.68 to 1.17) Fluvoxamine: -1.52 (-4.02 to 0.98) Paroxetine: -0.56 (-1.70 to 0.59) Sertraline: -0.41 (-1.84 to 1.02) Venlafaxine: -1.18 (-3.20 to 0.84) SRI monotherapy CV Congenital Defects, adjusted risk difference (95% CI) Citalopram: 2.28 (0.19 to 4.36) Fluoxetine: 0.08 (-0.54 to 0.70) Fluvoxamine: -0.55 (-1.45 to 0.36) Paroxetine: 0.12 (-0.38 to 0.62) Sertraline: -0.09 (-0.65 to 0.47) Venlafaxine: 0.01 (-0.77 to 0.79)	NR	NR

Author Year Country Study Design/Data Source Risk of Bias	7. Fetus/infant/child outcomes up to 12 months of age	8. Child outcomes after 12 months of age	9. Maternal Outcomes
Okun 2011[38] US PC Medium	NR	NR	Mean depression ratings: Hamilton Rating Scale for Depression, SSRI vs. No SSRI (depressed and non-depressed): Week 20: 6.6 vs. 5.1, p=0.01 Week 30: 6.5 vs. 4.1, p=0.0001 Week 36: 6.2 vs. 3.9, p=0.007 Hamilton Rating Scale for Depression, Atypical symptoms: Week 20: 4.0 vs. 3.6, p=0.27 Week 30: 4.2 vs. 3.4, p=0.04 Week 36: 4.0 vs. 3.4, p=0.07 Structured interview, Hamilton Rating Scale for Depression: Week 20: 10.5 vs. 8.7, p=0.03 Week 30: 10.6 vs. 7.5, p=0.0004 Week 36: 10.2 vs. 7.3, p=0.01 Atypical Symptoms/Structured interview, Hamilton Rating Scale for Depression: Week 20: 38.1 vs. 46.9, p=0.01 Week 30: 39.8 vs. 45.4, p=0.07 Week 36: 44.6 vs. 47.4, p=0.53

Author Year Country Study Design/Data Source Risk of Bias	7. Fetus/infant/child outcomes up to 12 months of age	8. Child outcomes after 12 months of age	9. Maternal Outcomes
Okun 2012[59] US PC Medium	ORs for pre-term birth compared to No MDD, No SSRI group. Week 20 No MDD, taking SSRI: OR, 4.15; 95% CI, 1.43 to 12.0 MDD, No SSRI: OR, 1.45; 95% CI, 0.43 to 4.88 MDD, taking SSRI: OR, 3.76; 95% CI, 1.04 to 13.6 Week 30 No MDD, taking SSRI: OR, 7.93; 95% CI, 2.44 to 25.7 MDD, No SSRI: OR, 1.36; 95% CI, 0.27 to 6.94 MDD, taking SSRI: OR, 5.00; 95% CI, 1.42 to 17.5	NR	NR
Palmsten 2012[60] Canada RC-LD Medium	NR	NR	Preeclampsia, adjusted RR vs unexposed (95% CI): (Model 4 - adjusted for delivery year, age, diabetes, multifetal gestation, obesity, primiparity, and physician visits) SSRI monotherapy: 1.22 (0.97-1.54) SSRI polytherapy: 1.28 (0.73-2.22) SNRI monotherapy: 1.95 (1.25-3.03) TCA monotherapy: 3.23 (1.87-5.59) Preeclampsia, adjusted RR for continuation vs. discontinuation (Model 4 - adjusted for delivery year, age, diabetes, multifetal gestation, obesity, primiparity, and physician visits) SSRI monotherapy: 1.32 (0.95, 1.84) SNRI monotherapy: 3.43 (1.77, 6.65) TCA monotherapy: 3.26 (1.04, 10.24)

Author Year Country Study Design/Data Source Risk of Bias	7. Fetus/infant/child outcomes up to 12 months of age	8. Child outcomes after 12 months of age	9. Maternal Outcomes
Pearson 2007[61] US Retrospective cohort Data/Source: [AD] Medium	Adjusted for tobacco use, marital status, maternal age, parity.	Exposed vs. Not Exposed N=252 Birth weight: mean (SD) 3.28 (.48) vs. 3.3 (.63) Gestational age wk: mean (SD) 39 (1.7) vs. 38.9 (2.3) Premature delivery: 10.7% vs. 10.1% Caesarean section: 16.7% vs. 26.8% Admission to SCN: 17.9% vs. 10.1% Timely SCN discharge: 73.3 % vs. 10.1% Neonatal outcomes SRIs vs. TCAs: SRIs N=42, TCAs N=37 Low birth weight: 2.4% vs. 5.4% Prematurity: 7.1% vs. 16.2% Admission to SCN: 11.9% vs. 29.7% Timely SCN discharge: 80% vs. 63.6%	NR
Pedersen 2009[62] Denmark PBD, LD Medium	Comparisons to unexposed infants, Adjusted OR (95% CI) Fluoxetine vs citalopram vs paroxetine vs sertraline vs >1 type of SSRI Minor malformations: 0.62(0.20 to 1.93) vs 0.79 (0.33 to 1.91) vs 1.43 (0.54 to 3.22) vs 0.76 (0.24 to 2.37) vs 1.08 (0.34 to 3.38) Cardiac malformations: 0.77 (0.19 to 3.11) vs 1.75 (0.78 to 3.93) vs 0.38 (0.22 to 3.55) vs 2.36 (0.97 to 5.72) vs 3.42 (1.40 to 8.34) Septal heart defects: 1.34 (0.33 to 5.41) vs 2.52 (1.04 to 6.10) vs 0.76 (0.11 to 5.43) vs 3.25 (1.21 to 8.75) vs 4.70 (1.74 to 12.7) Non-cardiac malformations: 1.08 (0.54 to 2.19) vs 0.83 (0.41 to 1.67) vs 1.59 (0.85 to 2.99) vs 1.18 (0.56 to 2.50) vs 0.95 (0.35 to 2.57)	NR	NR
Pedersen 2010[63] Denmark PC Medium	6 months, Adjusted OR Achievement of milestones, antidepressants vs. untreated depression Head control OR, 1.0; 95% CI, 0.2 to 6.1; Sits with straight back OR, 2.2; 95% CI, 1.0 to 4.8; Rolls from back to belly OR, 1.5; 95% CI, 1.0 to 2.1; Sits without support OR, 1.2; 95% CI, 0.8 to 1.7	19 months, Adjusted OR Antidepressants vs. untreated depression Going up stairs with support OR, 1.0; 95% CI, 0.50 to 2.05; Taking off socks and shoes when asked to OR, 1.1; 95% CI, 0.68 to 1.64; Drinking from ordinary cup without help OR, 3.4; 95% CI, 0.66 to 17.0	NR

Author Year Country Study Design/Data Source Risk of Bias	7. Fetus/infant/child outcomes up to 12 months of age	8. Child outcomes after 12 months of age	9. Maternal Outcomes
Pedersen 2013[64] (Pendersen, 2010) Denmark PBR Medium	NR	**Four and Five Year Olds** **Dichotomized SDQ score according to exposure during pregnancy** **ADs vs Untreated Depression AOR (95% CI)** Emotional symptoms 1.6 (0.8-8.9) Conduct problems 0.6 (0.3-1.3) Hyperactivity/inattention 1.8 (0.6-5.6) Peer problems 0.9 (0.2-4.8) Prosocial 0.5 (0.2-1.7) Total difficulties 1.3 (0.3-6.0) **Untreated Depression vs Unexposed AOR (95% CI)** Emotional symptoms 0.8 (0.2-3.1) Conduct problems 2.3 (1.2-4.5) Hyperactivity/inattention 0.8 (0.3-2.2) Peer problems 0.7 (0.2-2.4) Prosocial 3.0 (1.2-7.8) Total difficulties 0.8 (0.2-3.1) **Strengths and Difficulties Questionnaire score according to exposure during pregnancy AOR (95% CI)** **ADs vs Untreated Depression (Difference) (95% CI)** Emotional symptoms -0.3 (-0.7-0.1) Conduct problems - 0.1 (-0.5-0.3) Hyperactivity/inattention -0.2 (-0.7-0.4) Peer problems -0.1 (-0.4-0.2) Prosocial 0.1 (-0.4-0.5) Total difficulties -0.7 (-1.8-0.4) **Untreated Depression vs Unexposed (Difference) ACoeff (95% CI)** Emotional symptoms 0.5 (0.2-0.8) Conduct problems 0.3 (0.0-0.6) Hyperactivity/inattention 0.4 (-0.1-0.8) Peer problems 0.1 (-0.1-0.4) Prosocial -0.3 (-0.7-0.0) Total difficulties 1.2 (0.4-2.1) Including only women with normal Major Depression Inventory score at time of followup, untreated prenatal depression was associated with conduct problems, OR 2.3 (95% CI, 1.2–4.6). There was no statistically significant associations between specific behavioral problems in the subgroup of women with no psychiatric disease since childbirth and with normal Major Depression Inventory scores at followup.	NR

Author Year Country Study Design/Data Source Risk of Bias	7. Fetus/infant/child outcomes up to 12 months of age	8. Child outcomes after 12 months of age	9. Maternal Outcomes
Polen 2013[63] US PBD Medium	Adjusted odds ratios for infants exposed to venlafaxine Anencephaly 6.3 (1.5–20.2) Spina bifida 2.1 (0.4–7.6) Anotia or microtia - couldn't calculate Overall - Conotruncal heart defects 1.9 (0.6–5.3) D-Transposition of the great arteries- couldn't calculate Tetralogy of Fallot - couldn't calculate Overall - Septal heart defects 3.0 (1.4–6.4) Perimembranous ventricular septal defect 2.4 (0.8–6.7) Atrial septal defect, type 2 or not otherwise specified 3.1 (1.3–7.4) Ventricular septal defect-atrial septal defect association 3.1 (0.6–11.3) RVOTO defects 2.3 (0.6–6.6) Pulmonary valve stenosis 2.7 (0.8–7.9) LVOTO defects 3.3 (1.2–8.2) Hypoplastic left heart syndrome - couldn't calculate Coarctation of the aorta 4.1 (1.3–11.5) Cleft lip with or without cleft palate 1.5 (0.5–4.3) Cleft palate alone 3.3 (1.1–8.8) Anorectal atresia- couldn't calculate Esophageal atresia - couldn't calculate Hypospadias, 2nd/3rd degreed 2.3 (0.7–7.9) Any limb reduction defect 2.1 (0.4–7.6) Craniosynostosis 1.5 (0.3–5.4) Diaphragmatic hernia- couldn't calculate Gastroschisis 5.7 (1.8–15.9)	NR	NR

| Author
Year
Country
Study Design/Data Source
Risk of Bias	7. Fetus/infant/child outcomes up to 12 months of age	8. Child outcomes after 12 months of age	9. Maternal Outcomes
Rai 2013[66]
Sweden
CC
Low | NR | Adjusted OR (95% CI)
Autism spectrum disorder
Any antidepressant use: 1.90 (1.15-3.14)
Any antidepressant use with depression: 3.34 (1.50-7.47)
Any antidepressant use without depression: 1.61 (0.85-3.06)
Depression and no antidepressant use: 1.06 (0.68 to 1.66)
SSRIs: 1.65 (0.90-3.03)
Nonselective MRIs: 2.69 (1.04-6.06)

Autism spectrum disorder with intellectual disability
Any antidepressant use: 1.09 (0.41-2.88)
SSRIs: 1.01 (0.34-2.98)
Nonselective MRIs: 1.72 (0.20-15.03)
Any antidepressant use with depression: 1.81 (0.39-8.56)
Any antidepressant use without depression: 0.93 (0.27-3.21)
Depression and no antidepressant use: 1.06 (0.54 to 2.07)

Autism spectrum disorder without intellectual disability
Any antidepressant use: 2.54 (1.37-4.68)
SSRIs: 2.34 (1.09-5.06)
Nonselective MRIs: 2.93 (0.98-8.82)
Any antidepressant use with depression: 4.94 (1.85-13.23)
Any antidepressant use without depression: 2.10 (0.97-4.57)
Depression and no antidepressant use: 1.04 (0.57-1.92) | NR |

Author Year Country Study Design/Data Source Risk of Bias	7. Fetus/infant/child outcomes up to 12 months of age	8. Child outcomes after 12 months of age	9. Maternal Outcomes
Ramos 2008[67] Canada LD Medium	Adjusted ORs for risk of major congenital malformations Timing of antidepressant exposure: First trimester: OR, 1.10; 95%CI, 0.75 to 1.62 Second trimester: OR, 1.13; 95%CI, 0.59 to 2.17 Third trimester: OR, 0.86; 95%CI, 0.45 to 1.65 Duration of antidepressant use during first trimester: 1–30 days: OR,1.23; 95%CI, 0.77 to 1.98 31–60 days: OR, 1.03; 95%CI, 0.63 to 1.69 ≥61 days: OR, 0.92; 95%CI, 0.50 to 1.69 Class of antidepressant used during first trimester: Paroxetine: OR, 1.27; 95%CI, 0.78 to 2.06 Other SSRI: OR, 1.19; 95%CI, 0.71 to 1.97 Tricyclic antidepressant: OR, 0.78; 95%CI, 0.30 to 2.02 Other antidepressant: OR, 0.94; 95%CI, 0.51 to 1.75 Co-exposure: OR, 1.03; 95%CI, 0.44 to 2.41	NR	NR

| Author
Year
Country
Study Design/Data Source
Risk of Bias	7. Fetus/infant/child outcomes up to 12 months of age	8. Child outcomes after 12 months of age	9. Maternal Outcomes
Ramos 2010[68]
Canada
LD, supplemental questionnaire
Medium | Adjusted Risk Ratio for Small for GA (birth weight <10th percentile) by Trimester and class of antidepressant vs. no antidepressants:
First Trimester:
SSRIs: RR, 0.96; 95%CI, 0.74 to 1.25
Tricyclics: RR, 0.84; 95%CI, 0.44 to 1.58
Other antidepressants: RR, 1.17; 95%CI, 0.83 to 1.66
Co-exposure: RR, 0.83; 95%CI, 0.51 to 1.35

Second Trimester:
SSRIs: RR, 1.40; 95%CI, 0.96 to 2.02
Tricyclics: RR, 0.69; 95%CI, 0.18 to 2.60
Other antidepressants: RR, 2.25; 95%CI, 1.30 to 3.92
Co-exposure: RR, 3.48; 95%CI, 1.56 to 7.75

Third Trimester:
SSRIs: RR, 0.70; 95%CI, 0.48 to 1.01
Tricyclics: RR, 2.12; 95%CI, 0.58 to 7.72
Other antidepressants: RR, 0.47; 95%CI, 0.24 to 0.90
Co-exposure: RR, 0.33; 95%CI, 0.12 to 0.89

Adjusted Risk Ratio for Small for GA by class of antidepressant used during the second trimester in subset of cohort (N=938)
SSRIs: RR, 1.40; 95%CI, 0.73 to 2.67
Tricyclics: RR, 0.99; 95%CI, 0.13 to 7.37
Other antidepressants: RR, 2.41; 95%CI, 1.07 to 5.43
Co-exposure: RR, 3.28; 95%CI, 1.28 to 8.45 | NR | NR |

Author Year Country Study Design/Data Source Risk of Bias	7. Fetus/infant/child outcomes up to 12 months of age	8. Child outcomes after 12 months of age	9. Maternal Outcomes
Rampono 2009[69] Australia PC Medium	Gestational age at delivery, Median (IQR): Cases: 39 (38-40) Controls: 40 (39-40) p<0.05 No significant differences for obstetric outcomes (labor, presentation or delivery mode) or neonatal outcomes (need for resuscitation, birth weight, or head circumference) Neonatal Abstinence: Present in 5% of cases (4% SSRIs, 9% venlafaxine) Maximum neonatal abstinence score on day 1, Median (IQR): Cases: 2 (0-1.05) Controls: 0 (0-6) P<0.05 No other differences in mean or maximum NAS scores (days 1-3 Brazelton Neonatal Behavioral Assessment Scale, Mean (SD): Controls/Cases/SSRI/SNRI (higher score indicates better response): Habituation: 7.64 (0.84)/6.57 (1.60)/6.62 (1.80)/6.46 (1.65) Social-interactive: 7.29 (1.12)/6.22 (1.90)/6.10 (2.02)/6.49 (1.63) Motor: 6.13 (0.44)/5.35 (0.59)/5.38 (0.55)/5.27 (0.69) Range: 3.53 (0.75)/3.49 (0.58)/3.47 (0.61)/3.55 (0.52) Regulation: 6.26 (1.00)/5.96 (1.18)/5.91 (1.13)/6.09 (1.32) Autonomic: 6.20 (0.63)/5.51 (1.17)/5.52 (0.98)/5.47 (1.59) Reflexes: 0.75 (0.07)/0.73(0.09)/0.74 (0.08)/0.72 (0.11) P<0.05 for controls vs cases for habituation, social-interactive, and autonomic P<0.05 for controls vs SSRI vs SNRI for motor and autonomic	NR	NR

Author Year Country Study Design/Data Source Risk of Bias	7. Fetus/infant/child outcomes up to 12 months of age	8. Child outcomes after 12 months of age	9. Maternal Outcomes
Reebye 2002[70] Canada PC Medium	SSRI vs SSRI+ vs nonexposed Bayley scale at 2 months Mental development index Mean (SD): 98 (8.1) vs 93 (5.1) vs 96 (7.5) Psychomotor development index Mean (SD): 106 (5.4) vs 102 (6.3) vs 101 (7.9) Gestational age, wks Mean (SD): 39.5(1.2) vs 39.5 (1.3) vs 39.3 (1.4) Birthweight, g Mean (SD): 3364 (408) vs 3515 (452) vs 3414 (437)	NR	SSRI alone vs SSRI plus vs Non-exposed Maternal infant positive correlations at 3 months During Feeding 0.35 vs 0.32 vs 0.58 (p<0.01) sensitivity: 0.40 (p<0.05) vs 0.06 vs -0.02 During free play 0.40 (p<0.05) vs 0.61(p<0.05) vs 0.20 sensitivity: 0.20 vs 0.51(p<0.05) vs -0.13 negativity: -0.26 vs -0.72 (p<0.05) vs -0.08 Intercorrelations between parent variable and negative infant affect at 3 months SSRI Negative infant affect vs apathetic mood vs sober mood Feeding Positive maternal affect: -0.21 vs -0.17 vs 0.01 Free play Positive maternal affect: 0.04 vs -0.48 (p<0.05) vs -0.55 (p<0.05) Feeding sensitivity : -0.15 vs -0.08 vs -0.14 Free play sensitivity: -0.12 vs -0.38 (p<0.05) vs -0.17 Free play negativity: 0.25 vs 0.14 vs -0.05 SSRI + Negative infant affect vs apathetic mood vs sober mood Feeding Positive maternal affect:-0.57 (p<0.05) vs NR vs -0.26 Free play Positive maternal affect: -0.47 vs -0.23 vs -0.56 (p<0.05)

| Author
Year
Country
Study Design/Data Source
Risk of Bias	7. Fetus/infant/child outcomes up to 12 months of age	8. Child outcomes after 12 months of age	9. Maternal Outcomes
Reebye 2002[70]
Canada
PC
Medium
……..(Cont) | | | Feeding sensitivity : 0.00 vs NR vs -0.33
Free play sensitivity: -0.15 vs -0.55(p<0.05) vs -0.43
Free play negativity: 0.53 (p<0.05) vs 0.38 vs 0.54 (p<0.05)
Nonexposed:
Negative infant affect vs apathetic mood vs sober mood
Feeding Positive maternal affect: 0.35 vs -0.33 vs -0.39(p<0.05)
Free play Positive maternal affect: -0.18 vs -0.55(p<0.05) vs -0.28
Feeding sensitivity: 0.30 vs 0.14 vs -0.28
Free play sensitivity: -0.15 vs -0.27 vs 0.18
Free play negativity: 0.17 vs 0.31 vs -0.6 |

Author Year Country Study Design/Data Source Risk of Bias	7. Fetus/infant/child outcomes up to 12 months of age	8. Child outcomes after 12 months of age	9. Maternal Outcomes
Reis 2010[71] Sweden PBR Medium	Infant characteristics according to antidepressant use later in pregnancy: TCA/SSRI/SNRI, Adjusted OR (95% CI) Preterm birth (<37 weeks): 2.36 (1.89, 2.94)/1.46 (1.31, 1.63)/1.98 (1.49, 2.63) Low birthweight (<2500 gm): 1.39 (1.00, 1.95)/1.13 (0.97, 1.31)/1.87 (1.33, 2.64) High birthweight (>4500 gm): 0.62 (0.40, 0.95)/0.89 (0.70, 1.04)/0.80 (0.53, 1.38) Small for gestational age: 0.77 (0.45, 1.32)/1.01 (0.84, 1.22)/1.84 (1.20, 2.81) Large for gestational age: 1.12 (0.85, 1.48)/1.06 (0.93, 1.19)/1.23 (0.88, 1.72)

Neonatal diagnoses in infants born after maternal antidepressant use: Early use/Later use/Both early and later use, Adjusted OR (95% CI) Hypoglycemia: 1.33 (1.22, 1.45)/1.43 (1.31, 1.65)/1.56 (1.36, 1.79) Respiratory diagnoses: 1.34 (1.25, 1.44)/1.62 (1.47, 1.79)/1.65 (1.46, 1.85) CNS diagnoses: 1.31 (1.11, 1.56)/1.50 (1.19, 1.88)/1.49 (1.013, 1.97) Jaundice: 1.09 (1.01, 1.19)/1.13 (1.01, 1.27)/1.22 (1.06, 1.39) Intracerebral hemorrhage: 1.17 (0.77, 1.78)/1.28 (0.66, 2.23)/1.20 (0.52, 2.37) | NR | Maternal delivery diagnoses after use of antidepressants: Early use/Later use/Both early and later use, Adjusted OR (95% CI) Preexisting diabetes: 1.35 (1.19, 1.52)/1.32 (1.11, 1.58)/-- Chronic hypertension: 1.34(1.18, 1.52)/1.25 (1.04, 1.51)/-- Gestational diabetes: 1.37 (1.18, 1.58)/1.16 (0.93, 1.45)/1.37 (1.08, 1.75) Pre-eclampsia: 1.28 (1.19, 1.37)/1.38 (1.25, 1.53)/1.50 (1.33, 1.69) Hyperemesis: 1.45 (1.27, 1.66)/1.31 (1.07, 1.60)/1.59 (1.28, 1.96) Placenta previa: 1.36 (1.20, 1.55)/1.21 (1.00, 1.47)/1.38 (1.11, 1.72) Placenta abruption: 1.29 (1.14, 1.47)/1.05 (0.86, 1.29)/1.23 (0.99, 1.53) Premature rupture of membranes: 1.30 (1.18, 1.43)/1.36 (1.19, 1.56)/1.47 (1.26, 1.72) Bleeding before partus: 1.25 (1.10, 1.42)/1.15 (0.95, 1.39)/1.34 (1.09, 1.66) Bleeding during partus: 1.33 (1.20, 1.46)/1.45 (1.27, 1.65)/1.58 (1.36, 1.84) Bleeding after partus: 1.11 (1.03, 1.19)/1.02 (0.92, 1.14)/1.08 (0.95, 1.22) Induction of delivery: 1.29 (1.22, 1.35)/1.29 (1.19, 1.38)/1.29 (1.18, 1.41) Caesarean section: 1.38 (1.32, 1.44)/1.35 (1.27, 1.44)/1.74 (1.30, 1.51) |

Author Year Country Study Design/Data Source Risk of Bias	7. Fetus/infant/child outcomes up to 12 months of age	8. Child outcomes after 12 months of age	9. Maternal Outcomes
Salisbury 2011[72] US PC Medium	Non-MDD vs. MDD vs. MDD+SRI GA at birth: 39.48 vs. 39.66 vs. 38.99, F=3.6, p=0.03 Birth weight, g: 3,553.82 vs. 3,466.95 vs. 3,320, F=2.3, p=0.11 1 min-APGAR, % <8: 10.71% vs. 16.67% vs. 30.57%, x2=5.6, p=0.03 5 min-APGAR, %<9: 5.36% vs. 5.56% vs. 16.67%, x2 3.2, x2= 3.2, p=0.23 NICU network neurobehavioral scores, Non-MDD vs. MDD vs. MDD+SRI; Attention: 5.84 vs. 4.36 vs. 5.96, p=0.00 Quality of Movement: 4.63 vs. 4.82 vs. 4.27, p=0.05 Self-regulation: 5.50 vs. 5.47 vs. 5.27, p=0.67 Handling: 0.38 vs. 0.40 vs. 0.42, p=0.41 Arousal: 4.27 vs. 4.20 vs. 4.04, p=0.03 Excitability: 3.55 vs. 3.17 vs. 3.67, p=0.73 Lethargy: 3.02 vs. 4.24 vs. 3.34, p=1.00 Stress/abstinence signs, total: 0.08 vs. 0.08 vs. 0.11, p=0.10 Stress/abstinence signs, CNS: 0.05 vs. 0.0 vs. 0.13, p=0.00 Nonoptimal reflexes: 1.60 vs. 1.73 vs. 2.17, p=0.41 Asymmetrical reflexes: 0.33 vs. 0.50 vs. 0.56, p=0.72 Hypertonia: 0.05 vs. 0.04 vs. 0.16, p=0.05 Hypotonia: 0.16 vs. 0.05 vs. 0.23, p=0.49	NR	NR
Salkeld 2008[73] Canada CC-LD Low	NR	NR	Postpartum hemorrhage, multivariate OR (95% CI): 90-day exposure: SSRI: 1.30 (0.98–1.72) Non-SSRI: 1.12 (0.62–2.01) 30-day exposure: SSRI: 1.33 (0.94–1.89) Non-SSRI: 1.29 (0.58–2.84) 60-day exposure: SSRI: 1.40 (1.04–1.88) Non-SSRI: 1.11 (0.55–2.22) 180-day exposure: SSRI: 1.32 (1.03–1.70) Non-SSRI: 1.04 (0.61–1.75)

Author Year Country Study Design/Data Source Risk of Bias	7. Fetus/infant/child outcomes up to 12 months of age	8. Child outcomes after 12 months of age	9. Maternal Outcomes
Simon 2002[74] US RC-HCDB Low	Exposed vs unexposed: Adjusted difference (95% CI): Estimated gestational age (weeks): TCAs= -0.2 (-0.6 to 0.2); SSRIs= -0.9 (-1.3 to -0.5); SSRIs in 3rd trimester only= -0.7 (-1.3 to -0.1); SSRIs in 1st or 2nd trimesters only= -0.9 (-1.5 to -0.4) Birth weight (g): TCAs= -53 (-167 to 62); SSRIs= -172 (-299 to -46); SSRIs in 3rd trimester only= -148 (-343 to 48); SSRIs in 1st or 2nd trimesters only= -169 (-336 to -2) Head circumference (cm): TCAs= 0.0 (-0.5 to 0.4); SSRIs= 0.0 (-1.0 to 1.0) Adjusted OR (95% CI): Estimated gestational age ≤ 36 weeks: TCAs= 1.86 (0.83 to 4.17); SSRIs= 4.38 (1.57 to 12.22) Birth weight <2500 g: TCAs= 1.18 (0.42 to 3.28); SSRIs= 2.73 (0.92 to 8.09) Major malformation: TCAs= 0.82 (0.35 to 1.95); SSRIs=1.36 (0.56 to 3.30) Minor malformation: TCAs= 0.76 (0.37 to 1.58); SSRIs=1.14 (0.56 to 2.31) Genitourinary malformation: TCAs=0.66 (0.23 to 1.88); SSRIs=1.17 (0.39 to 3.56) Cardiac malformation: TCAs= 0.50 (0.05 to 5.53); SSRIs=NA (0 events in unexposed) Skeletal malformation: TCAs= 0.80 (0.21 to 3.0); SSRIs=0.24 (0.05 to 1.15) Vascular malformation: TCAs= 1.34 (0.30 to 6.06); SSRIs=1.15 (0.41 to 3.23) Craniofacial malformation: TCAs=1.26 (0.33 to 4.75); SSRIs=0.59 (0.14 to 2.52) Seizure disorder: TCAs=NA (0 events in unexposed): SSRIs=4.07 (0.45 to 36.73) Motor delay: TCAs=1.00 (0.14 to 7.17); SSRIs=1.1 3.07 (0.61 to 15.40) Speech delay: TCAs=1.00 (0.14 to 7.17); SSRIs=1.00 (0.14 to 7.18) Other motor abnormality: TCAs=0.49 (0.09 to 2.73); SSRIs=0.50 (0.09 to 2.73)	NR	NR

Author Year Country Study Design/Data Source Risk of Bias	7. Fetus/infant/child outcomes up to 12 months of age	8. Child outcomes after 12 months of age	9. Maternal Outcomes
Sit 2011[75] US PC Medium	OR for Preterm Birth by Maximum depression level: OR, 1.0; 95%CI, 0.8 to 1.2 ORs for Infant Peripartum Events identified on Peripartum Events Scale by Maximum depression level: > 1 peripartum event: OR, 1.0; 95% CI, 0.8 to 1.2 ≥1 peripartum event: OR, 1.0; 95%CI, 0.9 to 1.2	NR	NR
Smith 2013[76] US PC High	Specific to infant outcomes, birth weight, length, head circumference, neonatal intensive care admission, and 1 minute APGAR scores did not significantly differ between the exposed and unexposed infants Gestational age, weeks (se) 39.00 (0.97) vs. 38.00 (0.89), p=0.02 Weight, g (se) 3357.80 (426.76) vs. 3004.00 (569.10) p=0.06 Length, cm (se) 50.91 (2.61) vs. 49.75 (1.50) p=0.39 Head circumference, cm (se) 33.83 (1.67) vs. 33.40 (2.19) p=0.60 Apgar 1 min 8.49 (0.92) vs. 8.33 (1.21) p=0.70 5 min 8.97 (0.26) vs. 8.50 (1.22) p=0.01 NICU 4 (6.56%) vs. 1 (16.67%) p=0.38 There were no statistically significant differences in sleep patterns recorded by the Actiwatch between infants with more than one month of SRI exposure in the third trimester and control infants with no SRI exposure in pregnancy After adjusting for gestational age, tremulousness episodes per minute (0.009) vs.(0.003) (p=0.05).	NR	NR

Author Year Country Study Design/Data Source Risk of Bias	7. Fetus/infant/child outcomes up to 12 months of age	8. Child outcomes after 12 months of age	9. Maternal Outcomes
Stephansson 2013[77] Sweden PBR Medium	Exposure to SSRIs from 3 months before pregnancy until birth, adjusted OR (95% CI) Stillbirth: 1.17 (0.96, 1.41); P=0.12 Stillbirth, no previous psychiatric hospitalization: 1.07 (0.84, 1.36); P=0.59 Stillbirth, previous psychiatric hospitalization: 0.92 (0.66, 1.28); P=0.62 Neonatal death: 1.23 (0.96, 1.57); P=0.11 Neonatal death, no previous psychiatric hospitalization: 1.14 (0.84, 1.56); P=0.39 Neonatal death, previous psychiatric hospitalization: 0.89 (0.58, 1.39); P=0.62 Postneonatal death (28-364 days): 1.34(0.97, 1.86); P=0.08 Postneonatal death, no previous psychiatric hospitalization: 1.10 (0.71, 1.72); P=0.66 Postneonatal death, previous psychiatric hospitalization: 1.02 (0.61, 1.69); P=0.95 Exposure to SSRIs per trimester, adjusted OR (95% CI) Stillbirth/Neonatal death/Postneonatal death Unexposed: 1.0 (reference) T0: 1.19 (0.87, 1.65); P=0.28/1.04 (0.66, 1.64); P=0.86/1.28 (0.72, 2.26); P=0.40 T0-T1: 1.56 (1.06, 2.30); P=0.03/1.16 (0.61, 2.21); P=0.65/1.02 (0.42, 2.46); P=0.96 T0-T2: 1.11 (0.50, 2.48); P=0.80/1.135 (0.51, 3.62); P=0.55/2.06 (0.66, 6.39); P=0.821 T0-T3: 0.94 (0.53, 1.65); P=0.83/1.56 (0.86, 2.83); P=0.14/1.76 (0.79, 3.93); P=0.17 Other: 1.01 (0.70, 1.46); P=0.94/1.31 (0.85, 2.02); P=0.22/1.31 (0.72, 2.37); P=0.38	NR	NR

Author Year Country Study Design/Data Source Risk of Bias	7. Fetus/infant/child outcomes up to 12 months of age	8. Child outcomes after 12 months of age	9. Maternal Outcomes
Suri 2007[78] US PC Medium	Birth Outcome Means (unless otherwise specified) by antidepressant use, MDD, with antidepressants vs. MDD, no antidepressants vs. No psychiatric history, no antidepressants: GA, weeks: 38.5 vs. 39.4 vs. 39.7; F=6.0, p=0.004 Birth weight, kg: 3.28 vs. 3.39 vs. 3.36; F=0.47, p=0.63 Apgar, 1 minute: 7.7 vs. 8.2 vs. 8.0; F=1.2, p=0.32 Apgar, 5 minute: 8.8 vs. 9.0 vs. 8.9; F=1.7, p=0.02 Preterm birth: 14.3% vs. 0% vs. 5.3%: χ2=6.0, p=0.05 Special care nursery: 21% vs. 9% vs. 0%; χ2=1.8, p=0.40 Birth Outcome Means (unless otherwise specified) by Antidepressant Dose, High vs. Low-Medium vs. None: GA, weeks: 38.2 vs. 33.8 vs. 39.5; F=3.1, p=0.05 Birth weight, kg: 3.29 vs. 3.30 vs. 3.38; F=0.17, p=0.85 Apgar, 1 minute: 7.3 vs. 8.0 vs. 8.1; F=1.9, p=0.16 Apgar, 5 minute: 8.7 vs. 8.9 vs. 8.9; F==0.82, p=0.44 Preterm birth: 20% vs. 9% vs. 0%; χ2=4.3, p=0.12 Special care nursery: 26.7% vs. 17.1% vs. 7.1%; χ2=2.1, p=0.36	NR	NR

Author Year Country Study Design/Data Source Risk of Bias	7. Fetus/infant/child outcomes up to 12 months of age	8. Child outcomes after 12 months of age	9. Maternal Outcomes
Suri 2011[79] US PC Medium	Delivery Outcomes, MDD with antidepressants vs. MDD no antidepressants vs. No MDD GA, M weeks: 38.1 vs. 39.2 vs. 39.1; F=5.33, p<0.01 Preterm birth <37 weeks: 12% vs. 0% vs. 7%; F=3.34, p=0.19 Birth weight, kg: 3.3 vs. 3.4 vs. 3.3; F=0.46, p=0.63 Apgar, 1 minute, M: 7.8 vs. 8.2 vs. 8.0; F=0.75, p=0.48 Apgar, 5 minute, M: 8.8 vs. 8.9 vs. 9.0; F=1.83, p=0.17 Special care nursery, 18% vs. 12% vs. 0%; χ^2=4.88, p=0.09 Brazelton Neonatal Behavioral Assessment Scale, Mean scores, MDD with antidepressants vs. MDD no antidepressants vs. No MDD 1 Week of Age: Habituation: 5.90 vs. 7.1 vs. 6.06; F=0.58, p=0.56 Orientation: 4.68 vs. 4.84 vs. 5.01; F= 0.12, p=0.88 Motor: 5.15 vs. 5.31 vs. 5.03; F=0.51, p=0.61 Regulation of state: 5.39 vs. 5.67 vs. 4.61; F=2.12, p=0.13 Range of state: 3.29 vs. 3.68 vs. 3.47; F=0.79, p=0.46 Rapidity of buildup: 2.33 vs. 3.75 vs. 3.18; F=3.28, p=0.05, but NSD after Bonferroni correction Autonomic stability: 7.06 vs. 6.76 vs. 7.41; F=1.29, p=0.28 Reflexes: 2.32 vs. 1.86 vs. 1.86; F=0.70; p=0.50 6-8 Weeks of Age: Habituation: 6.04 vs. 4.50 vs. 8.75; F=2.16, p=0.16 Orientation: 6.17 vs. 6.87 vs. 6.84; F=1.17, p=0.32 Inanimate auditory: 4.93 vs. 6.10 vs. 6.64; F=4.35, p=0.02, but NSD after Bonferroni correction Motor: 5.89 vs. 6.20 vs. 5.94; F=0.97, p=0.39 Defense: 7.19 vs. 7.00 vs. 6.31; F=3.39, p=0.04, but NSD after Bonferroni correction Range of state: 3.14 vs. 3.25 vs. 3.42; F=0.38, p=0.68 Autonomic stability: 7.48 vs. 7.67 vs. 7.61; F=0.31, p=0.74 Reflexes: 3.13 vs. 2.46 vs. 1.92; F=1.65, p=0.20	NR	NR

Author Year Country Study Design/Data Source Risk of Bias	7. Fetus/infant/child outcomes up to 12 months of age	8. Child outcomes after 12 months of age	9. Maternal Outcomes
Ter Horst 2013[80] The Netherlands PD Medium	**Exposed to SSRIs** - incidence risk (IR) and incidence risk ration (IRR) (95% CI)) Anytime: IR = 0.61; IRR=1.20 (0.97– 1.49); IRR (adj)=1.17 (1.16– 1.18) Only 1st trimester: IR= 0.53; IRR=1.04 (0.73– 1.49); IRR (adj)=1.03 (0.98– 1.09) Only 2nd and 3rd trimester: IR= 0.64; IRR=1.26 (0.41– 3.91) At least 1st trimester: IR=0.61; IRR=1.20 (0.96– 1.51) IRR (adj)=1.18 (1.17–1.2) At least 2nd and 3rd trimester: IR=0.66; IRR=1.30 (0.95– 1.78) **Exposed to TCAs** Anytime: IR=0.56 IRR=1.10 (0.63– 1.94); IRR (adj)=1.07 (0.96– 1.19) Only 1st trimester: IR=0.59 IRR=1.16 (0.58– 2.32) Only 2nd and 3rd trimester - NA At least 1st trimester: IR=0.53; IRR =1.04 (0.58– 1.88) At least 2nd and 3rd trimester: IR=0.4; IRR=0.79 (0.25– 2.44) **Risk after exposure to possible confounders** In utero exposure to antibiotics: IR=1.08; IRR =1.08 (1.02–1.14) in utero exposure to benzodiazepines : IR=0.92; IRR =0.92 (0.81–1.05) Children with a mother aged > 30 at delivery: IR=1.04; IRR =1.04 (1.00–1.09) In utero exposure to insulin: IR=1.43; IRR =1.43 (1.08–1.89) In utero exposure to drugs for pulmonary disease: IR=1.1; IRR =1.10 (1.00–1.21)	NR	NR

Author Year Country Study Design/Data Source Risk of Bias	7. Fetus/infant/child outcomes up to 12 months of age	8. Child outcomes after 12 months of age	9. Maternal Outcomes
Toh 2009[81] US CC Medium	NR	NR	Any gestational hypertension, Adjusted RR (95% CI) No SSRI exposure: Reference SSRI exposure: 1.90 (1.35, 2.67) Discontinued SSRI exposure: 1.33 (0.78, 2.27) Continued SSRI exposure: 2.49 (1.62, 3.83) Gestational hypertension with preeclampsia, Adjusted RR (95% CI) SSRI exposure: 3.16 (1.89, 5.29) Discontinued SSRI exposure: 1.37 (0.50, 3.76) Continued SSRI exposure: 4.86 (2.70, 8.76) Gestational hypertension without preeclampsia, Adjusted RR (95% CI) SSRI exposure: 1.36 (0.85, 2.15) Discontinued SSRI exposure: 1.30 (0.69, 2.46) Continued SSRI exposure: 1.41 (0.74, 2.69)

Author Year Country Study Design/Data Source Risk of Bias	7. Fetus/infant/child outcomes up to 12 months of age	8. Child outcomes after 12 months of age	9. Maternal Outcomes
Ververs 2009[82] The Netherlands AD Medium	RRs, Healthcare utilization, vs. non-users >First 2 Weeks of Life GP visits, ≥1 Continuous: RR, 0.9; 95%CI, 0.5 to 1.6 Irregular: RR, 0.9; 95%CI, 0.7 to 1.4 Stoppers: RR, 1.3 ; 95%CI, 0.9 to 1.6 >Specialist visits, 1 Continuous: RR,1.3; 95%CI, 1.1 to 1.5 Irregular: RR, 1.2; 95%CI, 1.0 to 1.3 Stoppers: RR, 0.9 ; 95%CI, 0.8 to 1.1 >Specialist visits, ≥2 Continuous: RR, 2.4; 95%CI, 1.7 to 3.3 Irregular: RR, 0.8; 95%CI, 0.6 to 1.2 Stoppers: RR, 1.1; 95%CI, 0.8 to 1.4 >Specialist procedures, 1 Continuous: RR, 1.5; 95%CI, 1.2 to 1.8 Irregular: RR, 1.1; 95%CI, 1.0 to 1.3 Stoppers: RR, 0.9; 95%CI, 0.8 to 1.1 >Specialist procedures, ≥2 Continuous: RR, 1.7; 95%CI, 1.1 to 2.6 Irregular: RR, 1.2; 95%CI, 0.9 to 1.6 Stoppers: RR, 0.8 ; 95%CI, 0.5 to 1.1 >Diagnostic tests, 1 Continuous: RR, 1.1; 95%CI, 0.8 to 1.6 Irregular: RR, 1.1; 95%CI, 0.9 to 1.3 Stoppers: RR, 1.1; 95%CI, 0.9 to 1.3	NR	NR

Author Year Country Study Design/Data Source Risk of Bias	7. Fetus/infant/child outcomes up to 12 months of age	8. Child outcomes after 12 months of age	9. Maternal Outcomes
Ververs 2009[82] The Netherlands AD Medium ……..(Cont)	>Diagnostic tests, ≥2 Continuous: RR, 1.9; 95%CI, 1.4 to 2.5 Irregular: RR, 1.5; 95%CI, 1.2 to 1.9 Stoppers: RR, 0.9; 95%CI, 0.7 to 1.1 >Hospital admissions, 1 Continuous: RR,1.5; 95%CI,1.3 to 1.8 Irregular: RR, 1.2; 95%CI, 1.0 to 1.3 Stoppers: RR,1; 95%CI, 0.9 to 1.1 >Hospital admissions, ≥2 Continuous: RR,2.4; 95%CI, 1.8 to 3.1 Irregular: RR,1.4; 95%CI, 1.1 to 1.8 Stoppers: RR,0.8; 95%CI, 0.6 to 0.9 Drug prescriptions, ≥1 Continuous: RR, 0.5; 95%CI, 0.3 to 0.8 Irregular: RR, 0.9; 95%CI, 0.8 to 1.1 Stoppers: RR, 1; 95%CI, 0.9 to 1.2 First year of Life GP visits, 1 Continuous: RR, 1.0; 95%CI, 0.8 to 1.4 Irregular: RR, 1.0; 95%CI, 0.9 to 1.2 Stopper: RR, 1.1; 95%CI, 0.9 to 1.2 GP visits, ≥2 Continuous: RR, 1.5; 95%CI, 1.3 to 1.8 Irregular: RR, 1.2; 95%CI, 1.1 to 1.4 Stopper: RR, 1.3; 95%CI, 1.2 to 1.5		

Author Year Country Study Design/Data Source Risk of Bias	7. Fetus/infant/child outcomes up to 12 months of age	8. Child outcomes after 12 months of age	9. Maternal Outcomes
Ververs 2009[82] The Netherlands AD Medium ………(Cont)	Specialist visits, 1 Continuous: RR, 1.4; 95% CI, 1.1 to 1.8 Irregular: RR, 1.1; 95%CI, 0.9 to 1.3 Stopper: RR, 1.0; 95%CI, 0.9 to 1.2 Specialist visits, ≥2 Continuous: RR, 1.5; 95%CI, 1.2 to 1.9 Irregular: RR, 1.4; 95%CI, 1.2 to 1.6 Stopper: RR, 1.2; 95%CI, 1.1 to 1.4 Specialist procedures, 1 Continuous: RR, 1.6; 95%CI, 1.3 to 2.0 Irregular: RR, 1.1; 95%CI, 0.9 to 1.2 Stopper: RR, 1.1; 95%CI, 0.9 to 1.3 Specialist procedures, ≥2 Continuous: RR, 1.3; 95%CI, 0.9 to 1.7 Irregular: RR, 1.3; 95%CI, 1.1 to 1.5 Stopper: RR, 1.1; 95%CI, 0.9 to 1.3 Diagnostic tests, 1 to 2 Continuous: RR, 1.2; 95% CI, 0.9 to 1.6 Irregular: RR, 1.2; 95%CI, 0.9 to 1.4 Stopper: RR, 1.2; 95%CI, 0.9 to 1.4 Diagnostic tests, ≥3 Continuous: RR, 1.2; 95%CI, 0.8 to 1.6 Irregular: RR, 1.1; 95%CI, 0.9 to 1.4 Stopper: RR, 1.1; 95%CI, 0.9 to 1.3 Hospital admissions, 1 Continuous: RR, 2.2; 95%CI, 1.5 to 3.1 Irregular: RR, 1.1; 95%CI, 0.8 to 1.5		
Wilson 2011[83] US CC Medium	PPHN, Adjusted OR (95% CI) Use of SSRI after 20 weeks: 0 (0, 3.0)	NR	NR

Author Year Country Study Design/Data Source Risk of Bias	7. Fetus/infant/child outcomes up to 12 months of age	8. Child outcomes after 12 months of age	9. Maternal Outcomes
Wisner 2009[84] US Prospective cohort Medium	Minor' physical anomalies: Data available for 203 (85%) of infants. Neither first-trimester nor continuous exposure to SSRIs or depression was associated with a significant increase in the number of minor anomalies or theproportion of infants with three or more anomalies. No major malformations were observed. Infant birth weight: Adjusted P = 0.12 across groups; Proportion of infants birthweights < 10th or above 90th percentile (NSD across exp groups) (P not given), head circumference or birth length (NSD across exp groups) (P not given) Mean Infant Birthweight (N) mean kg, SD No SSRI, no depression (N = 130) 3.53, 0.5 Continuous SSRI exposure (N = 47) 3.36, 0.7 Continuous depression, no SSRI (N = 14) 3.22, 0.6 Partial SSRI exposure (N = 22) 3.39, 0.4 Partial depression, no SSRI (N = 22) 3.37, 0.6 Gestational Age: χ^2 = 14.06, df = 8, p=0.08 across groups Preterm Birth: χ^2 = 13.63, df = 4, p=0.009. across groups Adjusted Rate Ratios Continuous SSRI exposure (N=48) 5.43 1.98–14.84 Continuous depression, no SSRI (N=14) 3.71 0.98–14.13 Partial SSRI exposure (N=23) 0.86 0.11–6.92 Partial depression, no SSRI (N=22) 1.04 0.22–5.01 NICU admissions p=0.88 across groups Score >= 2 on Infant Subscale of Peripartum Events Scale: p=0.39 across groups; Post hoc Fisher's exact test indicated that the group with continuous SSRI exposure and the group with continuous depression and no SSRI exposure did not differ from each other and that both differed from the group with neither exposure.	NR	Weight gain: Adjusted P = 0.41 across groups Mean Weight gain (N), pounds, SD No SSRI, no depression (N = 82) 31.6, 13.0 Continuous SSRI exposure (N = 23) 28.6, 13.8 Continuous depression, no SSRI (N = 3) 17.7, 15.5 Partial SSRI exposure (N = 16) 31.4, 12.0 Partial depression, no SSRI (N = 18) 24.8, 16.2

Author Year Country Study Design/Data Source Risk of Bias	7. Fetus/infant/child outcomes up to 12 months of age	8. Child outcomes after 12 months of age	9. Maternal Outcomes
Wisner 2013[85] (Wisner 2009/Okun 2012) US PC Medium	All (N=178) vs. No exposure (N=100) vs. SSRI (N=47) vs. Depressed (N=31) Birth weight (g) (Mean (SD) 3,470 (577) vs. 3,563 (531) vs. 3,343 (626) vs. 3,366 (605) p= 0.052 (overall) Birth length (cm) (Mean (SD)) 51.1 (2.8) vs. 51.5 (2.7) vs. 50.2 (3.0) vs. 51.1 (2.7) p= 0.04 (overall) Birth head circumference (cm) (Mean (SD)) 34.6 (1.7) vs. 34.7 (1.7) vs. 34.3 (1.8) vs. 34.6 (1.6) p=0.36 (overall) <37 weeks gestation at delivery N(%) 17 (9.6) vs. 5 (5.0) vs. 9 (19.1) vs. 3 (9.7) vs p= 0.03 (overall) Sex N(%) Gender - Male 99 (55.6) vs. 64 (64.0) vs. 17 (36.2) vs. 18 (58.1) Gender - Female 79 (44.4) vs. 36 (36.0) vs. 30 (63.8) vs. 13 (41.9) p= 0.006 (for sex overall) Ever breast-fed N(%) 138 (77.5) vs. 83 (83.0) vs 35 (74.5) vs 20 (64.5) p= 0.09 (overall)	NR	NR
Wogelius 2006[86] Denmark PBR Medium	Congenital malformations, Adjusted OR (95% CI) Women who redeemed a prescription for an SSRI during 2nd and 3rd trimester All births: 1.34 (1.00, 1.79) >=37 weeks gestation: 1.23 (0.88, 1.72) <37 weeks gestation: 1.63 (0.85, 3.15) Women who redeemed a prescription for an SSRI during 1st trimester or 30 days before All births: 1.84 (1.25, 2.71) >=37 weeks gestation: 1.75 (1.14, 2.70) <37 weeks gestation: 1.77 (0.73, 4.32)	NR	NR

Author Year Country Study Design/Data Source Risk of Bias	7. Fetus/infant/child outcomes up to 12 months of age	8. Child outcomes after 12 months of age	9. Maternal Outcomes
Yonkers 2012[87] US Prospective Cohort [PC] Low	Risk of preterm birth: (term vs. preterm) Additionally Adjusted OR and 95% CI Major depressive episode, exposed 1.51 (0.60-3.8) Major depressive episode, unexposed .86 (0.44-1.7) No major depressive episode, exposed 1.50 (0.94-2.4) No major depressive episode, unexposed reference category Risk of early and late preterm birth: (term vs. preterm) Adjusted OR and 95% CI Early preterm birth N=59 Major depressive episode, exposed NA Major depressive episode, unexposed 0.86 (0.29-2.6) No major depressive episode, exposed 0.93 (0.35-2.4) No major depressive episode, unexposed reference category Late preterm birth N=166 Major depressive episode, exposed 3.14 (1.5-6.8) Major depressive episode, unexposed 1.34 (0.71-2.5) No major depressive episode, exposed 1.93 (1.2-3.2) No major depressive episode, unexposed reference category	NR	NR

| Author
Year
Country
Study Design/Data Source
Risk of Bias	7. Fetus/infant/child outcomes up to 12 months of age	8. Child outcomes after 12 months of age	9. Maternal Outcomes
Zeskind 2004[88]
US
Prospective cohort study/Data Source [PC, AD]
Medium | Gestational age, wk 38.66 (0.35) vs. 39.65 (0.20) P=.019
Birth weight, g 3453.53 (98.87) vs. 3297.35 (88.79) P=.25
Length, cm 51.06 (0.65) vs. 50.81 (0.43) P=.75
Head circumference, cm 33.87 (0.40) vs. 33.53 (0.40) P=.55

Neurobehavioral Outcomes:
Adjusted Mean (SE)
Tremulousness 2.32 (0.20) vs. 1.80 (0.20) P=.038
Behavioral states:
Number different: 2.53 (0.32) vs. 3.71 (0.32) P=.009
Number of changes:7.15 (2.34) vs. 16.56 (2.34) P=.005
Active sleep
Number of epochs: 94.66 (6.64) vs. 83.46 (6.64) P=.13
Number of bouts: 3.36 (0.44) vs. 6.58 (0.44) P=.001
Longest bout: 68.20 (6.37) vs. 49.80 (6.37) P=.03
Number of startles: 14.59 (2.70) vs. 9.85 (2.59) P=.13
Motor activity: 152.05 (21.25) vs. 106.51 (21.96) P=.08
Number of HRV rhythms: 1.98 (0.19) vs. 2.39 (0.19) P= .07 | NR | NR |

AD = administrative database; ADHD = attention deficit hyperactivity disorder; ASD = atrial septal defects; BMI = body mass index; BRS = Behavioral Rating Scale; CC = case control; CES-D = Center for Epidemiologic Studies Depression Scale; CGI-I = Clinical Global Impression scale - Improvement; CGI-S = Clinical Global Impression Scale - Severity; CI = confidence interval; CNS = central nervous system; CV = cardiovascular; DSM-IV = Diagnostic and Statistical Manual of Mental Disorders; Fourth Edition; ECG = electrocardiogram; ETOH = alcohol; FDA = US Food and Drug Administration; GA = gestational age; GI = gastrointestinal; GP = general practitioner; HAM-A = Hamilton Anxiety Rating Scale; HAM-D = Hamilton Depression Rating Scale; IQ = intelligence quotient; IQR = Interquartile range; ITT = intention to treat; LD = linked database; LMP = last menstrual period; MADRS = Montgomery-Asberg Depression Rating Scale; MDD = major depressive disorder; mDDD = multiple defined daily dose; MDI = Mental Development Index; MR = mental retardation; MRI = magnetic resonance imaging; NA = not applicable; NBDPS = National Birth Defects Prevention Study; NICU = neonatal intensive care unit; NR = not reported; NSAID = non steroidal anti inflammatory drug; NSD = no significant difference; OCD = obsessive compulsive disorder; OR = odds ratio; PBD = population-based database; PBR = population-based registry; PC = prospective cohort; PDD = pervasive developmental disorder; PDI = Psychomotor Development Index; PPHN = persistent pulmonary hypertension; PTSD = post-traumatic stress disorder; RR = relative risk; RRR = relative risk reduction; SCN = special care nursery; SD = standard deviation; SEIFA = Socio-Economic Indexes for Areas; SES = socio-economic status; SNRI = serotonin norepinephrine reuptake inhibitor; SRI = serotonin reuptake inhibitor; SSRI = selective serotonin reuptake inhibitor; TCA = tricyclic antidepressant; TUS = Teratogen Information Service; UK = United Kingdom; US = United States; VSD = ventricular septal defects

Evidence Table 2. Risk of bias assessment observational studies

Author Year Country	1. Unbiased patient selection?	2. Adequate exposure ascertainment?	3. Reasonable followup duration?	4. Acceptable levels of differential or overall high loss to followup?	5. Events adequately specified and defined?
Alwan 2007[1] US	Unclear; although patients with pre-gestational diabetes were not pre-specified to be excluded, they were ultimately excluded from the analyses (2.2% cases and 0.5 controls; $P<0.001$)	No, self-report 6 weeks to 2 years after delivery, without validation and no ultrasound to confirm gestational age	Yes	Yes; Yes	Yes
Alwan 2010[2] US	Unclear; consent rates NR; also, although patients with pre-gestational diabetes were not pre-specified to be excluded, they were ultimately excluded from the analyses (2.7% cases and 0.6% controls; $P<0.001$)	No, self-report 6 weeks to 2 years after delivery, without validation and method for confirming gestational age is NR	Yes	Yes, Yes	Yes
Andrade 2009[89] US	Yes	Unclear; pharmacy database; length of gestation not available, trimester of exposure based on estimates of gestational age	Yes	Yes	Yes
Bakker 2010[4] The Netherlands	Unclear; overall consent rate of 80%, but between-groups comparability NR	Unclear; prescription database verified by telephone interview with mother; but methods for confirming gestational age NR	Yes	Yes, Yes	Yes
Bakker 2010[4,5] The Netherlands	Unclear; consent rates NR for controls	Unclear; prescription database verified by telephone interview with mother; but methods for confirming gestational age NR	Yes	Unclear, completeness of data NR for controls	Yes
Ban 2012[6] UK	Yes	Unclear	Yes	Yes	Yes
Batton 2013[7] US	Yes	Yes	Yes	Yes	Yes
Berard 2007[8] Canada	Yes	Unclear; prescription database, no assessment of compliance; gestational age estimated by LMP	Yes	Unclear; completeness of data NR for controls	Yes
Berle 2004[90] Norway	Unclear, process for selecting control group NR	Yes, serum concentrations	Unclear, not specified	Unclear, NR	Yes
Bogen 2010[9] US (companion to Wisner 2009)	Yes	Yes	Yes	No overall=39% Yes differential	Yes

E-118

Author Year Country	1. Unbiased patient selection?	2. Adequate exposure ascertainment?	3. Reasonable followup duration?	4. Acceptable levels of differential or overall high loss to followup?	5. Events adequately specified and defined?
Boucher 2008[10] Canada	Unclear; comparison group from same population-base, but high potential for confounding by indication as comparison is AD exposed or not and depression diagnosis data NR	Unclear; data source is pharmacy database and no methods to overcome uncertainties, few exposure details reported, more concerning in context of narrow exposure window	Unclear, not specified	Yes	Yes
Bracken 1981[91] US	Yes	No; self-report without validation (only contacted prescriber in 10% of instances when further info was required)	Yes	Yes overall=13% No for differential: 24% vs 5.5%	No
Casper 2003[11] US	Unclear; time frame, number screened, consent rates NR	Unclear; self-report with no validation, but some prospective data and dosages reported	Yes	Unclear; participation rate NR	Yes
Chambers 1996[12] US	Unclear	Unclear (self-report, MR corroboration not mentioned)	Yes	Yes	Yes
Chambers 2006[13] US	Yes	Unclear; self-report based on structured telephone interview, no validation reported	Yes	Yes	Yes
Chun-Fai-Chan 2005[92] Canada	No - 1) could be a referral bias of some kind causing women to be recommended bupropion may differ by country or database 2) Comparison group was composed from only one of the three data sources	No - self report of exposure by patient with no confirmation	Yes	Unclear	Yes
Cole 2007[15] US	Yes	Unclear - drug dispensing data only	Yes	Yes	Yes
Cole 2007[14] US (Paroxetine in the first trimester)	Yes	Unclear; prescription database, gestational age estimated by earliest/latest conception	Yes	Unclear; completeness of data not clearly reported, but in Discussion indicates that greater frequency of charts that could not be abstracted in the 'other antidepressant' group	Yes

Author Year Country	1. Unbiased patient selection?	2. Adequate exposure ascertainment?	3. Reasonable followup duration?	4. Acceptable levels of differential or overall high loss to followup?	5. Events adequately specified and defined?
Colvin 2010[93] Australia	Yes	Unclear; first trimester exposure based on LMP	Yes (up to 6 years with definition in citation)	Unclear; missing data for 'general patient' category for 23 medicines with incomplete ascertainment	Yes
Colvin 2011[94] Australia	Unclear - only 80% of the claims data is captured by the PBS database	Unclear - only have drug dispensing data	Yes	Yes	Yes
Colvin 2012[16] Australia	Unclear - only 80% of the claims data is captured by the PBS database	Unclear - only have drug dispensing data	Yes	Yes	Yes
Costei 2002[95] Canada	Unclear; reasons for exclusions NR	No; no verification and no ultrasound.	Yes (presumed though not stated when f/u interview performed)	Unclear; completeness of data NR	No (not defined, parental report)
Croen 2011[17] US	Yes	Yes	Unclear; only 18% of autism diagnosis before age 3 this applies to both cases and controls	Unclear; reasons for exclusion of 122 of original 420 cases NR	Yes
Davidson 2009[18] Israel	Unclear (not stated)	Unclear (self-report only? "during entire pregnancy")	Yes	Yes	Yes
Davis 2007[19] US	Yes	Unclear; pharmacy database; length of gestation not available, trimester of exposure based on estimates of gestational age	Yes	Overall: 30 days=yes (11%), 365 days=no (42%) Differential: 30 days=unclear, 365 days=yes	Unclear; identified use of ICD-9 codes, but did not pre-specify which ones
De Vera 2012[96] Canada	Yes	Yes	Yes	Unclear; completeness of data NR	Yes
De Vries 2013[20] Australia	Yes	Unclear - not clear if they used self-report or medical records	Yes	Yes	Yes
Diav-Citrin 2008[97] Israel	Unclear	Unclear	Yes	Unclear	Yes
Djulus 2006[98] Canada	Unclear	Unclear	Yes	Unclear	Yes

E-120

Author Year Country	1. Unbiased patient selection?	2. Adequate exposure ascertainment?	3. Reasonable followup duration?	4. Acceptable levels of differential or overall high loss to followup?	5. Events adequately specified and defined?
Dubnov-Raz 2012[22] Israel	Unclear (not stated)	Unclear (self-report, "any stage")	Yes	Yes	Yes
Dubnov-Raz, 2012[21] Israel	Unclear (control group selected because of murmur and normal echo)	Unclear (method/dose/duration not stated--presumed self-report at onset of labor)	Yes	Yes	Yes
Einarson 2009[99] Canada	Unclear	Unclear	Yes	Unclear	Yes
Einarson 2009[100] Canada	Unclear (not stated)	No; no verification and no ultrasound.	Unclear (timing of f/u interview unknown)	Unclear; completeness of data NR	No (no method of assigning malformations reported)
Einarson 2010[101] Canada	Unclear (report number followed only)	Unclear (self-report only)	Yes	Unclear (not stated)	Yes
Einarson, 2003[102] Canada	Unclear (only reported # followed)	Unclear (self-report only)	Yes	Unclear (not stated)	Yes
Einarson, 2010[101] Canada	Unclear how group of 1245 exposed women was formed	No (self-report)	Yes	Unclear, completeness of data NR	No; definitions NR
Ericson 1999[103] Sweden	Unclear; population cohort but selection based on drug exposure only	Unclear - not described	Yes	Unclear	Yes
Ferreira 2007[24] Canada	Unclear; population cohort but selection based on drug exposure only	Unclear - not described	Yes	Yes	No
Figueroa 2010[25] US	Yes (data set)	No (prescriptions) prescription database without compliance data and gestation estimated by subtracting 93 days at a time from deliver date	Yes	Unclear	Yes
Galbally 2009[104] Australia	Unclear; very little description	No, appears to be self-report without validation	Yes	Yes	Yes
Galbally 2011[105] Australia (companion to Galbally 2009)	Unclear; very little description	No, appears to be self-report without validation	Yes	No - 25% overall, 30% in unexposed group and 18.5% in exposed group.	Yes - maternal depression and child development scales

E-121

Author Year Country	1. Unbiased patient selection?	2. Adequate exposure ascertainment?	3. Reasonable followup duration?	4. Acceptable levels of differential or overall high loss to followup?	5. Events adequately specified and defined?
Gorman 2012[26] US	Unclear; 2320 possible; 284 included - not clear how selected. Selection of control group unclear.	No - self report.	Yes	Yes	Yes
Grzeskowiak 2012[27] Australia	Unclear; population cohort but selection based on drug exposure only	Yes	Yes	Unclear	Yes
Hale 2010[106] US	Unclear (who, when, why?)	Unclear (self-report via survey)	Yes	Unclear; completeness of data NR	No (subjective, e.g. "low body temp")
Hanley 2013[28] Canada	Yes	Yes	Yes	Yes	Yes
Heikkinen 2002[29] Finland	Unclear (not stated how 11/10 chosen)	Unclear (self-report?)	Yes	Yes	Unclear
Jimenez-Solem 2012[30] Denmark	Yes	Unclear - drug dispensing data only	Yes	Yes	Yes
Jimenez-Solem, 2013, Denmark[31]	Yes	Yes	Yes	Yes	Yes
Jordan 2008[32] US	Yes	Yes	Yes	Yes	Yes
Kallen 2004[33] Sweden	Yes	Unclear; 39% timing not stated	Yes	Yes - see ref #14 for supplemental information	Yes
Kallen 2007[107] Sweden	Unclear; population cohort but selection based on drug exposure only	Unclear - exposure primarily self-report.	Yes	Unclear	Yes
Kallen 2007[34] Sweden	Unclear - we don't know if they were depressed or not	No - self-report	Yes	Yes	Yes
Kieler 2012[36] Sweden	Yes	Yes	Yes	Unclear	Yes
Kleiger-Grossmann 2011[108] Canada	Unclear - could be a referral bias of some kind causing women to be recommended escitalopram, may differ by country or database	No - self report of exposure by patient with no confirmation	Unclear - it is unclear if all major malformations (particularly cardiac) would have been detected at the time of followup	No - loss to followup is not reported	Yes

Author Year Country	1. Unbiased patient selection?	2. Adequate exposure ascertainment?	3. Reasonable followup duration?	4. Acceptable levels of differential or overall high loss to followup?	5. Events adequately specified and defined?
Klinger 2010[109] Israel	Yes	Unclear, self-report without verification	Yes	No (12% with NAS, 55% without)	Yes
Kornum 2010[37] Denmark	Unclear - we don't know if they were depressed or not	Yes	Yes	Yes	Yes
Kulin 1998[110] Canada	Unclear; recruitment time frame not reported, number excluded not reported.	No; self-report without validation, very little detail provided about dose, duration, etc.	Yes	No	No
Laine 2003[38] Finland	Unclear	Unclear - exposed mothers blood was analyzed for drug, but unexposed was not. No other verification methods.	Yes	Yes	Yes
Latendresse, 2011[39] US	Yes	Yes	Unclear	No. 20% excluded after initial enrolment	Yes
Lennestal 2007[40] Sweden	Yes - birth registries	No	Yes (delivery outcomes)	Unclear, completeness of data NR	Yes
Levinson-Castiel 2006[41] Israel	Yes	No, self-report with no verification	Yes	Yes	Yes
Lewis 2010[42] Australia	Yes	No – self-report only	Yes	Yes	Yes
Logsdon 2011[43] US	Yes	Unclear - drug levels taken only on those thought to be taking SSRs - not everyone.	Yes	Unclear - not reported and it looks like it could be as high as about 30%	Yes
Louik 2007[111] US	Unclear – about 40% of the eligible people refused to participate	No - self-report	Unclear	Yes	Yes
Lund 2009[44] Denmark	Yes	Unclear because self-report and no verification	Yes	Unclear	Yes
Malm 2011[45] Finland	Yes	Yes	Yes	Yes	Yes
Manakova 2011[112] Czech Republic	No. Only describes # followed but not the # eligible for the study	Unclear	Unclear	Unclear	No.

E-123

Author Year Country	1. Unbiased patient selection?	2. Adequate exposure ascertainment?	3. Reasonable followup duration?	4. Acceptable levels of differential or overall high loss to followup?	5. Events adequately specified and defined?
Marroun[23] 2012 The Netherlands	Yes	Yes	Yes	Yes	Yes
Maschi 2008[113] Italy	Yes	No, self-report and no validation and unclear about confirmation of gestational age	Yes	Unclear	No.
McElhatton 1996[114] UK	Unclear - unclear that they were including everyone who called	No - self-report	Yes	No – 16-20% loss to follow up	Yes
McFarland 2011[46] US	Yes	No - self-report	Yes	No	Yes
Merlob 2009[47] Israel	Yes	No - self-report	Yes	Yes	Yes
Misri 1991[115] Canada	Unclear; eligibility criteria described, but #'s and reasons for exclusions NR	Unclear, medications managed prospectively, but compliance NR	Yes	Unclear, NR	No
Misri 2006[48] Canada	Unclear: eligibility criteria NR	Unclear, NR	Yes	No (58% attrition in exposed group, 39% in control group)	Yes
Misri 2010[49] Canada	Unclear; eligibility criteria described, but #'s and reasons for exclusions NR	Unclear; methods NR	Yes	Yes overall, 19% loss to followup Unclear differential	Yes
Mulder 2011[50] The Netherlands	Unclear; participation required patient be identified by MD or midwife and comparability of between-groups consent rates NR	Unclear; self-report	Yes	No; overall high and study group higher than comparison group	Yes
Nakhai-Pour 2010[51] Canada	Yes	Yes	Yes	Yes	Yes
Nijenhuis 2012[116] The Netherlands	Yes database	Unclear; date of conception guessed. Exposure "calculated", unclear compliance. Used admin data base	Yes	Yes	Yes
Nordeng 2012[52] Norway	Yes	Unclear	Yes	Yes	Yes

Author Year Country	1. Unbiased patient selection?	2. Adequate exposure ascertainment?	3. Reasonable followup duration?	4. Acceptable levels of differential or overall high loss to followup?	5. Events adequately specified and defined?
Nulman 1997[117] Canada	Unclear; exclusions reported, similar consent rates, but inclusion based on self-report and recruitment time frame end date NR.	No; self-report without validation, very few exposure details reported	Yes	Yes	No for birth defects and perinatal complications, yes for neurobehavioral
Nulman 2002[118] Canada	Unclear; recruitment time frame end date NR, only reported # followed-up	No; self-report without validation, very little detail provided about dose, duration, etc.	Yes	Yes for Reynell, no for Baley (35% missing overall: 18% for fluoxetine group, 39% for TCA group and 505 for comparisons group); no for McCarthy (60% excluded from analysis overall; unclear about differential)	Yes
Nulman 2012[53] Canada	Unclear; although they demonstrated between-group balance in exclusions due to "unable to be located or refused participation", they didn't itemize which groups the 381 who did not meet the inclusion criteria came from	Unclear; self-report	Yes	Yes overall; LTFU higher in TCA group (19% vs 7%)	Yes
Oberlander 2002[54] Canada (2-day), Oberlander 2005[119] (2-month)	Unclear; "consecutive" recruitment, but criteria NR; 63% participation rate overall and between-group comparability in participation rate NR; notes this is part of a larger study, but no citation	Yes	Yes	Yes overall, no differential at 2 days (med=27% vs 12%=controls) and 2 months (17% vs 4%)	Yes
Oberlander 2004[120] Canada	Unclear; exposed cohorts enrolled consecutively, but unclear about controls	Yes, plasma levels	Yes	Yes	Yes
Oberlander 2006[55]	Yes	Unclear; no details about exposure	Yes	Yes	Yes

Author Year Country	1. Unbiased patient selection?	2. Adequate exposure ascertainment?	3. Reasonable followup duration?	4. Acceptable levels of differential or overall high loss to followup?	5. Events adequately specified and defined?
Oberlander 2007[121] (4-year followup to Oberlander 2005) Canada	Unclear (see Oberlander 2002)	Yes (see Oberlander 2002)	Yes	No for differential (SSRI=52%, control=39%); no for overall=48%	Yes
Oberlander 2008[56] Canada	Yes	Unclear - drug dispensing data only	Yes	Yes	Yes
Oberlander 2008[57] Canada	Unclear; inclusion criteria NR	Yes	Yes	Yes overall (14%); unclear for differential	Yes
Oberlander 2010[122] Canada	Unclear, eligibility criteria NR, described as a convenience sample, no time frame	Unclear, methods NR, but doses reported	Yes	Yes overall (23% after 3 years); between-groups NR	Yes
Okun 2011[58] US	Yes	Yes	Yes	Yes at week 20, no at weeks 30 (27%) and 36 (36%)	Yes
Okun 2012[59] US	Yes	Unclear	Yes	Yes	Yes
Palmsten 2012[60] Canada	Yes	Unclear; gestational age estimated as 280 days prior to estimated delivery date	Yes	Unclear; completeness of data NR	Yes
Pastuszak 1993[123] US	Unclear; recruitment time frame NR, only reported # followed up	No; self-report without validation, very few exposure details reported	Yes	Unclear; participation rate NR	No for birth defects, yes for pregnancy outcomes
Pawluski 2009[124] Canada	Unclear; insufficient information	Yes, serum concentrations	Yes	No. 30% missing data (14% in SSRI group vs 50% in non-SSRI group); but no differences between those with and without data	No for neonatal outcomes, yes for neonatal adaptation symptoms and maternal mood
Pearlstein 2006[125] US	Yes	Yes	Unclear; 12 weeks	Overall: No, Differential: No	Unclear

Author Year Country	1. Unbiased patient selection?	2. Adequate exposure ascertainment?	3. Reasonable followup duration?	4. Acceptable levels of differential or overall high loss to followup?	5. Events adequately specified and defined?
Pearson 2007[61] US	Unclear; only reported number enrolled	Unclear; methods NR	Yes	Yes, no LTFU	Yes
Pedersen 2009[62] Denmark	Yes	Unclear because database with no compliance data	Yes	Yes: overall, differential: unclear	Yes
Pedersen 2010[63] Denmark	Unclear; comparability of between-groups consent rates NR	Unclear; self-report, no verification	Yes	No for overall: 76% to 79% at 6m and 54% to 62% at 19m; Yes for differential	Yes
Pedersen 2013[64] (companion to Pendersen, 2010) Denmark	Unclear; comparability of between-groups consent rates NR	Yes	Yes	No for overall; Yes for differential	Yes
Polen 2013[65] US	No - The case group includes still births and elective terminations and the control group includes only live born infants	Unclear; self-report, no verification; method of gestational age ascertainment NR and that assessment of venlafaxine use differed for birth's between 1997-2005 and after 2005	Yes	Yes	Yes
Rai 2013[66] Sweden	Yes	Unclear - relies on self-report	Yes	Yes	Yes
Ramos 2008[126] Canada	Yes	Unclear; pharmacy data; gestational estimated by LMP date, but confirmed between two databases	Yes	Yes for differential; unclear for overall because nonresponders were less likely to be welfare recipients than responders	Yes
Ramos 2010[68] Canada	Yes	Unclear; pharmacy data; gestational estimated by LMP date, but confirmed between two databases	Yes	Yes	Yes
Rampono 2004[127] Australia	Unclear; only reported number enrolled	No; timing is an issue they were taking in 3rd trimester but could have been taking entire pregnancy	Yes	Yes	Yes

E-127

Author Year Country	1. Unbiased patient selection?	2. Adequate exposure ascertainment?	3. Reasonable followup duration?	4. Acceptable levels of differential or overall high loss to followup?	5. Events adequately specified and defined?
Reebye 2002[70] British Columbia	Unclear; exposed groups recruited during pregnancy and controls after delivery; unclear how decided who to approach	Unclear; not described, but prospective and dosages reported	Yes	No overall (24%); no differential (17% vs 33%)	Yes
Reis 2010[71] Sweden	Yes	Unclear	Yes	Yes	Yes
Rompono 2009 Australia	Unclear; only reported number enrolled	Yes; serum concentrations	Yes	No for overall (25%); unclear for differential	Yes
Salisbury 2011[72] US	Yes, eligibility criteria described and flow of patient selection described	Yes (TLFB Interview)	Yes - Delivery outcomes, NB assessments	Ratings are No for overall and unclear for differential	Yes
Salkeld 2008[73] Canada	Yes	Yes	Yes	Yes	Yes
Simon 2002[74] US	Yes	Yes	Yes	Yes	Yes
Sit 2011[75] US	Yes	Yes	Yes	No overall (only included 21 of original 48 from 'continuous SSRI exposure group, 44%); unclear differential	Yes
Sivojlezova 2005[128] Canada	Unclear	Unclear	Yes	Unclear	Yes
Smith 2013[76] US	Unclear - they "approached" only some of the women but it is not clear how they chose who to approach and there is a difference in age between those approached and not suggesting a possible selection bias; only 150 of 277 eligible women were approached	Yes	Yes	Yes	Yes
Stephansson 2013[77] Sweden	Yes	Unclear	Yes	Yes	Yes
Suri 2004[129] US	Unclear	Unclear	Yes	Yes	Yes

Author Year Country	1. Unbiased patient selection?	2. Adequate exposure ascertainment?	3. Reasonable followup duration?	4. Acceptable levels of differential or overall high loss to followup?	5. Events adequately specified and defined?
Suri 2007[78] US	Unclear; numbers and reasons for exclusions NR	Yes	Yes	No overall, 36% excluded from analysis; unclear about differential, NR	Yes
Suri 2011[79] US	Unclear; Higher participation rate in controls (79%) vs Group 1 (67%)	Yes	Yes	Yes	Yes
Ter Horst 2013[80] The Netherlands	Yes	Yes	Yes	Yes	Yes
Toh 2009[130] US/Canada	No (live-born, malformed excluded; since primary outcome GA, pre-term and weight, this may influence)	No (self-report, some attempt to verify with bottle, unclear what percent had GA by US)	Yes	Yes (95% overall, losses not described)	Yes
Toh 2009[81] US/Canada	Yes	No (self-report, some attempt to clarify with bottle, LMP and US as self-report)	Yes	Yes	No (high BP not defined)
Ververs 2009[82] The Netherlands	Yes	Unclear (pharmacy dispensing of "at least one" Rx)	Yes	Yes	Yes
Wen 2006[131] Canada	Yes	Yes	Yes	Unclear, completeness of data NR	Yes
Wichman 2009[132] US	Unclear (no info on diagnosis/severity)	Yes	Unclear (similar between groups, but just followed until discharge from birth hospitalization)	Yes	Yes
Wilson 2011[83] US	Unclear (not stated how identified in EMR, controls matched for GA only)	Yes	Yes	Yes	Yes
Wisner 2009[84]/Okun 2012[59] US	Yes	Yes, maternal serum levels	Yes	No overall, 27% missing data (54% delivery data, 46% missing congenital anomaly assessments); unclear differential as between-groups missing data NR	Yes

Author Year Country	1. Unbiased patient selection?	2. Adequate exposure ascertainment?	3. Reasonable followup duration?	4. Acceptable levels of differential or overall high loss to followup?	5. Events adequately specified and defined?
Wisner 2013[85] US (Wisner 2009/Okun 2012)	Yes	Unclear, serum samples not taken in unexposed group to confirm they weren't taking drugs	Yes	No, differential; No, overall	Yes
Wogelius 2006[86] Danish	Yes	Yes	Yes	Yes	Unclear (ICD-9 codes without verification)
Yonkers 2012[87] US	Yes	Unclear (self-report)	Yes	Yes	Yes
Zeskind 2004[88] US	Unclear (how cases and controls were chosen)	Yes	Yes	Yes	Unclear (exact age at which behavioral state monitored not given, just range of all; this is important as infants have very distinct behavior in first hours of life)

E-130

Author Year Country	6. Unbiased and accurate event ascertainment?	7. Free of selective outcome reporting?	8. Adequate handling of potential confounding variables?	Overall Risk of Bias Rating
Alwan 2007[1] US	Yes	Yes	Yes	Medium
Alwan 2010[2] US	Yes	Yes	Yes	Medium
Andrade 2009[89] US	Unclear; verification of hospital claims with medical charts was only possible in 72% overall; 71% among unexposed and 72% among	Yes	No; matched on age, but data on race, other exposures, meconium aspiration, and NSAID exposure NR; higher rates of diabetes and asthma in exposed group, no control for confounders	Medium
Bakker 2010[4] The Netherlands	Yes	Yes	Yes	Medium
Bakker 2010[5] The Netherlands	Unclear; ICD-9 or 10 codes, but no information about any verification	Yes	Yes	Medium
Ban 2012[6] UK	Unclear; use of electronic medical record but no validation	Yes	Yes	Medium
Batton 2013[7] US	Unclear - no mention of blinding.	Yes	Yes	Medium
Berard 2007[8] Canada	Unclear; ICD-9 codes, no verification	Yes	Yes	Medium
Berle 2004[90] Norway	Unclear; mothers rated infants using an invalidated symptom score form	Yes	Unclear; stated that groups did not differ with respect to demographic data, but data not shown and no adjustments	High
Bogen 2010[9] US (companion to Wisner 2009)	Yes	Yes	Yes	Medium
Boucher 2008[10] Canada	Unclear; blinding, assessor characteristics, accuracy of data collection NR	Yes	Yes	Medium
Bracken 1981[91] US	Yes	Yes	No, unable to adjust for covariates because of small numbers	High
Casper 2003[11] US	Yes	Yes	Unclear; no adjustment for more miscarriages in unmedicated group (54% vs 29%), but matched on numerous other variables	Medium
Chambers 1996[12] US	Unclear (blinding not stated for all outcomes)	Yes	Yes	Medium

E-131

Author Year Country	6. Unbiased and accurate event ascertainment?	7. Free of selective outcome reporting?	8. Adequate handling of potential confounding variables?	Overall Risk of Bias Rating
Chambers 2006[13] US	Unclear; blinded neonatologist, but pulmonary hypertension documented either by oxygen saturation or echocardiographic evidence and unclear how balanced the methods were between groups	Yes	Yes	Medium
Chun-Fai-Chan 2005[92] Canada	Unclear - assessors were not blinded to group allocation	Yes	Unclear	High
Cole 2007[15] US	Yes	Yes	Unclear - not all confounders were accounted for	Low
Cole 2007[14] US (Paroxetine in the first trimester)	Yes	Yes	Yes	Medium
Colvin 2010[93] Australia	Unclear (no blinding)	Yes	No (women with Rx may be different)	High
Colvin 2011[94] Australia	Unclear - included only live born infants	Yes	Yes	Medium
Colvin 2012[16] Australia	Unclear - included only live born infants	Yes	Yes	Medium
Costei 2002[95] Canada	No (self-report, no mention of corroboration, no blinding)		Yes (increased smokers in exposure group, but modeling accounted for this)	High
Croen 2011[17] US	Yes	Yes	Yes	Medium
Davidson 2009[18] Israel	Unclear (no blinding, SSRI group gets put in incubator; delays in discharge related to this?)	Yes	No (matched for GA only, no controlling)	Medium
Davis 2007[19] US	Yes for limb and eye anomalies and spina bifida for which ICD-9 codes were verified by chart review; unclear for others	Yes	Unclear; collected data on age but baseline comparability NR; race and other exposures data not available; parity not mentioned; control for confounders NR	Medium
De Vera 2012[96] Canada	Yes (although no blinding, tightly defined objective variable with cited validation; no increased visits to increase detection)	Yes	Yes	Low
De Vries 2013[20] Australia	Yes	Yes	Yes	Medium
Diav-Citrin 2008[97] Israel	Unclear	Yes	Yes	High

Author Year Country	6. Unbiased and accurate event ascertainment?	7. Free of selective outcome reporting?	8. Adequate handling of potential confounding variables?	Overall Risk of Bias Rating
Djulus 2006[98] Canada	Unclear	Yes	Yes	High
Dubnov-Raz 2012[22] Israel	Unclear (blinding?)	Yes	Yes	Medium
Dubnov-Raz, 2012[21] Israel	Yes for ECG outcomes, but other outcomes = unclear	Yes	No (matched for GA only, control group had audible murmur)	Medium
Einarson 2009[99] Canada	Unclear	Yes	Yes	High
Einarson 2009[100] Canada	Unclear; no blinding and based on maternal report. Attempts made to corroborate with treating physician, but no information about corroboration rate	Unclear; individual anomalies NR for the control group NR	Unclear (matched for age, tob, EtOH, but simple stats)	High
Einarson 2010[101] Canada	Unclear (asked MD, but it's not clear how many women gave permission or how many MDs responded)	Yes	Unclear (matched for maternal age, smoking, EtOH only); no group with depression; lack of knowing if ascertainment of the factors matched on was good (self-report)	High
Einarson, 2003[102] Canada	Unclear (assume self-report, no mention of blinding)	Yes	Unclear (matched, but does not appear to be adjusted for increased smokers in one group)	High
Einarson, 2010[101] Canada	Unclear; blinding NR, details of corroboration NR	Yes	Matched for age, smoking, alcohol use, timing of call, but results of matching NR and information based on self-report without verification	High
Ericson 1999[103] Sweden	Unclear	Yes	no	High
Ferreira 2007[24] Canada	Yes	Yes	Yes	Medium
Figueroa 2010[25] US	Unclear; no validation study of accuracy	Yes	Yes	Med
Galbally 2009[104] Australia	birth outcomes - no; depression - yes; withdrawal symptoms - yes	Yes	Unclear	High

E-133

Author Year Country	6. Unbiased and accurate event ascertainment?	7. Free of selective outcome reporting?	8. Adequate handling of potential confounding variables?	Overall Risk of Bias Rating
Galbally 2011[105] Australia (companion to Galbally 2009)	birth outcomes - no; depression and child development - yes	Yes	Unclear - control group matched but not stated for what characteristics	High
Gorman 2012[26] US	birth outcomes - no (self-report with unclear number confirmed by medical chart); breastfeeding outcomes - yes	Yes	Yes	Medium
Grzeskowiak 2012[27] Australia	Yes	Yes	Yes	Medium
Hale 2010[106] US	No (self-report, no blinding)	Unclear (hard to determine which participants are in reporting)	Yes	High
Hanley 2013[28] Canada	Yes	Yes	No - adjusts for some variables on our list, but not for education, which was different at baseline	Medium
Heikkinen 2002[29] Finland	Unclear (no mention of blinding)	Yes	No (no adjustment)	Medium
Jimenez-Solem 2012[30] Denmark	Unclear - no validation study described	Yes	Yes	Low
Jimenez-Solem, 2013, Denmark[31]	Unclear (methods for verifying the gestational age at death, and also unclear if national records are reliable)	Yes	Yes	Low
Jordan 2008[32] US	Unclear - obtained from medical charts where MD generally knew exposure status	Yes	No	Medium
Kallen 2004[33] Sweden	Yes	Yes	Unclear; other than paroxetine they didn't adjust for preterm birth or medical disorders such as diabetes (important for hypoglycemia)	Medium
Kallen 2007[107] Sweden	Unclear - ICD-10 code P293B; no validation cited	Yes	Yes	Medium
Kallen 2007[34] Sweden	Unclear - some data from 2005 is missing, may be screening women/fetuses with ultrasound more in women who take ADs	Yes	Yes	Medium
Kieler 2012[36] Sweden	Unclear - no validation of ICD codes	Yes	Yes	Low

Author Year Country	6. Unbiased and accurate event ascertainment?	7. Free of selective outcome reporting?	8. Adequate handling of potential confounding variables?	Overall Risk of Bias Rating
Kleiger-Grossmann 2011[108] Canada	Unclear - assessors were not blinded to group allocation	Yes	Yes	High
Klinger 2010[109] Israel	Yes	Yes	No, higher maternal age in NAS group and this was not controlled for (34 vs 32)	High
Kornum 2010[37] Denmark	No - 1) included only live born infants; 2) accuracy of coding and diagnosis is questioned on p.34; 3) detection bias x 2 sources	Yes	Yes	Medium
Kulin 1998[110] Canada	Yes for major malformations; no for others based on self-report alone	Yes	No; more tobacco use in SSRI group and other differences, no control for differences	High
Laine 2003[38] Finland	Unclear - blinding of outcome assessors intended but stated to not be maintained. Not clear what proportion unblinded	Yes	No	Medium
Latendresse, 2011[39] US	Unclear. No mention of blinding	Yes	Yes	Medium
Lennestal 2007[40] Sweden	Yes	Yes	Yes	Medium
Levinson-Castiel 2006[41] Israel	Unclear, unblinded assessors	Yes	Unclear, similar in age but no other confounders reported and no regression analysis	Medium
Lewis 2010[42] Australia	Unclear	Yes	No	Medium
Logsdon 2011[43] US	Yes	Yes	No - only race was controlled for	Medium
Louik 2007[111] US	Unclear - not clear how they confirmed specific diagnoses	Yes	Yes	High
Lund 2009[44] Denmark	Unclear, no mention of blinding	Yes	Yes	Medium
Malm 2011[45] Finland	Yes	Yes	Yes	Low
Manakova 2011[112] Czech Republic	No. No mention of blinding	Yes	Unclear	High

Author Year Country	6. Unbiased and accurate event ascertainment?	7. Free of selective outcome reporting?	8. Adequate handling of potential confounding variables?	Overall Risk of Bias Rating
Marroun 2012[23] The Netherlands	Yes	Yes	Yes	Low
Maschi 2008[113] Italy	No	Yes	Yes	High
McElhatton 1996[114] UK	Yes	Yes	No - no confounders are adjusted for	High
McFarland 2011[46] US	Yes	Yes	Unclear - they do not adjust for smoking status, comorbidities or other medications	Medium
Merlob 2009[47] Israel	No - cardiologists not blinded to exposure for last 2 years of study	Yes	No - they collected some of them and didn't adjust for them because the sample was too small and there was not matching to the control group	Medium
Misri 1991[115] Canada	Unclear, methods NR	Yes	NA, no between-groups comparison	High
Misri 2006[48] Canada	Yes	Yes	Unclear; similar in age, univariate control for depression and anxiety	Medium
Misri 2010[49] Canada	Unclear	Yes	Unclear, only controlled for age and # of children in home	Medium
Mulder 2011[50] The Netherlands	Unclear; blinding NR	Yes	Yes	Medium
Nakhai-Pour 2010[51] Canada	Yes	Yes	Yes	Low
Nijenhuis 2012[116] The Netherlands	Yes	Yes	No, no confounding variables reported or controlled for	High
Nordeng 2012[52] Norway	Yes	Yes	Yes	Medium
Nulman 1997[117] Canada	Yes for neurobehavioral in children (blind psychometrician, standardized instruments); unclear and perinatal complications (verified by pediatrician), but unclear for maternal outcomes	Yes	No; differences in gravidity, parity, previous abortions, SES, alcohol use and cigarette smoking not controlled for	High

Author Year Country	6. Unbiased and accurate event ascertainment?	7. Free of selective outcome reporting?	8. Adequate handling of potential confounding variables?	Overall Risk of Bias Rating
Nulman 2002[118] Canada	Yes	Yes	Unclear; multiple linear regression adjusted for differences in maternal depression duration, severity, # episodes, but not number of anxiolytic drugs	Medium for Reynell; High for others
Nulman 2012[53] Canada	Yes	Yes	Unclear; no control for higher gravidity (3 vs 2), previous therapeutic abortions (0.6 vs 0.3), light alcohol use (62% vs 55%) and cigarette smoking (45% vs 31%), lower SES in fluoxetine group (40 vs 46), or genetic factors; assessed based on self-report	High
Oberlander 2002[54] Canada (2-day), Oberlander 2005[119] Canada (2-month)	Yes	Yes	Unclear; no baseline differences in maternal age or depression, but no other material variables reported	Medium
Oberlander 2004[120] Canada	Unclear, partial blinding and respiratory symptoms not assessed in a standardized way, only when concern expressed	Yes	Unclear; only age reported and was balanced	High
Oberlander 2006[55] Canada	Yes	Yes	Yes	Medium
Oberlander 2007[121] Canada (4-year followup to Oberlander 2005 Canada)	Yes	Yes	Unclear; age was balanced between groups; regression models examined maternal mood, prenatal clonazepam exposure, a history of PNA, and umbilical cord drug levels as predictors of child behavior	High
Oberlander 2008[56]	Unclear - included only live born infants	Yes	Unclear - key confounders not accounted for	Medium
Oberlander 2008[57] Canada	Yes	Yes; perhaps exception of maternal mood	Unclear; no control for higher levels of depression and anxiety in exposed group.	Medium

Author Year Country	6. Unbiased and accurate event ascertainment?	7. Free of selective outcome reporting?	8. Adequate handling of potential confounding variables?	Overall Risk of Bias Rating
Oberlander 2010[122] Canada	Unclear; blinding NR	Yes	Unclear; methods for confounding variable ascertainment NR; no adjustment for some baseline differences; non-SSRI exposed group had higher education (18 yrs vs 15 yrs) and higher rates of 1-10 alcohol drinks (42% vs 24%)	High
Okun 2011[58] US	Unclear; blinding NR	Yes	No, no information about comparability of baseline characteristics between SSRI-exposed and non-exposed groups and no adjustment for confounders	Medium
Okun 2012[59] US	Unclear - they did not use objective tests of sleep latency or have sleep info pre-pregnancy	Yes	Unclear - they note because of the small sample size they were unable to control for all variables	Medium
Palmsten 2012[60] Canada	Unclear-no mention of blinding, wide range of ICD-9 code accuracy in validation study	Yes	Yes	Medium
Pastuszak 1993[123] US	Yes, self-report verified by written documentation by pediatrician	Yes	No; age matched, but higher parity in fluoxetine vs NTC and no control	High
Pawluski 2009[124] Canada	Unclear; blinding NR	Yes	Unclear; few characteristics reported, but similar at baseline	High
Pearlstein 2006[125] US	No blinding	Unclear	Unclear if matched for age, race. Baseline characteristics reported overall and not by group	High
Pearson 2007[61] US	Yes	Yes	Unclear; some differences that were not controlled for: exposed group had lower tobacco use (24% vs 54%) and more married women (97% vs 77%). Also exposed group had higher levels of missing data on tobacco use (40% vs 6%) and marital status (31% vs 10%)	Medium
Pedersen 2009[62] Denmark	No. Only includes live-born infants	Yes	Yes	Medium
Pedersen 2010[63] Denmark	Unclear; self-report, not verification; unblinded assessors	Yes	Unclear; adjusted for multiple factors, but all were measured based on self-report	Medium

Author Year Country	6. Unbiased and accurate event ascertainment?	7. Free of selective outcome reporting?	8. Adequate handling of potential confounding variables?	Overall Risk of Bias Rating
Pedersen 2013[64] (Pendersen, 2010) Denmark	Unclear; self-report, not verification; unblinded assessors	Yes	Unclear; adjusted for multiple factors, but all were measured based on self-report	Medium
Polen 2013[65] US	Yes	Yes	Yes	Medium
Rai 2013[66] Sweden	Yes	Yes	Yes	Low
Ramos 2008[126] Canada	Unclear; ICD-9 codes, no verification	Yes	Yes	Medium
Ramos 2010[68] Canada	Unclear - no data on how reliable database is for this	Yes	Yes; although don't have placental abnormalities or genetic issues which would contribute to both	Medium
Rampono 2004[127] Australia	Unclear; blinding NR	Yes	No; comparability of baseline characteristics NR, no analysis	High
Reebye 2002[70] Canada	Yes	Yes	Unclear; only difference was higher education for control mothers and no adjustment	Medium
Reis 2010[71] Sweden	Yes	Yes	Yes	Medium
Rompono 2009[69] Australia	Yes	Yes	Unclear; no adjustment for lower proportion of nulliparous (32% vs 56%) and higher proportion of hypertension (21% vs 6%) and alcohol use (24% vs 11%) in case group	Medium
Salisbury 2011[72] US	Yes	Yes	Yes	Medium (due to Loss to followup)
Salkeld 2008[73] Canada	Yes	Yes	Yes	Low
Simon 2002[74] US	Unclear - included only live born infants	Yes	Yes	Low
Sit 2011[75] US	Yes	Yes	Unclear; comparability of baseline characteristics NR between fluoxetine and short half-life agents groups, no adjustment	Medium
Sivojelezova 2005[128] Canada	Unclear	Yes	No	High

Author Year Country	6. Unbiased and accurate event ascertainment?	7. Free of selective outcome reporting?	8. Adequate handling of potential confounding variables?	Overall Risk of Bias Rating
Smith 2013[76] US	Yes	Yes	No - not assessed. There are only 6 people in the exposed group; % white is 100% in SRI group and only 67% in unexposed group	High
Stephansson 2013[77] Sweden	Yes	Yes	Yes	Medium
Suri 2004[129] US	Unclear	Yes	No	High
Suri 2007[78] US	Yes	Yes	Unclear; no significant differences in age or parity, other important confounders NR	Medium
Suri 2011[79] US	Yes	Yes	Unclear; no significant differences in age or parity, other important confounders NR	Medium
Ter Horst 2013[80] The Netherlands	Yes	Yes	Unclear - only used confounders related to lung disease, not any others specified by our TEP	Medium
Toh 2009[130] US/Canada	No	Yes	Yes (but confounding by depression could occur)	High
Toh 2009[81] US/Canada	No (self-report)	Yes	Yes	Medium
Ververs 2009[82] The Netherlands	Unclear (methods not described for how data obtained or verified)	Yes	No (no adjustment)	Medium
Wen 2006[131] Canada	Unclear. No mention of blinding	Yes	Yes	Medium
Wichman 2009[132] US	Unclear (no mention of blinding)	Yes	No (no adjustment)	High
Wilson 2011[83] US	Unclear (chart review, no blinding)	Yes	Unclear (matched for GA, confounding by depression)	Medium
Wisner 2009[84]/Okun 2012[59] US	Yes	Yes	Yes	Medium
Wisner 2013[85] US (Wisner 2009/Okun 2012)	Yes	Yes	Yes	Medium

Author Year Country	6. Unbiased and accurate event ascertainment?	7. Free of selective outcome reporting?	8. Adequate handling of potential confounding variables?	Overall Risk of Bias Rating
Wogelius 2006[86] Danish	Unclear (no blinding)	Unclear (3 most prevalent)	Yes	Medium
Yonkers 2012[87] US	Yes	Yes	Yes	Low
Zeskind 2004[88] US	Yes	Yes	Yes	Medium

AD = antidepressant; ETOH = alcohol; GA = gestational age; LMP = last menstrual period; MR = medical record; NA = not applicable; NB = newborn; NR = not reported; NSAID = nonsteroidal anti-inflammatory drug; SES = socio-economic status; SSRI = selective serotonin reuptake inhibitor; TCA = tricyclic antidepressant; UK = United Kingdom; US = United States

Evidence Table 3. Data abstraction of trials

Author Year Country Trial Name Risk of Bias	Population	Interventions	Age Ethnicity	Other Population Characteristics	Number Randomized
Appleby 1997[133] UK Medium	Inclusion Criteria: Depressed 6-8 weeks after childbirth. Score ≥ 10 on Edinburgh postnatal depression scale; Score ≥ 12 on the revised clinical interview schedule; satisfied research diagnostic criteria for major or minor depressive disorder. Exclusion Criteria: Inadequate English and living outside district. Chronic (>2 years) or resistant depression, current drug or alcohol misuse, severe illness requiring close monitoring or hospital admission, and breast feeding.	1) Fluoxetine + 1 CBT session 2) Fluoxetine + 6 CBT sessions 3) Placebo + 1 CBT session 4) Placebo + 6 CBT sessions Fluoxetine dose: NR Time Period: 12 wks	Mean age: 25 Ethnicity NR	Unplanned Pregnancy: 13.75% Major Depressive Disorder: 12.75% History of Postnatal Depression: 7.5% Family History of postnatal depression: 4%	87
Bloch 2012[134] Israel Medium	Age 18-45 years; criteria met during the screen and baseline visits for current major depressive disorder according to the Diagnostic and Statistical Manual of Mental Disorders, 4th Edition (DSM-IV), as assessed by the Structured Clinical Interview for DSM-IV Axis I disorders, and onset of the depressive episode starting within 2 months of parturition.	Three Treatment Groups 1) Sertraline+psychotherapy 2) Placebo+Psychotherapy Sertraline mean (SD) dose at 4 weeks: 65.0 (23.5)mg, at 8 weeks: 67.5 (24.5)mg Time Period: 8 wks	Mean age: NR Ethnicity: NR	Anxiety Diagnosis: 22.5% Past Depression: 22.5% Depression in Family: 37.5% Pregnancies: 1.4%	42
Misri, 2004[135] Canada Medium	Age 18-40 years; ≥18 on HAM-D, ≥ 20 on HAM-A and ≥ 12 on EPDS; delivered a healthy baby close to term (37-42 weeks) with a minimum birth weight of 2.5 kg; non smokers; willing to use adequate contraception during the study.	1. Paroxetine 2. Paroxetine+CBT Paroxetine max. dose: 50 mg Time period: 12 wks	Mean age: 30 White: 62.9% South Asian: 14.3% First Nations: 8.6% Mexican, Spanish, Indo-Canadian, Italian, South-American: 2.8% each	% of children previously born 1: 57% 2: 28.6% 3: 11.4% 4: 2.9% DSM diagnosis Depression only: 2.9% Depression+Anxiety: 34.3% Depression+Anxiety+Obsession: 31.4% Depression+Anxiety+OCD: 31.4%	35

E-142

Author Year Country Trial Name Risk of Bias	Population	Interventions	Age Ethnicity	Other Population Characteristics	Number Randomized
Morrell 2009[136] UK Medium	Inclusion Criteria: At-risk women (who returned a 6-week EPDS score ≥ 12 on the postal questionnaire), had an 8-week EPDS score ≥ 12 when the EPDS was repeated face-to-face by the HV at 8 weeks postnatally. Women eligible for the intervention were therefore defined by two EPDS score ≥ 12. The HV was allowed to provide the intervention to those women whom the HV felt might benefit from the intervention, irrespective of their EPDS score. Women were recruited if they were registered with participating GP practices, became 36 weeks pregnant during the recruitment phase of the trial, had a live baby and were on a collaborating HV's caseload for 4 months postnatally.	Primary comparison was between at-risk women randomized to Health Visitor training and women in practices randomized to provide Health Visitor usual care. Six Treatment Groups 1) Cognitive behavioral approach face-to-face 2) Cognitive behavioral approach postal 3) Person-centered approach face-to-face 4) Person-centered approach postal 5) Control (Health Visitor usual care)	Mean age: 30.9 (SD 5.4) Ethnicity: 93.3% White British	93.7% living with others, 6.3% living alone 47.1% first baby	101 clusters in 29 primary care trusts. 595

E-143

Author Year Country Trial Name Risk of Bias	Efficacy/Effectiveness Outcomes	Harms	Funding
Appleby 1997[133] UK Medium	**Revised Clinical Interview Schedule Score (Completer Analysis, N=61)** % difference in geometric mean scores (95% CI): Fluoxetine vs placebo: 4 weeks=37.1% (5.7% to 58.0%), 12 weeks=40.7% (10.9% to 60.6%); 6 CBT sessions vs 1 CBT session: 4 weeks=53.9% (2.3% to 131.2%), 12 weeks=38.7% (-9.2% to 111.7%) Change in geometric mean scores from baseline to 4 weeks/12 weeks (ITT): **Revised Clinical Interview Schedule** Fluoxetine+1 CBT session= -16.3/-22.7 Fluoxetine+6 CBT sessions= -16.9/-16.3 Placebo+1 CBT session= -10.4/-10.2 Placebo+6 CBT sessions= -13.7/-14.2 **Edinburgh postnatal depression scale** Fluoxetine+1 CBT session= -7.1/-9.5 Fluoxetine+6 CBT sessions= -9.7/-10.2 Placebo+1 CBT session= -8.1/-7.2 Placebo+6 CBT sessions= -6.6/6.9 **Hamilton score** Fluoxetine+1 CBT session= NR/-10 Fluoxetine+6 CBT sessions= NR/-8.9 Placebo+1 CBT session= NR/-5.9 Placebo+6 CBT sessions= NR/-8.9	NR	
Bloch 2012[134] Israel Medium	Sertraline+psychotherapy vs placebo+psychotherapy Change from baseline at 8 weeks, n=40 (p-values are NS presented as group by time interaction unless otherwise specified for MDRS, EPDS, CGI) Improvement in MADRS -13.86 vs -9.85, significant time effect p<0.0001 Improvement in EPDS: -9.75 vs -3.55, significant time effect p<0.0001 Improvement in CGI-S: -1.9 vs -1.5 Improvement in CGI-I: -2.00 vs -0.25 Response rates at 8 weeks MADRS or EPDS, n=40: 70% vs 55%, p=NS Remission rates at 8 weeks MADRS or EPDS, n=40, 65% vs 50%, p=NS	Hypomaniac switch in 10% (n=2) of patients in sertraline + psychotherapy group vs 0 in placebo	Independent investigator award for National Alliance on Research on Schizophrenia and Depression

Author Year Country Trial Name Risk of Bias	Efficacy/Effectiveness Outcomes	Harms	Funding
Misri, 2004[135] Canada Medium	Paroxetine vs Paroxetine +CBT Change from baseline (reduction) at final visit (P<0.01 for all) HAM-D: 17.6 vs 15.2 HAM-A: 14.3 vs 14.6 EPDS: 8.4 vs 10.2 YBOCS: 4.9 vs 9.1 CGI-I: 2.75 vs 2.59 % patients with reduction in symptom scores at final visit ≥50% score (p=NS between groups) HAM-D: 87.5 vs 78.9 HAM-A: 75.0 vs 84.2 EPDS: 61.5 vs 58.3 ≥60% score reduction in symptom scores at final visit (p=NS between groups) YBOCS: 80.0 vs 78.6 CGI (1=normal, not at all ill) (p=NS between groups) Depression (based on HAM_D): 75 vs 63.2 Anxiety (based on HAM-A): 75 vs 57.9 Obsessions and/or OCD (based on YBOCS): 80 vs 71.4	NR	Glaxo-Smithkline Canada

Author Year Country Trial Name Risk of Bias	Efficacy/Effectiveness Outcomes	Harms	Funding
Morrell 2009[136] UK Medium	Intervention vs control Proportion of at-risk women with a 6-month Edinburgh Postnatal Depression Scale score >=12 (Primary Outcome) 33.9% vs 45.6% OR, unadjusted: 0.62 (95% CI 0.40, 0.97); P=0.036 OR, adjusted for 6-week EPDS score: 0.64 (95% CI 0.40, 1.01); P=0.058 OR, adjusted for 6-week EPDS score, lives alone, history of postnatal depression, any life events: 0.60 (95% CI 0.38, 0.95); P=0.028 OR, adjusted for lives alone, history of postnatal depression, any life events: 0.57 (95% CI 0.36, 0.90); P=0.017 6-month outcomes: control vs intervention, adjusted mean difference in scores (95% CI) EPDS: -2.1 (-3.3, -0.9), P=0.001 SF-12 PCS: -1.7 (-3.6, 0.1), P=0.069 SF-12 MCS: 5.2 (2.5, 7.8), P=0.001 SF-6D: 0.03 (0.00, 0.06), P=0.025 CORE-OM well-being: -0.3 (-0.5, -0.2), P=0.001 CORE-OM risk: -0.0 (-0.1, 0.0), P=0.149 CORE-OM symptoms: -0.2 (-0.4, -0.1), P=0.005 CORE-OM functioning: -0.3 (-0.4, -0.1), P=0.001 CORE-OM total score: -0.2 (-0.4, -0.1), P=0.001 State anxiety: -3.9 (-6.6, -1.3), P=0.003 Trait anxiety: -3.7 (-6.1, -1.4), P=0.002 PSI parenting distress: 3.5 (1.3, 5.8), P=0.002 PSI PCDI: 2.1 (0.7, 3.5), P=0.003 PSI difficult child: 2.9 (1.7, 4.2), P=0.001 PSI total stress: 9.3 (137.3, 13.4), P=0.001	NR	Government (UK NHS)

CBT = cognitive behavioral therapy; CI = confidence interval; CGI-I = Clinical Global Impression scale - Improvement; CGI-S = Clinical Global Impression Scale - Severity; CORE-OM = Clinical Outcomes in Routine Evaluation ; DSM-IV = Diagnostic and Statistical Manual of Mental Disorders; Fourth Edition; HAM-A = Hamilton Anxiety Rating Scale; HAM-D = Hamilton Depression Rating Scale; ITT = intention to treat; MADRS = Montgomery-Asberg Depression Rating Scale; NR = not reported; OCD = obsessive compulsive disorder; OR = odds ratio; PCDI = Parent Child Dysfunctional Interaction; PSI = Parenting Stress Index; SD = standard deviation; UK = United Kingdom; US = United States

Evidence Table 4. Risk of bias assessment of trials

Author Year Country	Randomization adequate?	Allocation concealment adequate?	Groups similar at baseline?	Eligibility criteria specified?	Outcome assessors masked?	Care provider masked?
Appleby 1997[133] UK	Yes	Unclear	Placebo+1 session counseling younger	Yes	Yes to Drug/No to counseling	Yes to Drug/No to counseling
Bloch 2012[134] Israel	Yes	Unclear	Yes	Yes	Yes	Yes
Misri 2004[135] Canada	Yes	Unclear (no details given)	Yes	Yes	Unclear ((Yes at baseline, then for followup: "patient's progress was evaluated by the psychiatrist investigator who administered....)	NA
Morrell 2009[136] UK	Yes	Yes	Yes	Yes	Blinding not possible	Blinding not possible
Sharp 2010[137] UK	Yes	Yes	Yes	Yes	No	No
Wisner 2006[138] US	Yes	Unclear - it says randomized by a sequence generated by SPSS but it is unclear if people can see the whole list and so would know what the next assignment would be. If they knew the next assignment it would potentially introduce bias because they could change the order they enrolled a patient to get them into the group.	No - more non-white women were assigned to the sertraline group and no other baseline variables reported.	Yes	Yes	Unclear
Yonkers 2012[87] US	Yes	Unclear	Yes, mostly except IDS-SR score different between 2 groups, p<0.05	Yes	Yes	Yes

Author Year Country	Patient masked?	Intention-to-treat analysis	Maintenance of comparable groups	Acceptable levels of crossovers, adherence, and contamination?	Acceptable levels of overall attrition and between-group differences in attrition?	Overall Risk of Bias
Appleby 1997[133] UK	Yes except counseling	Yes	Yes	Unclear	Overall attrition 30%, acceptable between group differences in attrition	Medium
Bloch 2012[134] Israel	Yes	Yes	Yes	Yes for adherence and crossover, unclear for contamination	Yes	Medium
Misri 2004[135] Canada	No	Yes for all but EPDS	Yes	Unclear for all	Yes	Medium
Morrell 2009[136] UK	Blinding not possible	No, 418/595 included in primary statistical analysis. No imputation of missing data.	Yes	Unclear	Yes	Medium
Sharp 2010[137] UK	No	No, At 18 weeks 206/254 included in analysis[19% excluded]	Unclear	Adherence-No, Contamination: No, Crossover: unclear	At 18 weeks, overall attrition acceptable, between group differences: No>10%	High
Wisner 2006[138] US	Yes	Yes for primary, no for secondary	NA, not comparable at baseline	Unclear for all	No - there was 42% attrition in the sertraline group and 24% percent attrition in the nortriptyline group at 8 weeks. This is both high overall and differential attrition.	High
Yonkers 2012[87] US	Yes	No, 44.3% included in the analysis	Yes	High nonadherence: 37% (12 in treatment group, 14 in placebo), Other: unclear	Overall attrition 56%, acceptable between group differences in attrition	High

NA = not applicable; UK = United Kingdom; US = United States

Appendix E. References

1. Alwan S, Reefhuis J, Rasmussen SA, et al. Use of selective serotonin-reuptake inhibitors in pregnancy and the risk of birth defects. N Engl J Med. 2007 Jun 28;356(26):2684-92. PMID: 17596602.

2. Alwan S, Reefhuis J, Botto LD, et al. Maternal use of bupropion and risk for congenital heart defects. Am J Obstet Gynecol. 2010 Jul;203(1):52.e1-6. PMID: 20417496.

3. Andrade C. How to read a research paper: Reading between and beyond the lines. 2011;53(4):362-6. PMID: 2011438958. Language: English. Entry Date: 20120302. Revision Date: 20120622. Publication Type: journal article.

4. Bakker MK, Kerstjens-Frederikse WS, Buys CHCM, et al. First-trimester use of paroxetine and congenital heart defects: a population-based case-control study. Birth Defects Res Part A Clin Mol Teratol. 2010 Feb;88(2):94-100. PMID: 19937603.

5. Bakker MK, De Walle HEK, Wilffert B, et al. Fluoxetine and infantile hypertrophic pylorus stenosis: a signal from a birth defects-drug exposure surveillance study. Pharmacoepidemiol Drug Saf. 2010 Aug;19(8):808-13. PMID: 20572024.

6. Ban L, Tata LJ, West J, et al. Live and non-live pregnancy outcomes among women with depression and anxiety: A population-based study. PLoS ONE. 2012;7(8).

7. Batton B, Batton E, Weigler K, et al. In utero antidepressant exposure and neurodevelopment in preterm infants. Am J Perinatol. 2013;30(4):297-301.

8. Bérard A, Ramos É, Rey É, et al. First trimester exposure to paroxetine and risk of cardiac malformations in infants: The importance of dosage. Birth Defects Res B Dev Reprod Toxicol. 2007;80(1):18-27.

9. Bogen DL, Hanusa BH, Moses-Kolko E, et al. Are maternal depression or symptom severity associated with breastfeeding intention or outcomes? J Clin Psychiatry. 2010 Aug;71(8):1069-78. PMID: 20584521.

10. Boucher N, Bairam A, Beaulac-Baillargeon L. A new look at the neonate's clinical presentation after in utero exposure to antidepressants in late pregnancy. J Clin Psychopharmacol. 2008 Jun;28(3):334-9. PMID: 18480693.

11. Casper RC, Fleisher BE, Lee-Ancajas JC, et al. Follow-up of children of depressed mothers exposed or not exposed to antidepressant drugs during pregnancy. J Pediatr. 2003 Apr;142(4):402-8. PMID: 12712058.

12. Chambers CD, Johnson KA, Dick LM, et al. Birth outcomes in pregnant women taking fluoxetine. N Engl J Med. 1996 Oct 3;335(14):1010-5. PMID: 8793924.

13. Chambers CD, Hernandez-Diaz S, Van Marter LJ, et al. Selective serotonin-reuptake inhibitors and risk of persistent pulmonary hypertension of the newborn. N Engl J Med. 2006 Feb 9;354(6):579-87. PMID: 16467545.

14. Cole JA, Ephross SA, Cosmatos IS, et al. Paroxetine in the first trimester and the prevalence of congenital malformations. Pharmacoepidemiol Drug Saf. 2007 Oct;16(10):1075-85. PMID: 17729379.

15. Cole JA, Modell JG, Haight BR, et al. Bupropion in pregnancy and the prevalence of congenital malformations. Pharmacoepidemiol Drug Saf. 2007 May;16(5):474-84. PMID: 16897811.

16. Colvin L, Slack-Smith L, Stanley FJ, et al. Early morbidity and mortality following in utero exposure to selective serotonin reuptake inhibitors: a population-based study in Western australia. CNS Drugs. 2012;26(7):e1-e14. PMID: 2011592323.

17. Croen LA, Grether JK, Yoshida CK, et al. Antidepressant use during pregnancy and childhood autism spectrum disorders. Arch Gen Psychiatry. 2011 Nov;68(11):1104-12. PMID: 21727247.

18. Davidson S, Prokonov D, Taler M, et al. Effect of exposure to selective serotonin reuptake inhibitors in utero on fetal growth: potential role for the IGF-I and HPA axes. Pediatr Res. 2009 Feb;65(2):236-41. PMID: 19262294.

19. Davis RL, Rubanowice D, McPhillips H, et al. Risks of congenital malformations and perinatal events among infants exposed to antidepressant medications during pregnancy. Pharmacoepidemiol Drug Saf. 2007 Oct;16(10):1086-94. PMID: 17729378.

20. de Vries NKS, van der Veere CN, Reijneveld SA, et al. Early Neurological Outcome of Young Infants Exposed to Selective Serotonin Reuptake Inhibitors during Pregnancy: Results from the Observational SMOK Study. PLoS ONE. 2013;8(5).

21. Dubnov-Raz G, Juurlink DN, Fogelman R, et al. Antenatal use of selective serotonin-reuptake inhibitors and QT interval prolongation in newborns. Pediatrics. 2008 Sep;122(3):e710-5. PMID: 18762507.

22. Dubnov-Raz G, Hemila H, Vurembrand Y, et al. Maternal use of selective serotonin reuptake inhibitors during pregnancy and neonatal bone density. Early Hum Dev. 2012 Mar;88(3):191-4. PMID: 21890289.

23. El Marroun H, Jaddoe VWV, Hudziak JJ, et al. Maternal use of selective serotonin reuptake inhibitors, fetal growth, and risk of adverse birth outcomes. Arch Gen Psychiatry. 2012 Jul;69(7):706-14. PMID: 22393202.

24. Ferreira E, Carceller AM, Agogue C, et al. Effects of selective serotonin reuptake inhibitors and venlafaxine during pregnancy in term and preterm neonates. Pediatrics. 2007 Jan;119(1):52-9. PMID: 17200271.

25. Figueroa R. Use of antidepressants during pregnancy and risk of attention-deficit/hyperactivity disorder in the offspring. J Dev Behav Pediatr. 2010 Oct;31(8):641-8. PMID: 20613624.

26. Gorman JR, Kao K, Chambers CD. Breastfeeding among Women Exposed to Antidepressants during Pregnancy. J Hum Lact. 2012;28(2):181-8. PMID: 2011521514.

27. Grzeskowiak LE, Gilbert AL, Morrison JL. Neonatal outcomes after late-gestation exposure to selective serotonin reuptake inhibitors. J Clin Psychopharmacol . 2012;32(5):615-21.

28. Hanley GE, Brain U, Oberlander TF. Infant developmental outcomes following prenatal exposure to antidepressants, and maternal depressed mood and positive affect. Early Hum Dev. 2013;89(8):519-24.

29. Heikkinen T, Ekblad U, Kero P, et al. Citalopram in pregnancy and lactation. Clin Pharmacol Ther. 2002 Aug;72(2):184-91. PMID: 12189365.

30. Jimenez-Solem E, Andersen JT, Petersen M, et al. Exposure to selective serotonin reuptake inhibitors and the risk of congenital malformations: A nationwide cohort study. BMJ Open. 2012;2(3).

31. Jimenez-Solem E, Andersen JT, Petersen M, et al. SSRI Use During Pregnancy and Risk of Stillbirth and Neonatal Mortality. Am J Psychiatry. 2013 Mar 1;170(3):299-304

32. Jordan AE, Jackson GL, Deardorff D, et al. Serotonin reuptake inhibitor use in pregnancy and the neonatal behavioral syndrome. J Matern Fetal Neonatal Med. 2008 Oct;21(10):745-51. PMID: 19012191.

33. Kallen B. Neonate characteristics after maternal use of antidepressants in late pregnancy. Arch Pediatr Adolesc Med. 2004 Apr;158(4):312-6. PMID: 15066868.

34. Kallen BAJ, Otterblad Olausson P. Maternal use of selective serotonin re-uptake inhibitors in early pregnancy and infant congenital malformations. Birth Defects Res Part A Clin Mol Teratol. 2007 Apr;79(4):301-8. PMID: 17216624.

35. Kallen B, Olausson PO. Maternal use of selective serotonin re-uptake inhibitors and persistent pulmonary hypertension of the newborn. Pharmacoepidemiol Drug Saf. 2008 Aug;17(8):801-6. PMID: 18314924.

36. Kieler H, Artama M, Engeland A, et al. Selective serotonin reuptake inhibitors during pregnancy and risk of persistent pulmonary hypertension in the newborn: population based cohort study from the five Nordic countries. Bmj. 2012;344:d8012. PMID: 22240235.

37. Kornum JB. Use of selective serotonin-reuptake inhibitors during early pregnancy and risk of congenital malformations: updated analysis. Clin Epidemiol. 2010 Aug 9;2:29-36.

38. Laine K, Heikkinen T, Ekblad U, et al. Effects of exposure to selective serotonin reuptake inhibitors during pregnancy on serotonergic symptoms in newborns and cord blood monoamine and prolactin concentrations. Arch Gen Psychiatry. 2003 Jul;60(7):720-6. PMID: 12860776.

39. Latendresse G, Ruiz RJ. Maternal corticotropin-releasing hormone and the use of selective serotonin reuptake inhibitors independently predict the occurrence of preterm birth. J Midwifery Womens Health. 2011 Mar-Apr;56(2):118-26. PMID: 21429075.

40. Lennestal R, Kallen B. Delivery outcome in relation to maternal use of some recently introduced antidepressants. J Clin Psychopharmacol. 2007 Dec;27(6):607-13. PMID: 18004128.

41. Levinson-Castiel R, Merlob P, Linder N, et al. Neonatal abstinence syndrome after in utero exposure to selective serotonin reuptake inhibitors in term infants. Arch Pediatr Adolesc Med. 2006 Feb;160(2):173-6. PMID: 16461873.

42. Lewis AJ, Galbally M, Opie G, et al. Neonatal growth outcomes at birth and one month postpartum following in utero exposure to antidepressant medication. Aust N Z J Psychiatry. 2010 May;44(5):482-7. PMID: 20397792.

43. Logsdon MC, Wisner K, Sit D, et al. Depression treatment and maternal functioning. Depress Anxiety. 2011 Nov;28(11):1020-6. PMID: 21898714.

44. Lund N, Pedersen LH, Henriksen TB. Selective serotonin reuptake inhibitor exposure in utero and pregnancy outcomes.[Erratum appears in Arch Pediatr Adolesc Med. 2009 Dec;163(12):1143]. Arch Pediatr Adolesc Med. 2009 Oct;163(10):949-54. PMID: 19805715.

45. Malm H, Artama M, Gissler M, et al. Selective serotonin reuptake inhibitors and risk for major congenital anomalies. Obstet Gynecol. 2011 Jul;118(1):111-20. PMID: 21646927.

46. McFarland J, Salisbury AL, Battle CL, et al. Major depressive disorder during pregnancy and emotional attachment to the fetus. 2011;14(5):425-34.

47. Merlob P, Birk E, Sirota L, et al. Are selective serotonin reuptake inhibitors cardiac teratogens? Echocardiographic screening of newborns with persistent heart murmur. Birth Defects Res Part A Clin Mol Teratol. 2009 Oct;85(10):837-41. PMID: 19691085.

48. Misri S, Reebye P, Kendrick K, et al. Internalizing behaviors in 4-year-old children exposed in utero to psychotropic medications. Am J Psychiatry. 2006 Jun;163(6):1026-32. PMID: 16741203.

49. Misri S, Kendrick K, Oberlander TF, et al. Antenatal depression and anxiety affect postpartum parenting stress: a longitudinal, prospective study. Can J Psychiatry. 2010 Apr;55(4):222-8. PMID: 20416145.

50. Mulder EJ, Ververs FF, de Heus R, et al. Selective serotonin reuptake inhibitors affect neurobehavioral development in the human fetus. Neuropsychopharmacology. 2011 Sep;36(10):1961-71.

51. Nakhai-Pour HR, Broy P, Berard A. Use of antidepressants during pregnancy and the risk of spontaneous abortion. Cmaj. 2010 Jul 13;182(10):1031-7. PMID: 20513781.

52. Nordeng H, van Gelder MMHJ, Spigset O, et al. Pregnancy outcome after exposure to antidepressants and the role of maternal depression: results from the Norwegian Mother and Child Cohort Study. J Clin Psychopharmacol. 2012 Apr;32(2):186-94. PMID: 22367660.

53. Nulman I, Koren G, Rovet J, et al. Neurodevelopment of children following prenatal exposure to venlafaxine, selective serotonin reuptake inhibitors, or untreated maternal depression. 2012 Nov 1;169(11):1165-74. .

54. Oberlander TF, Eckstein Grunau R, Fitzgerald C, et al. Prolonged prenatal psychotropic medication exposure alters neonatal acute pain response. Pediatr Res. 2002 Apr;51(4):443-53. PMID: 11919328.

55. Oberlander TF, Warburton W, Misri S, et al. Neonatal outcomes after prenatal exposure to selective serotonin reuptake inhibitor antidepressants and maternal depression using population-based linked health data. Arch Gen Psychiatry. 2006 Aug;63(8):898-906. PMID: 16894066.

56. Oberlander TF, Bonaguro RJ, Misri S, et al. Infant serotonin transporter (SLC6A4) promoter genotype is associated with adverse neonatal outcomes after prenatal exposure to serotonin reuptake inhibitor medications. Mol Psychiatry. 2008 Jan;13(1):65-73. PMID: 17519929.

57. Oberlander TF, Warburton W, Misri S, et al. Major congenital malformations following prenatal exposure to serotonin reuptake inhibitors and benzodiazepines using population-based health data. Birth Defects Res Part B Dev Reprod Toxicol. 2008 Feb;83(1):68-76. PMID: 18293409.

58. Okun ML, Kiewra K, Luther JF, et al. Sleep disturbances in depressed and nondepressed pregnant women. Depress Anxiety. 2011 Aug;28(8):676-85. PMID: 21608086.

59. Okun ML, Luther JF, Wisniewski SR, et al. Disturbed sleep, a novel risk factor for preterm birth? J Womens Health (Larchmt). 2012 Jan;21(1):54-60. PMID: 21967121.

60. Palmsten K, Setoguchi S, Margulis AV, et al. Elevated risk of preeclampsia in pregnant women with depression: depression or antidepressants? Am J Epidemiol. 2012 May 15;175(10):988-97. PMID: 22442287.

61. Pearson KH, Nonacs RM, Viguera AC, et al. Birth outcomes following prenatal exposure to antidepressants. J Clin Psychiatry. 2007 Aug;68(8):1284-9. PMID: 17854255.

62. Pedersen LH, Henriksen TB, Vestergaard M, et al. Selective serotonin reuptake inhibitors in pregnancy and congenital malformations: population based cohort study. Bmj. 2009;339:b3569. PMID: 19776103.

63. Pedersen LH, Henriksen TB, Olsen J. Fetal exposure to antidepressants and normal milestone development at 6 and 19 months of age. Pediatrics. 2010 Mar;125(3):e600-8. PMID: 20176667.

64. Pedersen L, Henriksen T, Bech B, et al. Prenatal antidepressant exposure and behavioral problems in early childhood - A cohort study. Acta Psychiatrica Scandinavica. 2013 Feb;127(2):126-35. PMID: Peer Reviewed Journal: 2013-00954-005.

65. Polen KND, Rasmussen SA, Riehle-Colarusso T, et al. Association between reported venlafaxine use in early pregnancy and birth defects, national birth defects prevention study, 1997-2007. Birth Defects Res A Clin Mol Teratol. 2013;97(1):28-35. PMID: 23281074

66. Rai D, Lee BK, Dalman C, et al. Parental depression, maternal antidepressant use during pregnancy, and risk of autism spectrum disorders: population based case-control study. BMJ. 2013 2013-04-19 12:14:20;346.

67. Ramos E, Ofori B, Oraichi D, et al. Antidepressant therapy during pregnancy: an insight on its potential healthcare costs. Can J Clin Pharmacol. 2008;15(3):e398-410. PMID: 18953084.

68. Ramos E, St-Andre M, Berard A. Association between antidepressant use during pregnancy and infants born small for gestational age. Can J Psychiatry. 2010 Oct;55(10):643-52. PMID: 20964943.

69. Rampono J, Simmer K, Ilett KF, et al. Placental transfer of SSRI and SNRI antidepressants and effects on the neonate. Pharmacopsychiatry. 2009 May;42(3):95-100. PMID: 19452377.

70. Reebye P, Morison SJ, Panikkar H, et al. Affect expression in prenatally psychotropic exposed and nonexposed mother-infant dyads. Infant Ment Health J. 2002 Jul;23(4):403-16.

71. Reis M, Kallen B. Delivery outcome after maternal use of antidepressant drugs in pregnancy: an update using Swedish data. Psychol Med. 2010 Oct;40(10):1723-33. PMID: 20047705.

72. Salisbury AL, Wisner KL, Pearlstein T, et al. Newborn neurobehavioral patterns are differentially related to prenatal maternal major depressive disorder and serotonin reuptake inhibitor treatment. Depress Anxiety. 2011 Nov;28(11):1008-19. PMID: 21898709.

73. Salkeld E, Ferris LE, Juurlink DN. The risk of postpartum hemorrhage with selective serotonin reuptake inhibitors and other antidepressants. J Clin Psychopharmacol. 2008 Apr;28(2):230-4. PMID: 18344737.

74. Simon GE, Cunningham ML, Davis RL. Outcomes of prenatal antidepressant exposure. Am J Psychiatry. 2002 Dec;159(12):2055-61. PMID: 12450956.

75. Sit D, Perel JM, Wisniewski SR, et al. Mother-infant antidepressant concentrations, maternal depression, and perinatal events. J Clin Psychiatry. 2011 Jul;72(7):994-1001. PMID: 21824458.

76. Smith MV, Sung A, Shah B, et al. Neurobehavioral assessment of infants born at term and in utero exposure to serotonin reuptake inhibitors. Early Hum Dev. 2013;89(2):81-6. PMID: 22999988

77. Stephansson O KHHB, et al. Selective serotonin reuptake inhibitors during pregnancy and risk of stillbirth and infant mortality. JAMA. 2013;309(1):48-54. PMID: 23280224

78. Suri R, Altshuler L, Hellemann G, et al. Effects of antenatal depression and antidepressant treatment on gestational age at birth and risk of preterm birth. Am J Psychiatry. 2007 Aug;164(8):1206-13. PMID: 17671283.

79. Suri R, Hellemann G, Stowe ZN, et al. A prospective, naturalistic, blinded study of early neurobehavioral outcomes for infants following prenatal antidepressant exposure. J Clin Psychiatry. 2011 Jul;72(7):1002-7. PMID: 21672498.

80. Ter Horst PGJ, Bos HJ, De Jong-Van De Berg LTW, et al. In utero exposure to antidepressants and the use of drugs for pulmonary diseases in children. Eur J Clin Pharmacol. 2013;69(3):541-7. PMID: 22815049

81. Toh S, Mitchell AA, Louik C, et al. Selective serotonin reuptake inhibitor use and risk of gestational hypertension. Am J Psychiatry. 2009 Mar;166(3):320-8. PMID: 19122006.

82. Ververs TF, van Wensen K, Freund MW, et al. Association between antidepressant drug use during pregnancy and child healthcare utilisation. Bjog. 2009 Nov;116(12):1568-77. PMID: 19681852.

83. Wilson KL, Zelig CM, Harvey JP, et al. Persistent pulmonary hypertension of the newborn is associated with mode of delivery and not with maternal use of selective serotonin reuptake inhibitors. Am J Perinatol. 2011 Jan;28(1):19-24. PMID: 20607643.

84. Wisner KL, Sit DKY, Hanusa BH, et al. Major depression and antidepressant treatment: impact on pregnancy and neonatal outcomes. Am J Psychiatry. 2009 May;166(5):557-66. PMID: 19289451.

85. Wisner KL, Bogen DL, Sit D, et al. Does Fetal Exposure to SSRIs or Maternal Depression Impact Infant Growth? Am J Psychiatry. 2013 May 1;170(5):485-93. PMID: 23511234

86. Wogelius P, Norgaard M, Gislum M, et al. Maternal use of selective serotonin reuptake inhibitors and risk of congenital malformations. Epidemiology. 2006 Nov;17(6):701-4. PMID: 17028507.

87. Yonkers KA, Norwitz ER, Smith MV, et al. Depression and serotonin reuptake inhibitor treatment as risk factors for preterm birth. Epidemiology. 2012;23(5):677-85. PMID: 22627901.

88. Zeskind PS, Stephens LE. Maternal selective serotonin reuptake inhibitor use during pregnancy and newborn neurobehavior. Pediatrics. 2004 Feb;113(2):368-75. PMID: 14754951.

89. Andrade SE, McPhillips H, Loren D, et al. Antidepressant medication use and risk of persistent pulmonary hypertension of the newborn. Pharmacoepidemiol Drug Saf. 2009 Mar;18(3):246-52. PMID: 19148882.

90. Berle JO, Steen VM, Aamo TO, et al. Breastfeeding during maternal antidepressant treatment with serotonin reuptake inhibitors: infant exposure, clinical symptoms, and cytochrome p450 genotypes. J Clin Psychiatry. 2004 Sep;65(9):1228-34. PMID: 15367050.

91. Bracken MB, Holford TR. Exposure to prescribed drugs in pregnancy and association with congenital malformations. Obstet Gynecol. 1981;58(3):336-44.

92. Chun-Fai-Chan B, Koren G, Fayez I, et al. Pregnancy outcome of women exposed to bupropion during pregnancy: a prospective comparative study. Am J Obstet Gynecol. 2005 Mar;192(3):932-6. PMID: 15746694.

93. Colvin L, Slack-Smith L, Stanley FJ, et al. Linking a pharmaceutical claims database with a birth defects registry to investigate birth defect rates of suspected teratogens. Pharmacoepidemiol Drug Saf. 2010;19(11):1137-50.

94. Colvin L, Slack-Smith L, Stanley FJ, et al. Dispensing patterns and pregnancy outcomes for women dispensed selective serotonin reuptake inhibitors in pregnancy.[Erratum appears in Birth Defects Res A Clin Mol Teratol. 2011 Apr;91(4):268]. Birth Defects Res Part A Clin Mol Teratol. 2011 Mar;91(3):142-52. PMID: 21381184.

95. Costei AM, Kozer E, Ho T, et al. Perinatal outcome following third trimester exposure to paroxetine. Arch Pediatr Adolesc Med. 2002 Nov;156(11):1129-32. PMID: 12413342.

96. De Vera MA, Bérard A. Antidepressant use during pregnancy and the risk of pregnancy-induced hypertension. Br J Clin Pharmacol. 2012;74(2):362-9.

97. Diav-Citrin O, Shechtman S, Weinbaum D, et al. Paroxetine and fluoxetine in pregnancy: a prospective, multicentre, controlled, observational study. Br J Clin Pharmacol. 2008 Nov;66(5):695-705. PMID: 18754846.

98. Djulus J, Koren G, Einarson TR, et al. Exposure to mirtazapine during pregnancy: a prospective, comparative study of birth outcomes. J Clin Psychiatry. 2006 Aug;67(8):1280-4. PMID: 16965209.

99. Einarson A, Choi J, Einarson TR, et al. Rates of spontaneous and therapeutic abortions following use of antidepressants in pregnancy: results from a large prospective database. Journal of obstetrics and gynaecology Canada : JOGC 2009;31(5):452-6.

100. Einarson A, Choi J, Einarson TR, et al. Incidence of major malformations in infants following antidepressant exposure in pregnancy: results of a large prospective cohort study. Can J Psychiatry. 2009 Apr;54(4):242-6. PMID: 19321030.

101. Einarson A, Choi J, Einarson TR, et al. Adverse effects of antidepressant use in pregnancy: an evaluation of fetal growth and preterm birth. Depress Anxiety. 2010;27(1):35-8. PMID: 19691030.

102. Einarson A, Bonari L, Voyer-Lavigne S, et al. A multicentre prospective controlled study to determine the safety of trazodone and nefazodone use during pregnancy. Canadian J. of Psychiatry. 2003;48(2):106-10.

103. Ericson A, Kallen B, Wiholm B. Delivery outcome after the use of antidepressants in early pregnancy. Eur J Clin Pharmacol. 1999 Sep;55(7):503-8. PMID: 10501819.

104. Galbally M, Lewis AJ, Lum J, et al. Serotonin discontinuation syndrome following in utero exposure to antidepressant medication: prospective controlled study. Aust N Z J Psychiatry. 2009 Sep;43(9):846-54. PMID: 19670058.

105. Galbally M, Lewis AJ, Buist A. Developmental outcomes of children exposed to antidepressants in pregnancy. Aust N Z J Psychiatry. 2011 May;45(5):393-9. PMID: 21314237.

106. Hale TW, Kendall-Tackett K, Cong Z, et al. Discontinuation syndrome in newborns whose mothers took antidepressants while pregnant or breastfeeding. Breastfeed Med. 2010 Dec;5(4):283-8. PMID: 20807106.

107. Kallen B. The safety of antidepressant drugs during pregnancy. Expert Opin Drug Saf. 2007 Jul;6(4):357-70. PMID: 17688379.

108. Klieger-Grossmann C, Weitzner B, Panchaud A, et al. Pregnancy outcomes following use of escitalopram: a prospective comparative cohort study. J Clin Pharmacol. 2012 May;52(5):766-70. PMID: 22075232.

109. Klinger G, Frankenthal D, Merlob P, et al. Long-term outcome following selective serotonin reuptake inhibitor induced neonatal abstinence syndrome. J Perinatol. 2011 Sep;31(9):615-20. PMID: 21311497.

110. Kulin NA, Pastuszak A, Sage SR, et al. Pregnancy outcome following maternal use of the new selective serotonin reuptake inhibitors: a prospective controlled multicenter study. JAMA. 1998 Feb 25;279(8):609-10. PMID: 9486756.

111. Louik C, Lin AE, Werler MM, et al. First-trimester use of selective serotonin-reuptake inhibitors and the risk of birth defects. N Engl J Med. 2007 Jun 28;356(26):2675-83. PMID: 17596601.

112. Manakova E, Hubickova L. Antidepressant drug exposure during pregnancy. CZTIS small prospective study. Neuroendocrinol Lett. 2011;32 Suppl 1:53-6. PMID: 22167208.

113. Maschi S, Clavenna A, Campi R, et al. Neonatal outcome following pregnancy exposure to antidepressants: a prospective controlled cohort study. Bjog. 2008 Jan;115(2):283-9. PMID: 17903222.

114. McElhatton PR, Garbis HM, Elefant E, et al. The outcome of pregnancy in 689 women exposed to therapeutic doses of antidepressants. A collaborative study of the European Network of Teratology Information Services (ENTIS). Reprod Toxicol. 1996 Jul-Aug;10(4):285-94. PMID: 8829251.

115. Misri S, Sivertz K. Tricyclic drugs in pregnancy and lactation: a preliminary report. Int J Psychiatry Med. 1991;21(2):157-71. PMID: 1894455.

116. Nijenhuis CM, ter Horst PGJ, van Rein N, et al. Disturbed development of the enteric nervous system after in utero exposure of selective serotonin re-uptake inhibitors and tricyclic antidepressants. Part 2: Testing the hypotheses. Br J Clin Pharmacol. 2012 Jan;73(1):126-34. PMID: 21848990.

117. Nulman I, Rovet J, Stewart DE, et al. Neurodevelopment of children exposed in utero to antidepressant drugs. N Engl J Med. 1997 Jan 23;336(4):258-62. PMID: 8995088.

118. Nulman I, Rovet J, Stewart DE, et al. Child development following exposure to tricyclic antidepressants or fluoxetine throughout fetal life: a prospective, controlled study. Am J Psychiatry. 2002 Nov;159(11):1889-95. PMID: 12411224.

119. Oberlander TF, Grunau RE, Fitzgerald C, et al. Pain reactivity in 2-month-old infants after prenatal and postnatal serotonin reuptake inhibitor medication exposure. Pediatrics. 2005 Feb;115(2):411-25. PMID: 15687451.

120. Oberlander TF, Misri S, Fitzgerald CE, et al. Pharmacologic factors associated with transient neonatal symptoms following prenatal psychotropic medication exposure. J Clin Psychiatry. 2004 Feb;65(2):230-7. PMID: 15003078.

121. Oberlander TF, Reebye P, Misri S, et al. Externalizing and attentional behaviors in children of depressed mothers treated with a selective serotonin reuptake inhibitor antidepressant during pregnancy. Arch Pediatr Adolesc Med. 2007 Jan;161(1):22-9. PMID: 17199063.

122. Oberlander TF, Papsdorf M, Brain UM, et al. Prenatal effects of selective serotonin reuptake inhibitor antidepressants, serotonin transporter promoter genotype (SLC6A4), and maternal mood on child behavior at 3 years of age. Arch Pediatr Adolesc Med. 2010 May;164(5):444-51. PMID: 20439795.

123. Pastuszak A, Schick-Boschetto B, Zuber C, et al. Pregnancy outcome following first-trimester exposure to fluoxetine (Prozac). JAMA. 1993;269(17):2246-8.

124. Pawluski JL, Galea LAM, Brain U, et al. Neonatal S100B protein levels after prenatal exposure to selective serotonin reuptake inhibitors. Pediatrics. 2009 Oct;124(4):e662-70. PMID: 19786426.

125. Pearlstein TB, Zlotnick C, Battle CL, et al. Patient choice of treatment for postpartum depression: a pilot study. Arch Women Ment Health. 2006 Nov;9(6):303-8. PMID: 16932988.

126. Ramos E, St-Andre M, Rey E, et al. Duration of antidepressant use during pregnancy and risk of major congenital malformations. Br J Psychiatry. 2008 May;192(5):344-50. PMID: 18450657.

127. Rampono J, Proud S, Hackett LP, et al. A pilot study of newer antidepressant concentrations in cord and maternal serum and possible effects in the neonate. Int J Neuropsychopharmcol. 2004 Sep;7(3):329-34. PMID: 15035694.

128. Sivojelezova A, Shuhaiber S, Sarkissian L, et al. Citalopram use in pregnancy: prospective comparative evaluation of pregnancy and fetal outcome. Am J Obstet Gynecol. 2005 Dec;193(6):2004-9. PMID: 16325604.

129. Suri R, Altshuler L, Hendrick V, et al. The impact of depression and fluoxetine treatment on obstetrical outcome. Arch Women Ment Health. 2004 Jul;7(3):193-200. PMID: 15241665.

130. Toh S, Mitchell AA, Louik C, et al. Antidepressant use during pregnancy and the risk of preterm delivery and fetal growth restriction. J Clin Psychopharmacol. 2009 Dec;29(6):555-60. PMID: 19910720.

131. Wen SW, Yang Q, Garner P, et al. Selective serotonin reuptake inhibitors and adverse pregnancy outcomes. Am J Obstet Gynecol. 2006 Apr;194(4):961-6. PMID: 16580283.

132. Wichman CL, Moore KM, Lang TR, et al. Congenital heart disease associated with selective serotonin reuptake inhibitor use during pregnancy. Mayo Clin Proc. 2009;84(1):23-7. PMID: 19121250.

133. Appleby L, Warner R, Whitton A, et al. A controlled study of fluoxetine and cognitive-behavioural counselling in the treatment of postnatal depression. Bmj. 1997 Mar 29;314(7085):932-6. PMID: 9099116.

134. Bloch M, Meiboom H, Lorberblatt M, et al. The effect of sertraline add-on to brief dynamic psychotherapy for the treatment of postpartum depression: a randomized, double-blind, placebo-controlled study. J Clin Psychiatry. 2012 Feb;73(2):235-41. PMID: 22401479.

135. Misri S, Reebye P, Corral M, et al. The use of paroxetine and cognitive-behavioral therapy in postpartum depression and anxiety: a randomized controlled trial. J Clin Psychiatry. 2004 Sep;65(9):1236-41. PMID: 15367052.

136. Morrell CJ, Warner R, Slade P, et al. Psychological interventions for postnatal depression: cluster randomised trial and economic evaluation. The PoNDER trial. Health Technol Assess. 2009 1-153, 2009 Jun;13(30):iii-iv. PMID: 19555590.

137. Sharp DJ, Chew-Graham C, Tylee A, et al. A pragmatic randomised controlled trial to compare antidepressants with a community-based psychosocial intervention for the treatment of women with postnatal depression: the RESPOND trial. Health Technol Assess. 2010 1-153, 2010 Sep;14(43):iii-iv. PMID: 20860888.

138. Wisner KL, Hanusa BH, Perel JM, et al. Postpartum depression: a randomized trial of sertraline versus nortriptyline. J Clin Psychopharmacol. 2006 Aug;26(4):353-60. PMID: 16855451.